AF674780

Advances, Breakthroughs, Controversies & Dilemmas in ART

Advances, Breakthroughs, Controversies & Dilemmas in ART

Editors

Manisha Takhtani Kundnani
MD FNB FNUS
Infertility and Reproductive Medicine Specialist
Scientific Director and Chief Fertility Consultant
Fertility Square—The IVF Clinic
Mumbai, Maharashtra, India

Sulbha Arora
MD DNB
Clinical Director and Senior Consultant
Department of Reproductive Medicine
Nova IVF Fertility
Mumbai, Maharashtra, India

Foreword

Hrishikesh D Pai

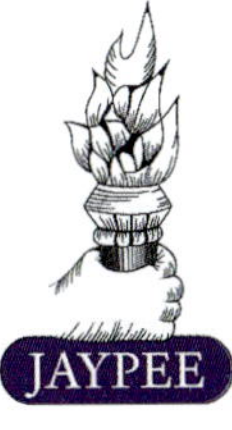

JAYPEE BROTHERS MEDICAL PUBLISHERS
The Health Sciences Publisher
New Delhi | London

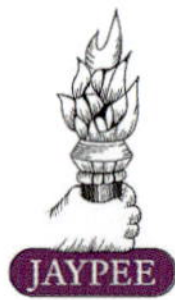

Jaypee Brothers Medical Publishers (P) Ltd

Headquarters

Jaypee Brothers Medical Publishers (P) Ltd
EMCA House, 23/23-B
Ansari Road, Daryaganj
New Delhi 110 002, India
Landline: +91-11-23272143, +91-11-23272703
+91-11-23282021, +91-11-23245672
Email: jaypee@jaypeebrothers.com

Corporate Office

Jaypee Brothers Medical Publishers (P) Ltd
4838/24, Ansari Road, Daryaganj
New Delhi 110 002, India
Phone: +91-11-43574357
Fax: +91-11-43574314
Email: jaypee@jaypeebrothers.com

Overseas Office

JP Medical Ltd.
83, Victoria Street, London
SW1H 0HW (UK)
Phone: +44 20 3170 8910
Fax: +44 (0)20 3008 6180
Email: info@jpmedpub.com

Website: www.jaypeebrothers.com
Website: www.jaypeedigital.com

Inquiries for bulk sales may be solicited at: jaypee@jaypeebrothers.com

Advances, Breakthroughs, Controversies & Dilemmas in ART

First Edition: **2024**

ISBN: 978-93-5696-885-1

Printed at: Samrat Offset Pvt. Ltd.

Dedicated to

Our mentors, who have been the guiding light always;
Our colleagues, who are superb role models;
Our fellows, who dare us to think more boldly;
Our students, who challenge us to be better teachers each day;
Our nurses, who encourage us to put patients' needs first;
Our families, whose love and support make our endeavors possible;
and
Our patients, who inspire us to strive for excellence.

Contributors

Akanksha Mishra
BSC MSC MS in Clinical Embryology (Oxford)
Chief Embryologist
Department of Embryology
Janini IVF
New Delhi, India

Anand Nanavati
DNB MRCOG (UK) Fellowship in IVF and Infertility (UK)
Clinical Director
Department of IVF
Create IVF and Fertility Centre
Mumbai, Maharashtra, India

Aneesha M Grover
DNB MSc Clinical Embryology, Diploma Clinical ART
Consultant
Department of Reproductive Medicine
Nova IVF Fertility
New Delhi, India

Anu Chawla
MRCOG MD DNB FICOG FRM FMAS
Director
Department of Reproductive Medicine
London Fertility Clinic
London, UK

Ashish Kale
MD DNB FICS FICOG DEPS
Director and Lead IVF Consultant
Ashakiran Hospitals and Asha IVF Centre
Pune, Maharashtra, India

Ashwini Kale
DNB DGO FICMCH
Director
Ashakiran Hospital and ASHA IVF Centre
Pune, Maharashtra, India

Aswati Nair
MD FNB
Senior Fertility Consultant
Nova IVF Fertility
New Delhi, India

Avantika Sharma
MBBS MS CIMP
Founder, Director and Senior Consultant
Department of Obstetrics and Gynecology
Lifeaid Medical Centre
Gurugram, Haryana, India

Charumati V Pekhale
MBBS DGO DNB
Consultant
Department of IVF
Nova IVF Fertility
Nasik, Maharashtra, India

Dimple Jain
MBBS DNB FCPS DGO MNAMS
Consultant
Department of Obstetrics and Gynecology
Currae Hospital, Fortis Hospital, and Oscar Hospital
Thane, Maharashtra, India

Divya Bansal
MSc (Biotechnology)
Senior Embryologist
Janini IVF
New Delhi, India

Durga G Rao
MBBS DGO MRCOG
Medical Director
Department of IVF
Oasis Fertility
Hyderabad, Telangana, India

Garima Sharma
MBBS MS DNB Fellow Reproductive Medicine
Senior Consultant and Medical Director
Department of Fertility Center
Evacare
Mumbai, Maharashtra, India

Gorakh G Mandrupkar
MBBS DGO FCPS FICOG MSc
Consultant
Department of Reproductive Medicine
Director
Mandrupkar Clinic, Islampur
Angel IVF
Pune, Maharashtra, India

Jwal Banker
MS DNB
Consultant
Department of ART
Banker IVF and Women's Hospital
Ahmedabad, Gujarat, India

Jyoti Pandey
MBBS MS MRCOG FRM
Consultant
Department of Reproductive Medicine
CIFAR Fertility and IVF Centre
Gurugram, Haryana, India

Jyoti Tripathi
DNB DRM (Germany)
Consultant Fertility Specialist
Department of IVF
Nova IVF Fertility
Indore, Madhya Pradesh, India

Kavya MP
MSc (Clinical Embryology)
Embryologist
Department of Embryology
Archish Fertility and IVF
Bengaluru, Karnataka, India

Kedar N Ganla
MBBS MD DGO DFP FCPS
Consultant
Department of Reproductive Medicine
Ankoor Fertility Clinic
Mumbai, Maharashtra, India

Keshav Malhotra
MBBS MCE FICRM
Lab Director
Department of Reproductive Medicine
Rainbow IVF
Agra, Uttar Pradesh, India

Kriti Sharma
MS FRM
Clinical Associate
Department of IVF
Create IVF and Fertility Centre
Mumbai, Maharashtra, India

Krishna Chaitanya Mantravadi
MBBS GRS MCE (Australia)
Scientific Head and Consultant Embryologist
Department of IVF
Oasis Fertility
Hyderabad, Telangana, India

Manish Banker
MD
Director and Consultant
Banker IVF and Women's Hospital
Ahmedabad, Gujarat, India

Manisha Nandi
MS FRM DRME (Germany)
Consultant Gynecologist
Department of Reproductive Medicine
Indira IVF
Udaipur, Rajasthan, India

Manisha Takhtani Kundnani
MD FNB FNUS
Infertility and Reproductive Medicine Specialist
Scientific Director and Chief Fertility Consultant
Fertility Square—The IVF Clinic
Mumbai, Maharashtra, India

Manjiri Valsangkar
MS (Obs & Gyne)
Director
Bhide Hospital IVF Centre
Pune, Maharashtra, India

Mohit Rajendra Saraogi
MD DNB DGO FCPS MNAMS Fellow ICOG
Director
Department of Infertility
Saraogi Hospital and Iris IVF Centre
Mumbai, Maharashtra, India

Monica Uppal
MS
Clinical Fellow
Department of Obstetrics and Gynecology
Altius Hospital
Bengaluru, Karnataka, India

Mugdha Parasnis
DNB
Head
Department of Reproductive Medicine
KEM Hospital
Pune, Maharashtra, India

Mukesh Gupta
MD DNB PGDPC
Founder Director
Le'Nest Hospital
Mumbai, Maharashtra, India

Navin Desai
MS (Human Clinical Embryology) MS (Biotechnology) MS (Business)
Co-Founder
Archish Fertility and IVF
Bengaluru, Karnataka, India

Pankaj Kaingade
PhD (Reproductive Biology)
Founder and Scientific Director
Department of Research and Development
ReproHelix Labs
Kolhapur, Maharashtra, India

Parul Arora
MD DNB
Consultant
Department of ART
Banker IVF and Women's Hospital
Ahmedabad, Gujarat, India

Pinky R Shah
DGO DNB FNB
Medical Director
Department of IVF
Dhiraj Vansh Fertility Centre, Dhule
Fertility Specialist
Sewa Superspecialty Hospital
Dhule, Maharashtra, India

Pooja Patil
MSc
Senior Embryologist
Department of IVF
Fertility Square—The IVF Clinic
Mumbai, Maharashtra, India

Pratik Tambe
MD FICOG FICRM
ART Consultant and Gyne Endoscopic Surgeon
Department of Obstetrics and Gynecology
Ashirwad IVF
Mumbai, Maharashtra, India

Pritimala Gangurde
MBBS DNB MRM
Medical Director
Department of IVF
Pearl Fertility and IVF
Mumbai, Maharashtra, India

Priyanka H Vora
MBBS DGO DFP FCPS
Consultant
Department of Reproductive Medicine
Ankoor Fertility Clinic
Mumbai, Maharashtra, India

Puneet Rana Arora
MBBS MS FRCOG MSc (Reproduction & Development, UK)
Senior Gynecologist and Founder
Department of Gynecology and Reproductive Medicine
CIFAR (Centre of Infertility and Assisted Reproduction)
Gurugram, Haryana, India

R Sujatha
PhD
Head
Department of Embryology
Nova IVF Fertility
Chennai, Tamil Nadu, India

Rahul Ramesh Salve
MBBS MD (Biochemistry) PGD (CEART)
Cluster Head
Department of Clinical Embryology
Nova IVF Fertility
Thane, Maharashtra, India

Rahul Wani
DNB DGO MBBS LLM LLB PGDMLS
Medicolegal Consultant
Department of Obstetrics
Archana Maternity Nursing Home
Navi Mumbai, Maharashtra, India

Rakshya Parajuli
MBBS MD (Obs & Gyne) Fellowship in Reproductive Endocrinology and Infertility
Fellow
Department of Obstetrics and Gynecology
Postgraduate Institute of Medical Education and Research
Chandigarh, India

Rana Choudhary
MBBS DNB DGO DFP FCPS Masters in Reproductive Medicine (UK) Diploma in ART (Germany) FCPS FICOG FICMCH
Consultant
Department of Reproductive Medicine
Ankoor Fertility Clinic
Mumbai, Maharashtra, India

Richa Sharma
MBBS MS FNB FRM
Fertility Consultant
Mumbai, Maharashtra, India

Rishina Bansal
MSc (Clinical Embryology) MS (Biotechnology)
Co-Founder
Archish Fertility and IVF
Bengaluru, Karnataka, India

Rohit Gutgutia
MBBS DGO
Medical Director
Department of IVF
Nova IVF
Kolkata, West Bengal, India

Runa Acharya
MD DNB FRM
Clinical Director
Department of Fertility
Medicover Fertility
Hyderabad, Telangana, India

S Lavanya
MSc (Clinical Embryology)
Junior Embryologist
Department of Embryology
Archish Fertility and IVF
Bengaluru, Karnataka, India

Sanket Pisat
MBBS MS DNB FICOG
Gyne Endoscopic Surgeon
Akanksha Maternity and Surgical Hospital
Mumbai, Maharashtra, India

Sayali Kandari
PhD MS
Clinical Director
Akruti IVF Centre LLP, Mumbai
CEO
Cellsure Biotech and Research Centre
Thane, Maharashtra, India

Seema Pandey
MD FICOG FRM
Director and Chief Consultant
Reproductive Medicine and IVF
Eva Fertility and Seema Hospital, Azamgarh
Vanshati Fertility, Lucknow
Uttar Pradesh, India

Shalini Gainder
MD Diploma MIS FMAS
Professor
Department of Obstetrics and Gynecology
Postgraduate Institute of Medical Education and Research
Chandigarh, India

Sheetal Sawankar
MBBS DNB MNAMS FICOG DRM (UK) MRM (Germany)
Founder and Director
Department of IVF
Avisa IVF and Fertility Center
Mumbai, Maharashtra, India

Shefali Bansal Madhav
MD
Director and IVF Specialist
Newlife Fertility Centre
Siliguri, West Bengal, India

Shrutika Thakkar
MS DNB DRM (Germany) MRM (UK)
Director
MedAnsh Multispeciality Hospital, Mumbai
Consultant Gynecologist and Fertility Specialist
Jupiter Hospital
Thane, Maharashtra, India

Sonia Malik
DGO MD FICOG FIAMS
Chief Clinical Mentor
Department of Infertility and IVF
Nova Southend Fertility and IVF
New Delhi, India

Sulbha Arora
MD DNB
Clinical Director and Senior Consultant
Department of Reproductive Medicine
Nova IVF Fertility
Mumbai, Maharashtra, India

Sunita Arora
MBBS MD FICOG
Clinical Head and Senior Consultant
Department of IVF
Fortis la Femme Hospital, Bloom IVF Centre
New Delhi, India

Suyesha Khanijao
MBBS DNB
IVF Specialist, Obstetrician and Gynecologist and Cosmetic Gynecologist
Department of Obstetrics and Gynecology
Angel's Hope, Sawan Neelu Angel's Hospital
New Delhi, India

Vikash Kumar
MS DNB MCh (Urology)
Head
Department of Urology
Bhaktivedanta Hospital and Research Institute
Mumbai, Maharashtra, India

Foreword

The inception of in vitro fertilization (IVF) in 1978, marked by the birth of Louise Brown, propelled fertility science to unprecedented heights. And since then, IVF and other assisted reproductive techniques have become a prominent solution for addressing infertility problems across the globe. There have been multiple new advancements and breakthroughs in the last few decades which have revolutionized the treatment strategies and have resulted in tremendous increase in the success rates.

In a quest to maximize outcomes, the field is shaped and changed constantly by advances in science and cutting-edge innovations. A number of fresh techniques are continuously being introduced every now and then to further increase the plateaued success rates. However, many of these are not always scientifically sound and are surrounded by controversies and dilemmas. Additionally, there are many difficult situations like poor ovarian response (POR), empty follicle, or failed fertilization which are challenging for the clinicians and frustrating for the patients.

The book ***A**dvances, **B**reakthroughs, **C**ontroversies & **D**ilemmas in ART* is a unique effort by the editors to compile all the latest advancements in the field of assisted reproductive technology (ART) including topics like artificial intelligence and time lapse, as well as covering in detail the various difficult and confusing situations in day-to-day practice. The chapters are written in a lucid and comprehensive manner so that the readers will enjoy reading it. The contributing authors are masters of the topic they have contributed. The manuscripts are therefore rich not only in the recent evidence but also with the vast experiences of the author; hence, they are full of practical tips and points which the readers will find extremely beneficial. I am sure the book will be a ready reckoner for both the students and clinicians to update their knowledge on evidence-based management of infertility.

I congratulate Manisha and Sulbha for their outstanding work to collate, edit, and publish such an exclusive book and for this unique contribution to our specialty.

Hrishikesh D Pai
MD FRCOG (UK-HON) FCPS FICOG MSc (USA)
Founder and Medical Director
Bloom IVF Group
Consultant Gynecologist
Lilavati Hospital IVF Center
Mumbai, Maharashtra, India
Professor of Reproductive Medicine
DY Patil University, Navi Mumbai
Past President FOGSI (2022–2023)
Trustee, FIGO Asia Oceania (2023–2025)

Preface

"The beginning of knowledge is the discovery of something we do not understand".

—**Frank Herbert**

The field of assisted reproduction has seen dramatic advancements since its inception. Multiple new technologies have been introduced in the last few decades for efficient patient management and to enhance success rates. Though the introduction of new technologies has led to significant improvement in patient care, it has also led to many controversies and debates surrounding the subject.

A*dvances,* ***B****reakthroughs,* ***C****ontroversies &* ***D****ilemmas in ART* is a unique effort to compile the major advancements and breakthroughs in this ever-growing field of assisted reproduction technology (ART). The book also simultaneously deals with various controversies, challenges, and difficult situations creating dilemmas. The contents of the book are exclusive and different from the other available textbooks on infertility, making it an interesting and productive read.

The book is divided into three sections: *Section 1* covers the recent advances and breakthroughs in the field of in vitro fertilization (IVF) and assisted reproduction; *Section 2* deals with all the difficult and challenging situations encountered in day-to-day practice; and *Section 3* deals with the various debates and dilemmas in the field of assisted reproduction. An addendum at the end will update the readers about the current ART laws in India.

The chapters are written by none other than stalwarts in the field from across the country and have been drafted in a manner that it will serve as a ready reckoner not only for the novice consultants but also for seasoned experts. The book will also be a guide for the students appearing for infertility super specialty examinations and for the gynecologists aspiring to learn infertility.

We sincerely hope that the book will be as rewarding for the readers as it has been for us to put together.

Wish you all a happy and prolific reading.

Manisha Takhtani Kundnani
Sulbha Arora

Contents

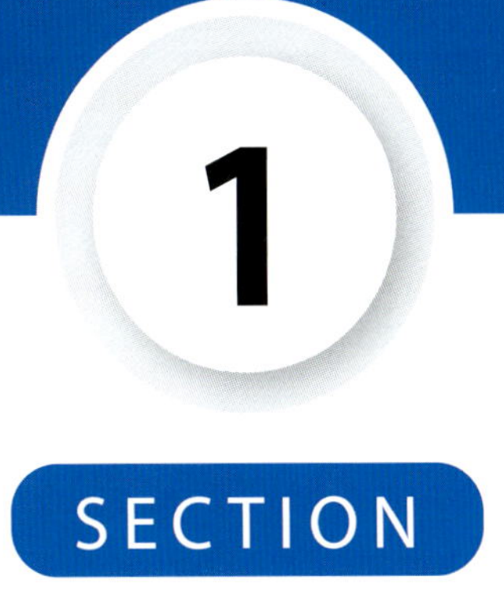

SECTION

Advances and Breakthroughs in Assisted Reproduction

Chapter

Artificial Intelligence in Assisted Reproductive Technology: The Future is Here

Richa Sharma

INTRODUCTION

Artificial intelligence (AI) as an official term first appeared at the Dartmouth conference in 1956. AI is already in use in various industries with ongoing research, such as in the transport and automotive industry, solving financial problems and facilitating face and speech recognition. AI has been gaining traction in the clinical setting in specialties such as nephrology, cardiology, ophthalmology, and primary care.

The number of treatment cycles in assisted reproductive technology (ART) is increasing steadily worldwide. Even though there have been gradual improvements in the success rate, one-third of the ART cycles result in a live birth and only 5% of the aspirated oocytes have the competence to develop into a child, which indicates that there is potential for improvement in the important steps in ART treatments, improving the efficiency and decreasing the complications.

Artificial intelligence is a strong technological wave providing the ability for a machine to perform cognitive functions, such as perceiving, reasoning, learning, and interacting. AI is quickly gaining traction in human reproduction and embryology. Advances in AI applications are constantly promoted by the increasing amount of data available in reproductive medicine. Despite some potential pitfalls, making decisions for infertility patients based on the analysis of medical data is the optimal clinical approach. To reduce the gap between research and clinical practice, we need to focus on combining ART and AI development.

Artificial intelligence and machine learning (ML) are new concepts in the field of medicine and more so in ART. Several studies have applied ML in ART, some of them focusing on clinical relevance, while others concern AI methodological aspects. Being a latest addition in ART, it definitely needs a large database and studies before making it part of clinical practice as a routine, which needs more transparent, comparable, and reproducible results and strong interdisciplinary collaborations to embark on the safety and implantation of the same.

In this chapter, we aim to shed light on the latest breakthroughs of AI in in vitro fertilization (IVF) stimulation and examine the potential of these technologies to transform the field. We will briefly review the technology, extensively review existing literature, and discuss how an AI-enabled future of controlled ovarian stimulation (COS) may come to fruition. We will also discuss the role of validation in these technologies and their potential limitations. By integrating AI into the field of reproductive medicine, we expect increased access to fertility services through higher-value clinical care, leading to more successful and efficient fertility treatments.

WHAT IS ARTIFICIAL INTELLIGENCE?

Artificial intelligence is a broad term for technologies, which mimic human intelligence for varied tasks such as image recognition and decision-making and it has been clubbed in various fields, which can help clinicians and add to the field of medicine **(Fig. 1)**.

Machine learning is a subset of AI that uses statistical modeling, which helps to analyze data patterns and generate predictive outputs without explicit coding or instructions. Applications of AI have ranged from predicting disease outcomes and identifying optimal treatment plans to automating administrative tasks and enhancing patient engagement. Thus it has a wide spectrum of benefits and will shape the future of medicine, which needs both scientific and technology investment as well as orientation of the doctors, scientists, healthcare workers, and awareness among the masses **(Fig. 2 and Flowchart 1)**.

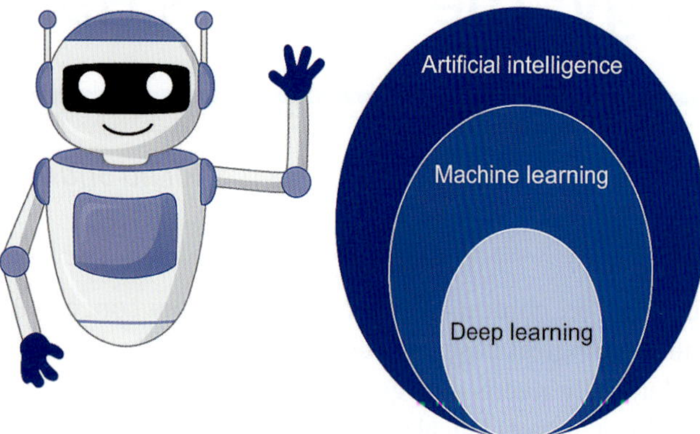

Fig. 1: Hierarchy of information processing theories in the computer science field. Artificial intelligence (AI) is an umbrella term attributed to the primary objective within the field of computer science to develop machines with intelligence. Machine learning describes approaches to achieve AI that learns from experience without explicit programming. Deep learning is a form of machine learning that utilizes artificial neural networks to extract, process, and predict information by learning from examples. It is commonly applied in the scientific field, in particular, in image classification.

ROLE OF ARTIFICIAL INTELLIGENCE IN ASSISTED REPRODUCTIVE TECHNOLOGIES

With the exponential growth of the fertility industry, how AI will smoothen the process and add to its significance is a burning topic of discussion these days so via this chapter we aim to cover the same **(Flowchart 2)**.

Reproductive experts can determine the best treatment for the individual infertility of patients by incorporating AI: ML and deep learning (DL).

It has been >45 years of ART with many new innovations being done to improve patient outcomes and increase operational efficiency through the application of new technologies, which include AI tools and ML.[1,2]

Although still in its infancy, the field of AI in reproductive medicine has benefited from increased research and investment from both the scientific and technology communities.[3]

Assisted Reproductive Technology Software

Artificial intelligence-based ART software covers the entire workflow of IVF treatments, from the time of first appointment of the patient until the final discharge

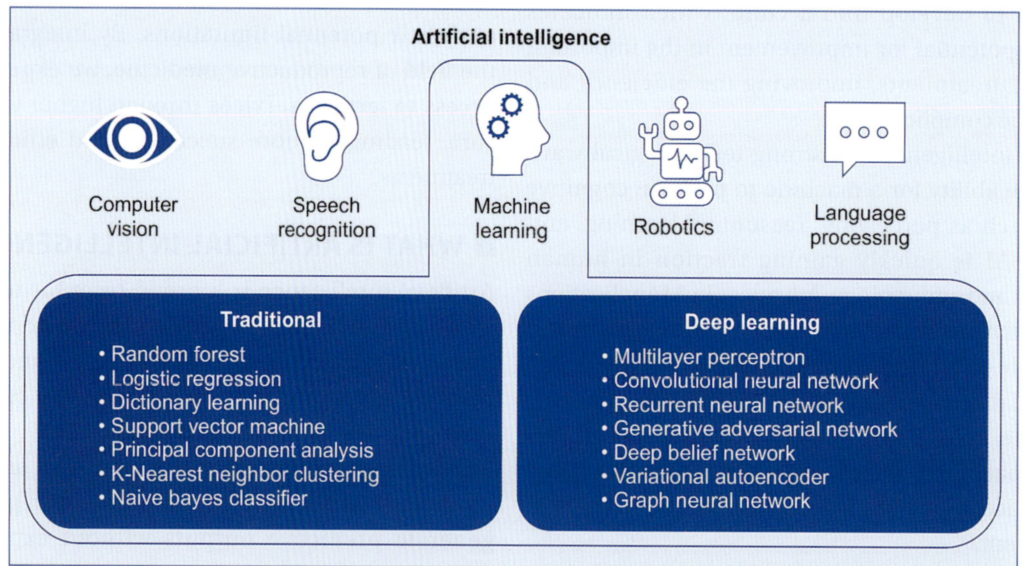

Fig. 2: Subfields defined by artificial intelligence; machine learning is the most relevant field for the current development of artificial intelligence system for the clinic. Machine learning can further be split into traditional machine learning methods and deep learning. Note that the subfields are not mutually exclusive; most of them rely heavily on machine learning, such as computer vision and language processing.

Flowchart 1: Development of a machine learning model: To implement a machine learning model at the clinic, at first a clinically relevant aim should be defined, and data must be collected in line with this aim. The collected data should then be stored in an appropriate format so that the machine learning algorithm can process it. The stored data should be split into training, validation, and testing partitions to ensure a robust and thorough evaluation. In the optimal case, the testing dataset is provided from an independent source (different clinic, new patients). These parts are then used to build a model that is in line with the medical goal. After the model is built, it should be thoroughly evaluated to verify its generalized ability and to avoid unintended biases. Once the model has been thoroughly tested, it can be implemented in the clinic. The model should be continuously monitored and tested while in production and as the circumstances required are updated.

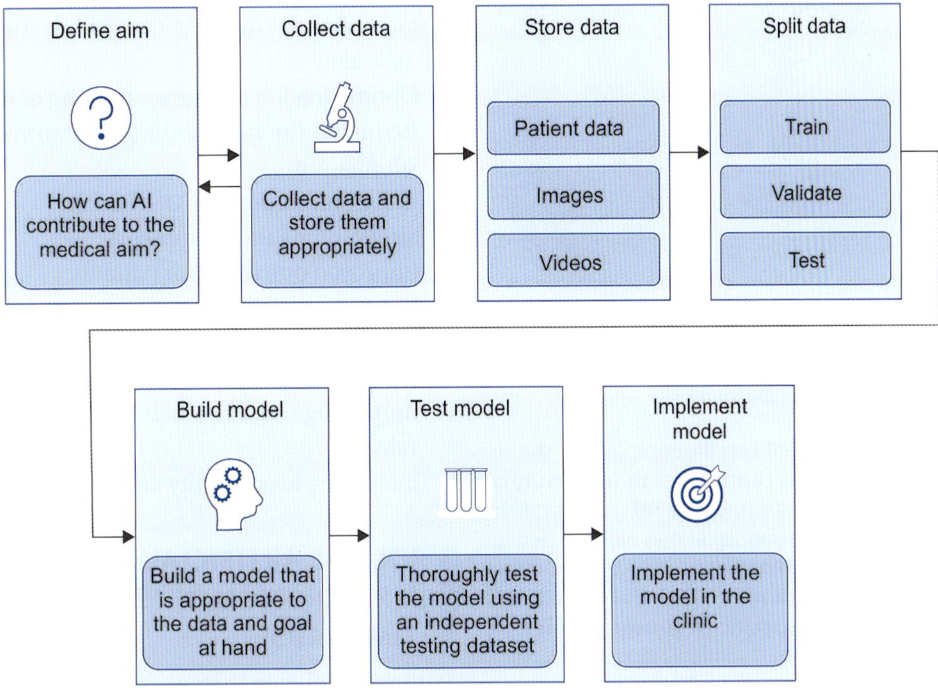

Flowchart 2: Usage of artificial intelligence (AI) in reproductive medicine.

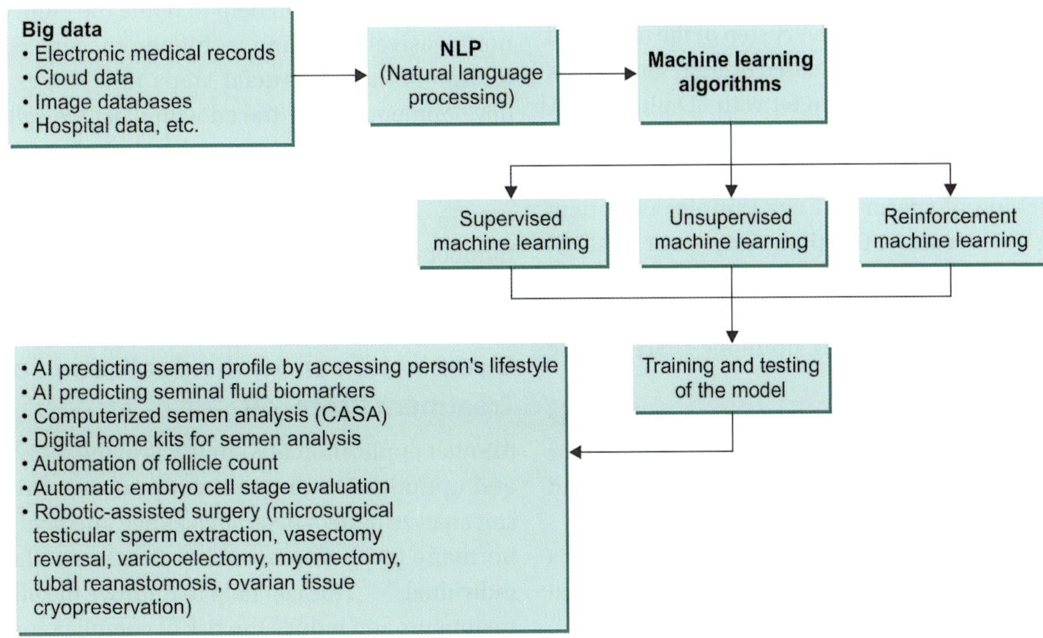

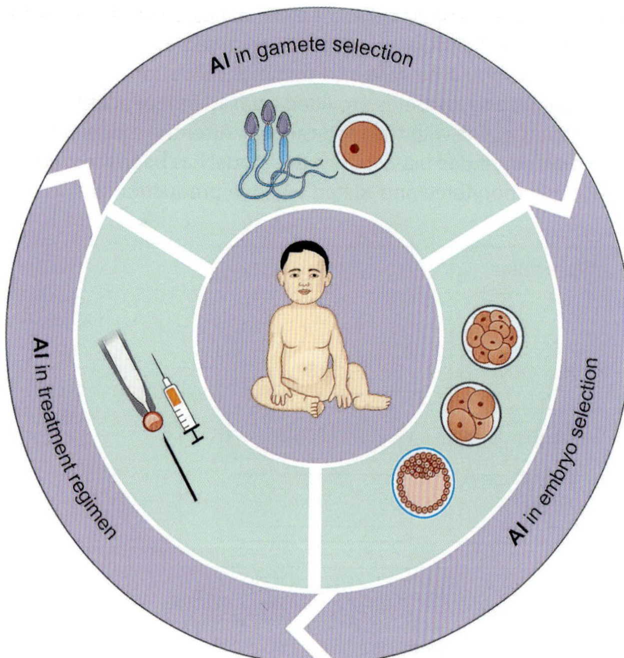

Fig. 3: Emerging role of artificial intelligence (AI) in the in vitro fertilization (IVF) clinic; AI represents an opportunity for technological advancement to improve IVF success. It is multifaceted in its capability. For example, AI may aid in selecting the best oocyte and sperm combination as well as predicting embryo quality. Furthermore, AI may assist the clinician in developing an optimal patient-specific treatment regimen to improve IVF success.

summary, everything is recorded, reported, analyzed, and automatized. An electronic system keeps the verification and matching data software on every step of the treatment [anti-Müllerian hormone (AMH)-based ovarian stimulation, measurements of follicular diameter with 3D ultrasound, sperm test, oocyte collection, oocyte tracking, embryo selection, preimplantation genetic screening (PGS)] and aids in matching of sperm and egg samples of patient undergoing IVF treatment without any error with AI system optimized **(Fig. 3)**.

The AI ART software also defines the dose of recombinant follicle-stimulating hormone (FSH) before the ovarian stimulation.

The AI ART software can analyze in detail all the information by automatic measurements of follicular diameter with 3D ultrasound to monitoring the cycle and human chorionic gonadotropin (hCG) triggering.

Synchronization of computer-aided sperm analysis (CASA) systems with AI ART software permits optimal selection of sperms for ART.

ROLE OF ARTIFICIAL INTELLIGENCE IN CONTROLLED OVARIAN STIMULATION IN VITRO FERTILIZATION

Role of AI in COS is a growing area of research and the purpose is to improve both the outcomes and efficiency of IVF.[4-6]

Various aspects where AI can add to the efficiency[7-12] of IVF include:

- Optimizing the dosage and timing of medications
- Reducing the likelihood of overstimulation or under stimulation
- Individualization of COS (ICOS)
- Streamlining the IVF process
- Improved outcomes for patients
- Providing quick services to more patients with greater efficiency and accuracy adding to precision value by reducing human errors and variability
- Improving clinical efficiency and adding to financial value
- Increasing accessibility and approachability to care.

ROLE OF ARTIFICIAL INTELLIGENCE IN PREDICTION OF EMBRYO QUALITY (TIME LAPSE)

Artificial intelligence has a role in prediction of embryo quality. In traditional IVF, embryologists visually examine embryos and the process can be subjective and prone to human error. This can help to refine the embryo selection noninvasively, leading to higher success rates for IVF treatments as all crucial steps and stages of embryo development can be traced with what we call time-lapse microscopy (TLM), hence predicting embryo development and implantation potential with about 70–77% accuracy, if an in vitro fertilized embryo has a normal or abnormal number of chromosomes (according to a new study from researchers at Weill Cornell Medicine).[13-15]

Optimization and Individualization of Treatment Protocols

Another application of AI in IVF is in the individualization and optimization of treatment protocols. AI algorithms can analyze patient data, such as age, medical history, and hormone levels to personalize treatment plans for each individual.[16-18] This can help to improve the efficacy of IVF treatments and reduce the risk of complications.

Artificial Intelligence-powered Microscopes to Track Sperms

Artificial intelligence is also being used in the development of new IVF technologies. For example, researchers are developing AI-powered microscopes[19-21] that can automatically identify and track sperm cells, which could help to improve the accuracy of IVF procedures.

ROLE OF ARTIFICIAL INTELLIGENCE IN UTERINE FACTORS

Artificial intelligence determines the uterine and endometrial conditions suitable for proper implantation by uploading ultrasound images into the system.[22,23]

Preimplantation Genetic Testing for Aneuploid Status

Preimplantation genetic testing (PGT) is now a widely applied procedure in genetic practices and ART, with more than one-third of ART centers in United States (US) already utilizing PGT technology. The current selection process of embryos with the highest developmental potential requires further improvement, as significant proportion of transferred euploid embryos still fail to result in an ongoing clinical pregnancy. To avoid a potential damage of embryo biopsy procedures, one of the important challenges will be the development of noninvasive approaches to PGT.[24-28]

How Does the Artificial Intelligence System Function?

The system can review a massive amount of data, far more than any human could ever process, including hundreds of images from each embryo. The growth patterns from these images are then related to whether each embryo developed into an ongoing pregnancy.

The predictive success of the AI system was tested by repeating the comparison against the outcomes of a separate group of embryos. The results showed a predictive value that is a significant improvement on any system that had previously been used in human embryology.[29-31]

What Are the Potential Benefits for Patients? (Table 1)

Artificial intelligence helps to select the right embryo more efficiently so that women going through IVF can conceive more quickly and thus lessen the strain of infertility on themselves and their families.[32-36]

TABLE 1: Steps toward adoption of artificial intelligence (AI) in the in vitro fertilization (IVF) clinic.

Hurdles	*Requirements to develop AI in the infertility service*
• Most clinics are too small in isolation to have sufficient data for AI • Limited computing power and data storage • Discrepancy in recorded and reported patient characteristics and reproductive outcomes between clinics • Variation between studies in the input parameters used for AI to predict reproductive outcomes	• Consortia to develop standardized and detailed recording and reporting of patient data • Multiclinic sharing of anonymized patient data • Increased computing power and data storage • Consensus on input parameters used in AI for predicting reproductive outcomes • Rigorous, high-quality, multicenter, peer-reviewed validation studies for AI algorithms

CONCLUSION

Emerging role of AI and ML in the IVF clinic represents an opportunity for technological advancement to improve IVF success. AI may assist the clinician in developing an optimal patient-specific treatment regimen to improve IVF success.

The limitations are often small datasets and the use of AI algorithms not specifically designed for the fertility clinic. Large open datasets and methods specifically developed and tailored for use in context with ART could lead to better results and understanding. For AI to significantly impact ART, the model must be developed in the context of clinical practice. Critical steps are proper evaluation and testing of AI systems in relation to outcomes and regulations, a better understanding of the technical aspects, and determination of the performance of AI models regarding practical value in the clinic.

In addition, it is important to standardize the use of AI in ART to enable more transparent, comparable, and reproducible results. To succeed with implementing AI as a valuable tool in the fertility clinic, a strong interdisciplinary collaboration is required between researchers in ART and AI as well as the clinical staff. In addition, there is a need for large-scale randomized controlled trials where several clinics are involved in testing the external validity of the algorithms before defining AI systems that are sufficiently robust for safe clinical implementation.

REFERENCES

1. Niederberger C, Pellicer A, Cohen J, Gardner DK, Palermo GD, O'Neill CL, et al. Forty years of IVF. Fertil Steril 2018; 110:185-324.e5.
2. Davenport T, Kalakota R. The potential for artificial intelligence in healthcare. Future Healthc J. 2019;6:94-8.
3. Albertini DF. The making and managing of a niche for artificial intelligence in reproductive medicine. J Assist Reprod Genet. 2023;40:211-2.
4. Hariton E, Chi EA, Chi G, Morris JR, Braatz J, Rajpurkar P, et al. A machine learning algorithm can optimize the day of trigger to improve in vitro fertilization outcomes. Fertil Steril. 2021;116:1227-35.
5. Letterie G, Mac Donald A. Artificial intelligence in in vitro fertilization: a computer decision support system for day-to-day management of ovarian stimulation during in vitro fertilization. Fertil Steril. 2020;114:1026-31.
6. Fanton M, Nutting V, Solano F, Maeder-York P, Hariton E, Barash O, et al. An interpretable machine learning model for predicting the optimal day of trigger during ovarian stimulation. Fertil Steril. 2022;118:101-8.
7. Kriegeskorte N, Golan T. Neural network models and deep learning. Curr Biol. 2019;29:R231-R236.
8. Deo RC. Machine learning in medicine. Circulation. 2015;132:1920-30.
9. Geras KJ, Mann RM, Moy L. Artificial intelligence for mammography and digital breast tomosynthesis: current concepts and future perspectives. Radiology. 2019;293: 246-59.
10. Trang NTH, Long KQ, An PL, Dang TN. Development of an artificial intelligence-based breast cancer detection model by combining mammograms and medical health records. Diagnostics (Basel). 2023;13:346.
11. Kim EY, Kim YJ, Choi WJ, Jeon JS, Kim MY, Oh DH, et al. Concordance rate of radiologists and a commercialized deep-learning solution for chest X-ray: real-world experience with a multicenter health screening cohort. PLoS One. 2022;17:e0264383.
12. Ström P, Kartasalo K, Olsson H, Solorzano L, Delahunt B, Berney DM, et al. Artificial intelligence for diagnosis and grading of prostate cancer in biopsies: a population-based, diagnostic study. Lancet Oncol. 2020;21:222-32.
13. Fleuren LM, Klausch TLT, Zwager CL, Schoonmade LJ, Guo T, Roggeveen LF, et al. Machine learning for the prediction of sepsis: a systematic review and meta-analysis of diagnostic test accuracy. Intensive Care Med. 2020;46(3):383-400.
14. Gaieski DF, Carr B, Toolan M, Ciotti K, Kidane A, Flaada D, et al. Can an end-to-end Telesepsis solution improve the severe sepsis and septic shock management Bundle-1 metrics for sepsis patients admitted from the emergency department to the hospital? Crit Care Explor. 2022;4:e0767.
15. Yuan Z, Yuan M, Song X, Huang X, Yan W. Development of an artificial intelligence based model for predicting the euploidy of blastocysts in PGT-A treatments. Sci Rep. 2023;13:2322.
16. Letterie G. Three ways of knowing: the integration of clinical expertise, evidence-based medicine, and artificial intelligence in assisted reproductive technologies. J Assist Reprod Genet. 2021;38:1617-25.
17. McLernon DJ, Raja EA, Toner JP, Baker VL, Doody KJ, Seifer DB, et al. Predicting personalized cumulative live birth following in vitro fertilization. Fertil Steril. 2022;117:326-38.
18. Wang CW, Kuo CY, Chen CH, Hsieh YH, Su ECY. Predicting clinical pregnancy using clinical features and machine learning algorithms in in vitro fertilization. PLoS One. 2022;17:e0267554.
19. Nelson SM, Fleming R, Gaudoin M, Choi B, Santo-Domingo K, Yao M. Antimullerian hormone levels and antral follicle count as prognostic indicators in a personalized prediction model of live birth. Fertil Steril. 2015;104:325-32.
20. Choi B, Bosch E, Lannon BM, Leveille MC, Wong WH, Leader A, et al. Personalized prediction of first-cycle in vitro fertilization success. Fertil Steril. 2013;99:1905-11.
21. Banerjee P, Choi B, Shahine LK, Jun SH, O'Leary K, Lathi RB, et al. Deep phenotyping to predict live birth outcomes in in vitro fertilization. Proc Natl Acad Sci U S A. 2010;107:13570-5.
22. Jun SH, Choi B, Shahine L, Westphal LM, Behr B, ReijoPera RA, et al. Defining human embryo phenotypes by cohort-specific prognostic factors. PLoS One. 2008;3:e2562.
23. Wald K, Hariton E, Morris JR, Chi EA, Jaswa EG, Cedars MI, et al. Changing stimulation protocol on repeat conventional ovarian stimulation cycles does not lead to improved laboratory outcomes. Fertil Steril. 2021;116:757-65.
24. Howles CM, Saunders H, Alam V, England P; FSH Treatment Guidelines Clinical Panel. Predictive factors and a corresponding treatment algorithm for controlled ovarian stimulation in patients treated with recombinant human follicle stimulating hormone (follitropin alfa) during assisted reproduction technology (ART) procedures. An analysis of 1378 patients. Curr Med Res Opin. 2006;22:907-18.
25. Olivennes F, Trew G, Borini A, Broekmans F, Arriagada P, Warne DW, et al. Randomized, controlled, open-label, non-inferiority study of the CONSORT algorithm for individualized dosing of follitropin alfa. Reprod Biomed Online. 2015;30:248-57.
26. Fanton M, Cho JH, Baker VL, Loewke K. A higher number of oocytes retrieved is associated with an increase in fertilized oocytes, blastocysts, and cumulative live birth rates. Fertil Steril. 2023;119:762-9.
27. Abbara A, Vuong LN, Ho VNA, Clarke SA, Jeffers L, Comninos AN, et al. Follicle size on day of trigger most likely to yield a mature oocyte. Front Endocrinol (Lausanne). 2018;9:193.
28. Liang X, Fang J, Li H, Yang X, Ni D, Zeng F, et al. CR-Unet-based ultrasonic follicle monitoring to reduce diameter variability and generate area automatically as a novel biomarker for follicular maturity. Ultrasound Med Biol. 2020;46:3125-34.

29. Sun H, Gong TT, Jiang YT, Zhang S, Zhao YH, Wu QJ. Global, regional, and national prevalence and disability-adjusted life-years for infertility in 195 countries and territories, 1990–2017: results from a Global Burden of Disease Study, 2017. Aging (Albany NY). 2019;11:10952-91.
30. VerMilyea M, Hall JMM, Diakiw SM, Johnston A, Nguyen T, Perugini D, et al. Development of an artificial intelligence-based assessment model for prediction of embryo viability using static images captured by optical light microscopy during IVF. Hum Reprod. 2020;35:770-84.
31. Muehlematter UJ, Daniore P, Vokinger KN. Approval of artificial intelligence and machine learning-based medical devices in the USA and Europe (2015–20): a comparative analysis. Lancet Digit Health. 2021;3(3):e195-e203.
32. Van Laere S, Muylle KM, Cornu P. Clinical decision support and new regulatory frameworks for medical devices: are we ready for it?—A viewpoint paper. Int J Health Policy Manag. 2021;11:3159-63.
33. US Food and Drug Administration. (2019). Proposed regulatory framework for modifications to artificial intelligence/machine learning (AI/ML)-based software as a medical device (SaMD).
34. Kort J, Behr B. Biomechanics and developmental potential of oocytes and embryos. Fertil. Steril 2017;108(5): 738-41.
35. Wakimoto Y, Fukui A, Kojima T, Hasegawa A, Shigeta M, Shibahara H. Application of computer-aided sperm analysis (CASA) for detecting sperm-immobilizing antibody. Am J Reprod Immunol 2018;79(3).
36. Zaninovic N, Irani M, Meseguer M. Assessment of embryo morphology and developmental dynamics by time-lapse microscopy: is there a relation to implantation and ploidy? Fertil Steril. 2017;108(5):722-9.

Time-lapse Monitoring: Will it Change the Assisted Reproductive Technology Outcomes?

R Sujatha

INTRODUCTION

Embryo selection using time-lapse imaging (TLI) technique involves a specialized incubation system with an inbuilt camera, which takes frequent images of embryos in culture and these images are converted into a time-lapse video. This technology enables viewing and documentation of embryo growth and development at multiple time points, which can be used for ranking and selection of embryos. TLI offers the benefit of stable culture conditions, since embryos are not taken out of the incubator for assessment and embryo quality is scored based on annotations of morphology and morphokinetic parameters.

Time-lapse imaging has two advantages, both of which may play a potential role in improving success rates in in vitro fertilization (IVF). The first and foremost advantage is the stable environment provided to the embryo in terms of limited exposure to changes in temperature, pH, and osmolarity. Throughout the IVF process, gametes and embryos are transferred between dishes and their development is assessed at specified times.[1] Exposure to external conditions will alter culture media pH and temperature, thereby creating metabolic stress, which in turn might affect the growth and quality of embryos.[2] In culturing embryos to blastocyst stage, where the embryo spends longer time in culture compared to cleavage stage embryos, the stress is even more pronounced. In time-lapse systems, embryos are assessed within the incubator without disturbing culture conditions.

The second advantage is access to various morphokinetic parameters, such as timing of cell divisions and intervals between different cell cycles, throughout the culture period, which may help in selecting embryos with the highest implantation potential. In the conventional method of embryo assessment, embryos are taken out from the incubator and manually checked at fixed time points once per day. Dynamics of embryo development and crucial information on events such as reverse cleavage, abnormal cell divisions, and direct cleavage may be missed.

Different types of incubator systems are applied in time-lapse microscopy: Open system, where the camera and dishes with embryos are placed inside a regular box incubator, or closed system where there is a complete integration of camera into a smaller incubator.[3] In the case of the latter, embryos can be kept inside the time-lapse system after fertilization until day 5 or 6, without being taken out of the incubator even once for assessment during the entire culture period.

This chapter provides an overview of embryo assessment in TLI, efficiency and limitations of the system, its utility as a deselection tool, and safety and prospects.

EMBRYO ASSESSMENT: CONVENTIONAL METHOD VERSUS TIME-LAPSE IMAGING

Several scoring features have been identified over the last few decades and the most common ones which were associated with increased pregnancy rate and implantation rates are early cleavage rate, blastomere number and size, number of nuclei in blastomeres, embryo fragmentation rate, trophectoderm morphology, and blastocoel expansion.[4] However, all these parameters have been confounded by several factors and offer no significant predictive power on IVF outcome.

In time-lapse systems, algorithms are created based on morphokinetic variables, which are the morphologic and cleavage features, such as pronuclear appearance, disappearance, time to division to 2 cells, 3 cells, cleavage cycle, duration between two cell phases, etc., assessed at specific checkpoints during culture period using large datasets.[5-7] Morphokinetic characteristics are then correlated to outcomes such as implantation rate or live birth rate. Different authors have different explanations to these terminologies and several embryo scoring algorithms (ESAs) have been published to correlate morphokinetic characteristics with blastulation, implantation, and or pregnancy rates.

EFFICIENCY OF TIME-LAPSE IMAGING

Some of the most common algorithms are Eeva™ (Early Embryo Viability Assessment) and KIDS (Known Implantation Data Score). Eeva is an FDA (Food and Drug Administration)-approved software, which predicts blastulation rates by assessing cell division timings namely P2 (time between cytokinesis 1 and 2) and P3 (time between cytokinesis 2 and 3). However, results so far suggest that Eeva™ showed no advantage in blastocyst prediction and embryo selection on comparison with manual assessment.[8] KIDScore is based on six annotations (the number of pronuclei, time from insemination to pronuclei fading at the 1-cell stage, time from insemination to the 2-cell stage, time from insemination to the 3-cell stage, time from insemination to the 5-cell stage, and time from insemination to the 8-cell stage).[9] Barrie et al. compared six ESAs to a large set of known implantation embryos, and none of these ESAs crossed an AUC [area under the receiver operating characteristic (ROC) curve] of 0.65 (0.54–0.63), which indicates poor predictive value.[10] It has been shown that most predictive algorithms were developed from small databases, which limits their routine application in all assisted reproduction laboratories.[11]

Several studies have reported improvement of outcome using time-lapse algorithms. Ongoing pregnancy rate per transfer was found to be statistically increased in the time-lapse group compared with the control group.[12] In another randomized sibling study, in which embryo transfers were done only with euploid embryos, it was observed that ongoing pregnancy rates were significantly increased when embryo selection was done based on morphokinetic scores (68.9% vs. 40.5%, respectively, $p = 0.019$).[13] These studies were found to be associated with several problems, such as different culture conditions for the study and intervention groups, nonsegregation of day 5 and day 3, and single- and double-embryo transfers. These issues make it difficult to attribute the benefit observed to time-lapse system.

Nine randomized controlled trials (RCTs) involving 2,955 couples were analyzed in the recent Cochrane meta-analysis on time-lapse technology[14] and the quality of evidence favoring TLI was graded as very low to low. It was concluded that there is insufficient good-quality evidence of outcomes between time-lapse and traditional systems. No study has been published as of today on comparison of cumulative live birth rates.

All evidence for embryo selection using still TLI images, compared with conventional incubation and assessment, was of low quality. In cycles involving conventional incubation and assessment, live birth or ongoing pregnancy rate was found to be 35%, and the rates in TLI with conventional morphological assessment using still TLI images was between 27% and 40%. Miscarriage rate in cycles in conventional incubation was 4%, compared to 4–14% in conventional morphological assessment of still TLI images.

Evidence was found to be of low quality in studies comparing embryo selection using TLI software (group A) compared with conventional assessment of still TLI images (group B). Ongoing pregnancy rate in group B was 47% compared to a range of 22–52% in group A. Miscarriage rate in group B was 5%, compared to a range of 4–15% in group A.

In case of embryo selection utilizing TLI software (group A) compared with conventional incubation and assessment (group B), it was found that there were lower rates of miscarriage in the cycles of group A. It was also observed that live birth rate in group B is 48%, in comparison to a range of 46–55% in group A. Miscarriage rate with conventional incubation is 11% whereas in the TLI was in the range of 5–10%. Evidence was found to be of low quality in this comparative analysis.

LIMITATIONS OF TIME-LAPSE IMAGING

Major concerns or potential bias in interpreting time-lapse algorithms are as follows. Embryo developmental parameters depend on culture conditions, media, incubator parameters such as temperature, and gas levels, low O_2, and it is difficult to extrapolate algorithms from one laboratory to another.[15,16] Annotations of the kinetic data are time-consuming, and it is likely that there is a lot of interpersonal variation among embryologists, influencing the calculated score. Due to these reasons, predictive value of morphokinetic parameters for implantation has not been confirmed in multicenter studies so far.[17,18] Some of the commonly used scoring algorithms based on known implantation data of individual embryos appear biased due to the exclusion of double-embryo transfer cycles, which resulted in singleton pregnancy. If the data on nonimplanting embryos are included, would the algorithms be different is the question, which has not been addressed until now. Different software are used in different time-lapse systems, and scoring is based on variable algorithms, making comparison between them less informative.

BENEFICIAL UTILITY OF TIME-LAPSE IMAGING

Even though there is inconclusive evidence on the utilization of TLI in improving pregnancy rates, there are other possibilities where TLI could be of benefit. One such advantage would be to deselect embryos. It has been shown that abnormal cleavage patterns, such as direct cleavage from single cell to three cells and reverse cleavage, which is due to blastomere fusion, or failed cytokinesis, negatively affects embryo quality. During conventional embryo assessment, these events are most probably missed. Deselection of these embryos was shown to improve implantation.[19,20]

Another advantage of TLI is it provides a tool for research, teaching, standardizing assessment, facilitating laboratory workflows, and quality control. Embryo morphology and timing of growth are documented diligently without removing embryos from the incubator. This further reduces exposure to unfavorable environment. It also helps in increased understanding of "embryo growth behavior" (such as cleavage pattern) and compares culture conditions for example O_2 levels, pH, temperature, specific growth patterns, and outcome. In addition, time-lapse data might help in the validation of different embryo scoring systems and man power training.[21]

TIME-LAPSE IMAGING AND ASSESSMENT OF PLOIDY STATUS OF EMBRYOS

Assessing ploidy status of embryos before embryo transfer is gaining considerable importance lately based on the logic that exclusive euploid embryo transfer should increase implantation rates and/or decrease missed abortion rates, thereby increasing live birth. This has not been proved conclusively, as IVF pregnancy depends on multiple factors. STAR trial, the most recent and largest RCT including 661 treatment cycles, found no difference in ongoing pregnancy rate between the PGT-A group and the control group.[22] Miscarriage rates ($p = 0.90$) were not found to be different between both the groups. Cycles were cancelled in 17% of the patients in the PGT-A group (compared to 5% in the control group) as there were no euploid blastocysts. Current techniques for performing PGT-A are invasive, where cells are removed from the embryos, influencing success rates. It has been proposed to assess embryos' ploidy status using morphokinetic patterns. Selected morphokinetic parameters have been found to be associated with ploidy status of the embryo in few independent studies.[23,24] A large cohort study did not find any association between early (up to the 8-cell stage) morphokinetic parameters and aneuploidy.[25] In selected female age-groups, late kinetic parameters such as tSB (time for start of blastulation), tEB (time for initiation of expansion of the blastocyst), and tEB-tSB (the time difference between these two events) were found to be predictive of euploidy. It was found that chances of having a euploid blastocyst were 1.5 times higher when tSB is <96.2 hours. In these cycles, deselection of dysmorphic embryos further enhanced this predictive value.[26] Until more comparative data between embryo biopsy and TLI selection emerges, it must be assumed that TLI annotations depend on patient characteristics and laboratory conditions and cannot be used to confirm ploidy status of embryos.

PROSPECTS OF TIME-LAPSE IMAGING AND EMBRYO SELECTION

Data from time-lapse systems helps in deep machine learning, where analysis of entire time-lapse videos can be used to generate accurate, positive prediction models. One example for this application is the study, where 8,836 embryos were cultured in a time-lapse system and the videos were used to test and build a model, which could predict fetal heart pregnancy with an AUC of 0.93 [95% confidence interval (CI): 0.92–0.94].[27] More work is underway in this area where TLI can be used to select highest quality embryos.

CONCLUSION

Time-lapse imaging offers stable culture conditions and excellent information on many parameters, which may eventually prove to have an impact in the selection of embryos and lead to improvement of pregnancy rates. However, currently evidence is not conclusive to show that embryo selection through TLI is more accurate or predictive than conventional manual morphological selection. Though data from several individual studies show a positive trend toward the usage of TLI, it has been difficult to replicate the benefit across patient population and different laboratories.

REFERENCES

1. Alpha Scientists in Reproductive Medicine and ESHRE Special Interest Group of Embryology. The Istanbul consensus workshop on embryo assessment: proceedings of an expert meeting. Hum Reprod. 2011;26:1270-83.
2. Swain JE, Carrell D, Cobo A, Meseguer M, Rubio C, Smith GD. Optimizing the culture environment and embryo manipulation to help maintain embryo developmental potential. Fertil Steril. 2016;105:571-87.
3. Virtolife. [online] Available from http://www.fertilitech.com/en-GB/Home.aspx [Last accessed April, 2024].
4. Jiang X, Cai J, Liu L, Liu Z, Wang W, Chen J, et al. Does conventional morphological evaluation still play a role in predicting blastocyst formation? Reprod Biol Endocrinol. 2022;20(1):68.
5. Ciray HN, Campbell A, Agerholm IE, Aguilar J, Chamayou S, Esbert M, et al. Proposed guidelines on the nomenclature and annotation of dynamic human embryo monitoring by a time-lapse user group. Hum Reprod. 2014;29:2650-60.
6. Wong CC, Loewke KE, Bossert NL, Behr B, De Jonge CJ, Baer TM, et al. Non-invasive imaging of human embryos before embryonic genome activation predicts development to the blastocyst stage. Nat Biotechnol. 2010;28:1115-21.
7. Meseguer M, Herrero J, Tejera A, Hilligsøe KM, Ramsing NB, Remohí J. The use of morphokinetics as a predictor of embryo implantation. Hum Reprod. 2011;26:2658-71.
8. Conaghan J, Chen AA, Willman SP, Ivani K, Chenette PE, Boostanfar R, et al. Improving embryo selection using a computer-automated time-lapse image analysis test plus day 3 morphology: results from a prospective multicenter trial. Fertil Steril. 2013;100:412-9.e5.
9. Gazzo E, Peña F, Valdéz F, Chung A, Bonomini C, Ascenzo M, et al. The Kidscore™ D5 algorithm as an additional tool to morphological assessment and PGT-A in embryo selection: a time-lapse study. JBRA Assist Reprod. 2020;24(1):55-60.
10. Barrie A, Homburg R, McDowell G, Brown J, Kingsland C, Troup S. Examining the efficacy of six published time-lapse imaging embryo selection algorithms to predict implantation to demonstrate the need for the development of specific, in-house morphokinetic selection algorithms. Fertil Steril. 2017;107:613-21.
11. Petersen BM, Boel M, Montag M, Gardner DK. Development of a generally applicable morphokinetic algorithm capable of predicting the implantation potential of embryos transferred on Day 3. Hum Reprod. 2016;31(10):2231-44.
12. Rubio I, Galán A, Larreategui Z, Ayerdi F, Bellver J, Herrero J, et al. Clinical validation of embryo culture and selection by morphokinetic analysis: a randomized, controlled trial of the EmbryoScope. Fertil Steril. 2014;102: 1287-94.
13. Yang Z, Zhang J, Salem SA, Liu X, Kuang Y, Salem RD, et al. Selection of competent blastocysts for transfer by combining time-lapse monitoring and array CGH testing for patients undergoing preimplantation genetic screening: a prospective study with sibling oocytes. BMC Med Genomics. 2014;7:38.
14. Armstrong S, Bhide P, Jordan V, Pacey A, Marjoribanks J, Farquhar C. Time-lapse systems for embryo incubation and assessment in assisted reproduction. Cochrane Database Syst Rev. 2019;5:CD01132.
15. Ciray HN, Aksoy T, Goktas C, Ozturk B, Bahceci M. Time-lapse evaluation of human embryo development in single versus sequential culture media—a sibling oocyte study. J Assist Reprod Genet. 2012;29:891-900.
16. Basile N, Morbeck D, Garcia-Velasco J, Bronet F, Meseguer M. Type of culture media does not affect embryo kinetics: a time-lapse analysis of sibling oocytes. Hum Reprod. 2013; 28:634-41.
17. Ahlstrom A, Park H, Bergh C, Selleskog U, Lundin K. Conventional morphology performs better than morphokinetics for prediction of live birth after day 2 transfer. Reprod Biomed Online. 2016;33:61-70.
18. Liu Y, Feenan K, Chapple V, Matson P. Assessing efficacy of day 3 embryo time-lapse algorithms retrospectively: impacts of dataset type and confounding factors. Hum Fertil (Camb). 2019;22:182-90.
19. Athayde Wirka K, Chen AA, Conaghan J, Ivani K, Gvakharia M, Behr B, et al. Atypical embryo phenotypes identified by time-lapse microscopy: high prevalence and association with embryo development. Fertil Steril. 2014;101:1637-48.
20. Rubio I, Kuhlmann R, Agerholm I, Kirk J, Herrero J, Escribá MJ, et al. Limited implantation success of direct-cleaved human zygotes: a time-lapse study. Fertil Steril. 2012;98: 1458-63.
21. ESHRE Working group on Time-lapse technology; Apter S, Ebner T, Freour T, Guns Y, Kovacic B, Le Clef N, et al. Good practice recommendations for the use of time-lapse technology[†]. Hum Reprod Open. 2020;2020(2):hoaa008.
22. Munné S, Kaplan B, Frattarelli JL, Child T, Nakhuda G, Shamma FN, et al.; STAR Study Group. Preimplantation genetic testing for aneuploidy versus morphology as selection criteria for single frozen-thawed embryo transfer in good-prognosis patients: a multicenter randomized clinical trial. Fertil Steril. 2019;112(6):1071-9.
23. Kramer YG, Kofinas JD, Melzer K, Noyes N, McCaffrey C, Buldo-Licciardi J, et al. Assessing morphokinetic parameters

via time lapse microscopy (TLM) to predict euploidy: are aneuploidy risk classification models universal? J Assist Reprod Genet. 2014;31:1231-42.

24. Vera-Rodriguez M, Chavez SL, Rubio C, Reijo Pera RA, Simon C. Prediction model for aneuploidy in early human embryo development revealed by single-cell analysis. Nat Commun. 2015;6:7601.
25. Rienzi L, Capalbo A, Stoppa M, Romano S, Maggiulli R, Albricci L, et al. No evidence of association between blastocyst aneuploidy and morphokinetic assessment in a selected population of poor-prognosis patients: a longitudinal cohort study. Reprod Biomed Online. 2015; 30:57-66.
26. Desai N, Goldberg JM, Austin C, Falcone T. Are cleavage anomalies, multinucleation, or specific cell cycle kinetics observed with time-lapse imaging predictive of embryo developmental capacity or ploidy? Fertil Steril. 2018;109: 665-74.
27. Tran D, Cooke S, Illingworth PJ, Gardner DK. Deep learning as a predictive tool for fetal heart pregnancy following time-lapse incubation and blastocyst transfer. Hum Reprod. 2019;34:1011-8.

Chapter

Implementing Total Quality Management in Assisted Reproductive Technology: Role of Witnessing and Beyond

Sayali Kandari

INTRODUCTION

In vitro fertilization (IVF) has revolutionized reproductive medicine, offering hope to couples facing infertility challenges. The success of IVF procedures relies on intricate processes within the laboratory setting. Management is the core component of a successful IVF procedure.

The component and principles of total quality management (TQM) can significantly enhance efficiency, reduce errors, and improve success rates. This chapter explores the integration of TQM in IVF laboratories. Electronic witnessing has now become a quality parameter judging the IVF center's quality process. However, we emphasize that without a working TQM active in an IVF laboratory, electronic witnessing system (EWS) is limited in protecting patients from unforced errors.

It is hence, this chapter's motive to explain the significance of implementing TQM in a laboratory alongside manual or electronic witnessing to improve high-quality services to patients undergoing fertility treatments.

TOTAL QUALITY MANAGEMENT IN HEALTH CARE

Total quality management is a comprehensive management philosophy focusing on continuous improvement, customer satisfaction, and the involvement of all organizational members.[1] In the context of IVF laboratories, TQM encompasses processes, personnel, and technology to ensure the highest quality services.[2]

Embryology laboratories are an essential part of an assisted reproductive technology (ART) clinic. There are some recommendations already discussed by the European Society of Human Reproduction for key performance indicators (KPIs) in IVF laboratories.[3]

Implementing TQM in an IVF laboratory involves streamlining processes for clinical setting that is outpatient department (OPD), surgical setting that is inpatient department (IPD), all andrology and embryology procedures, preimplantation genetic procedures, diagnostic laboratory, handling finances, and regulatory as well as medicolegal mandatory requirements.

The important thing is that emphasis should be placed on optimizing workflows, minimizing variability, and maintaining consistency throughout each step of the procedure.[4]

It should be noted that TQM recognizes the importance of well-trained and motivated personnel. For it to run smoothly, continuous training programs for embryologists, technicians, and support staff are essential to enhance skills, reduce errors, and promote a culture of quality.

There are four basic steps to TQM:

1. Quality planning (QP)
2. Quality control (QC)
3. Quality assurance (QA)
4. Quality improvement (QI)

Total quality management is sometimes confused with QC and QA; there are major differences between the three quality plans:

- QC is an activity designed to ensure that a specific element within the laboratory is functioning correctly.

  Some QC activity involves, documenting laboratory parameters every day, ambient temperature and humidity, or temperature readings on display, and an external measuring instrument on a daily chart.
- QA is designed to identify problems or errors within the defined work processes and standard operating procedures (SOPs).

Quality assurance involves using QC parameters and designing audits internally to assure quality is within acceptable ranges of outcomes. KPI monitoring in an IVF laboratory is a QA activity.

- TQM is a comprehensive monitoring process designed not only to detect and eliminate problems, but also to enhance a laboratory's performance by exploring innovation and developing flexibility and effectiveness in all processes.

Total quality management indicators needed should be objective, relevant to the laboratory and clinical program, and measure a broad range of specific events or aspects of treatment that reflect the quality of care.

Threshold values for each of the indicators should be based on how the specific protocols used in the laboratory impact the outcomes and the nature of the indicators on quality of care.

TOTAL QUALITY MANAGEMENT IN ASSISTED REPRODUCTIVE TECHNOLOGY SERVICES (FIG. 1)

The ultimate test of any QC process has to begin with the main critical measure of the performance of the care provided. In a fertility clinic that must be clinical pregnancy rate for IVF laboratories and live birth rate per treatment cycle for the complete fertility unit.

An ongoing record of the results of fertilization, cleavage, and embryo development provide the best short-term evidence of good QC. Daily records in the form of a laboratory logbook or electronic database are essential, summarizing details of patients and outcome of laboratory procedures: age, cause of infertility, stimulation protocol, number of oocytes retrieved, semen analysis, sperm preparation details, insemination time, fertilization, cleavage, embryo transfer, and cryopreservation.

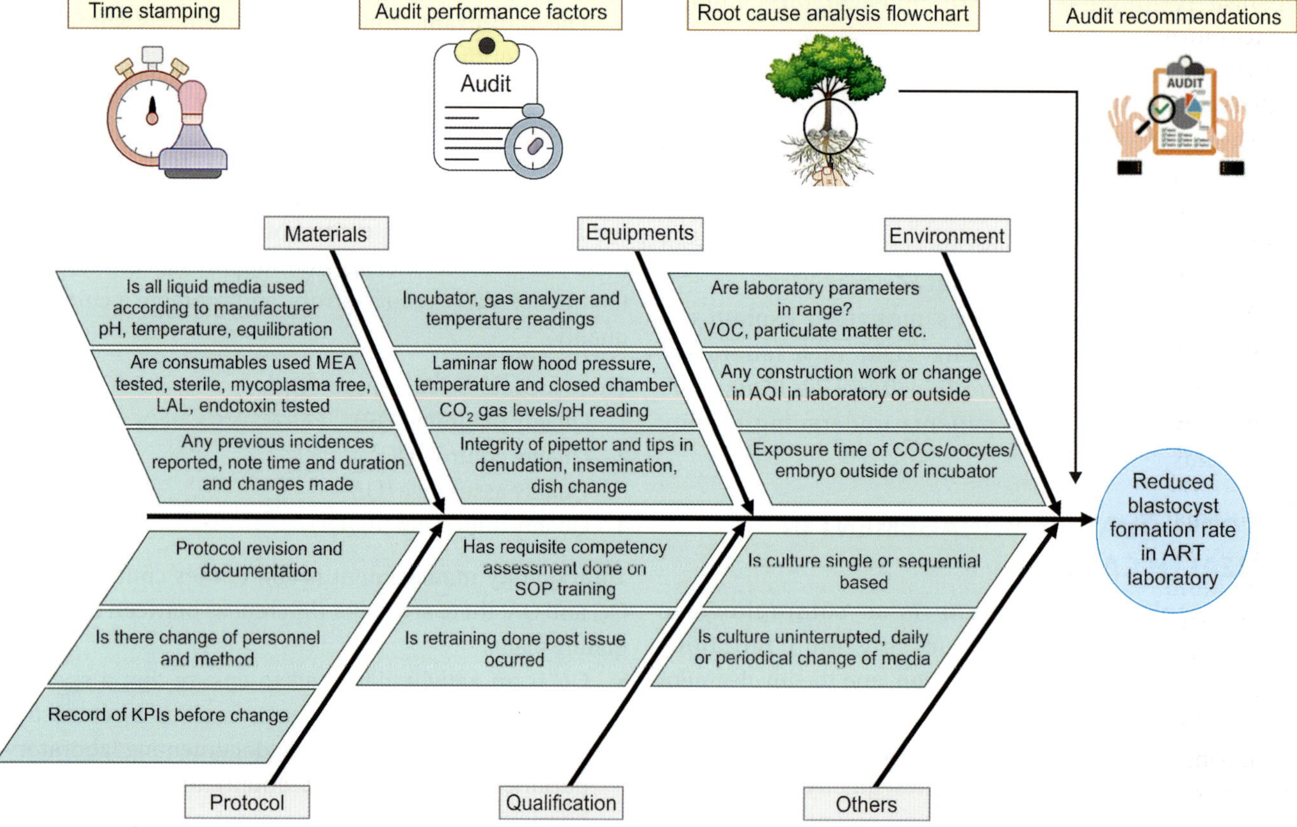

Fig. 1: Root cause analysis for evaluating lowered QA (KPI parameters) in an ART laboratory. All parameters within scope are analyzed for deviations and nonconformances noted. Audits internal and external serve the purpose of documenting and collecting data preventively and proactively in a TQM program. (AQI: air quality index; ART: assisted reproductive technology; COCs: combined oral contraceptives; KPI: key performance indicators; LAL: limulus amebocyte lysate; MEA: mouse embryo assay; QA: quality assurance; SOP: standard operating procedure)

Details of media and oil batches and all consumables that come into contact with gametes and embryos must also be recorded for reference, and the introduction of any new methods or materials must be documented. It is essential that all records are reviewed on a regular basis.

Implementing QC measures, such as regular equipment calibration, monitoring environmental conditions, and maintaining strict aseptic techniques, is critical for ensuring result reliability and minimizing the risk of contamination.

Incorporating cutting-edge technologies, such as time-lapse imaging and noninvasive embryo assessment tools, allows for real-time monitoring and improves the selection of viable embryos, contributing to increased success rates.[5]

ROLE OF WITNESSING SYSTEMS

Witnessing systems have emerged in the last decade to ameliorate the medicolegal issues arising out of dealing with human gametes and the very real risk of gamete mix ups owing to handling large volumes in a single laboratory, nonconformances in labeling by laboratory staff and unforced medical errors of clinical, reception, and other staff handling patients which could lead to labeling errors.

The entire process includes the period of stimulation and responding to the drugs, to getting mature eggs, the insemination via conventional IVF or intracytoplasmic sperm injection (ICSI), vitrification, or thawing or preimplantation genetic testing (PGT).

Assisted reproductive technology clinical processes are defined in three phases described here.

1. Preanalytical phase (e.g., patient identification, labeling, and clinical and laboratory plan of action)
2. Analytical phase (laboratory procedures; oocyte retrieval, insemination, cryopreservation, etc.)
3. Postanalytical phase (e.g., recording videos, photos of embryos and gametes, and reporting results).

To minimize and prevent mix-ups[6] from happening, appropriate authorities such as the Human Fertilization and Embryology Authority (HFEA) in 2003[7] and later the European Society of Human Reproduction and Embryology (ESHRE)[8] have recommended the use of manual double witnessing protocols in IVF clinics. This method involves verification of patient ID mentioned on dishes during the IVF procedure by a second person (double witnessing), in order to reduce possible human errors.[9]

On the other hand, there is also the increased risk of work interruptions and distractions by an additional human witness, which further led to the development of a proper standardized witnessing protocol known as the electronic witnessing system (EWS).[9,10]

Electronic witnessing system is based on the principal of monitoring critical work during different stages in the IVF laboratory and reducing the risks of sample errors by tagging all plasticware used for a particular patient in the IVF laboratory with either adhesive barcode stickers or adhesive radio frequency identification (RFID) labels which are identified by readers connected to a computer.[10,11] These systems eliminate the need for a second human witness and allows embryologists to monitor and trace matching events from sperm preparation up to embryology procedures thus minimizing mismatch errors while improving patient care and sample management. The system also eliminates work interruptions and distractions, thereby reducing the risk of sample mismatches.[9,12] By incorporating EWS in the IVF laboratory, embryologists would not face any possible "accidents" like working on more than one patient's biological sample at a time, or the potential omission of a key step during the procedure, ensuring that the SOP is followed.[13]

A few strong guidelines developed by international societies currently guide us to reduce risk of errors and catastrophe in IVF laboratories.

Regulatory bodies HFEA in the United Kingdom and the ESHRE have set up good practice guidelines to minimize these errors.

In India, we grapple with basic QC tasks in multitude of centers and a consistent comprehensive TQM is the need of the hour.

The highest priority is now to be designated in inculcating internal and external audit for minimizing and preventing reoccurrence of errors in IVF laboratories.

Current EWSs have begun to become more flexible and more amenable to Indian ART laboratories; however, due to their international origins, most still fail to understand and identify the unique problems we encounter in Indian context such as lack of trained personnel, need for translated documents for many housekeeping or entry level local staff as well as training which is kept in scope of ART units making it an implementation hurdle to cross.

Potential risky errors like mismatches can result in legal consequences against the embryologist and ART clinic, further destroying their reputation. To best avoid these mix-ups from happening, EWS alongside manual double witnessing would be a good choice to incorporate especially in busy ART clinics.[13] Though EWS is a boon to modern day busy IVF clinics, there is an unspoken risk of printing wrong labels or attaching a wrong label to plasticware in the IVF laboratory.

Total quality management hence is not an option but a requirement to reduce risk and error across the entire ART patient work flow.

ACCREDITATION: OPTIONS, CHALLENGES, OUTCOMES

ISO 9001:2000

ISO 9001 standards is a quality management requirement. It provides a framework to the organization to set quality standardized objectives and workflow ensuring that every procedure is followed, thereby minimizing potential mishaps, while guaranteeing quality performance and safety to the employees and patients.[14]

ISO 15189 has more standardization.[15] It is an international QMS guideline for medical laboratories that extends beyond equipment, personnel, addressing, and resolving complaints to other important aspects of the center like patient identification; sample collection, examination, and preparation; and appropriate interpretation and reporting of patient's sample/procedure results.[14,16]

It is the accreditation that is closest to ART services; however, most ISO 15189[17] components deal with diagnosis versus treatment which is completely counter to ART laboratory goals. There are many parts of ISO 15189 that do not apply and are hence tedious and unnecessary for fertility centers.

INDIAN SOCIETY OF ASSISTED REPRODUCTION ACCREDITATION

Currently, the Indian Society of Assisted Reproduction (ISAR) provides accreditation to fertility laboratories. These programs have created a baseline level of services; however, the penetration of the program is lower than desired and there is a lack of effective industry-oriented auditing that should be conducted by personnel privy to the fertility process in toto.[18]

Currently, we are working closely with ISAR to update the accreditation to include the TQM modules and upgrade quality management services to the Indian fertility treatment providers via the IVFCHECK© program.

NATIONAL ACCREDITATION BOARD FOR HOSPITALS ACCREDITATION

The National Accreditation Board for Hospitals (NABH) is a government regulated body that accredits hospitals registered in India. However, the scope and implementation of NABH is mainly in the medical insurance mandated sector provided by government or private players which are highly cost-controlled, and India's fertility industry is currently paid out-of-pocket by patients.[19]

INTERNATIONAL ACCREDITATIONS

The College of American Pathologists provides certification to Indian diagnostic providers; however, penetration in ART laboratories does not exist. The biggest hurdle is cost per certification as the workload of ART laboratories is fragmented between private players and it is unsustainable to invest every year in these accreditations, valuable though they are, they are currently not for small to medium ART laboratories.[20]

The Reproductive Technology Accreditation Committee (RTAC) is a professional group of the Board of the Fertility Society of Australia and penetration exists in multiple Asia-Pacific countries. However, RTAC was unable to find foothold in India due to the primary factor of cost of implementation including charges for international auditors and although valuable, remains out of reach of Indian fertility providers.[21]

IVFCHECK©

A TQM program developed with the Indian fertility services market at heart, the salient points and provisions are the following:

- IVF unit-wise SOP mapping
- Process mapping development
- Internal IVF audit management
- External audits
- Root cause analysis (RCA) and plan-do-check-action (PDCA)
- Medicolegal checklists
- Regulatory checklists
- Embryologist and staff competency training.

With the advent of the ART BILL 2021,[22] quality management in India has to be addressed in the context of the regulation and supervision of ART clinics and banks.

The Act aims to ensure safe and ethical practices in ART services for addressing reproductive health issues related to infertility, disease, or social and medical concerns.

The appropriate authorities, such as the National Board and State Boards, have the power to investigate complaints against ART clinics or banks and recommend modifications to rules and regulations based on changes in technology or social conditions. The National Registry, established under the Act, collects data that can be utilized by the National Board for policy-making, guideline development, and identifying new research areas in assisted reproduction and related fields. The Central Government can issue directions to the National Board, National Registry, and appropriate authorities to ensure the sovereignty, integrity, security, and public order of India.

Overall, the National Registry shall collect data related to the enrolment of individuals and couples, as well as data that supports policy-making, research, and the regulation of ART clinics and banks in India.[17]

FUTURE DIRECTIONS

Continuous improvement and a patient-centric approach are both essential to the current surviving and thriving of fertility centers in India.

Regular audits, competency assessments, and external quality assessment with a TQM focused approach shall lead IVF laboratories in India to compliance with established protocols, identify areas for improvement, and contribute to ongoing quality enhancement.

It is now time to encourage open communication with employees, management, clinical, nursing teams, counselors, embryologists and patients, addressing concerns, and continuously adapting processes to enhance the overall patient experience and optimize results.

Implementing TQM in IVF laboratories may face challenges such as resistance to change, financial constraints, and the need for ongoing staff training. Overcoming these challenges requires commitment from leadership, a robust training infrastructure, and a focus on long-term benefits.

CONCLUSION

By implementing QC as per quality management standards, a fertility clinic can perform their tasks with mental peace. The total quality management system (TQMS) makes tasks easier and more efficient, which is linked with the clinic's productivity, profitability, and medicolegal compliance.

It provides tools to monitor what to do, leading the way for continuous improvement of the service. High-quality robust metrics involving the various dimensions of care, effectiveness, safety, patient-centeredness, efficiency, timelines, and equity are the need of the hour for Indian ART centers and we hope that the new era and our work ushers in a quality management era of fertility industry in India.

REFERENCES

1. Dale BG. Managing Quality, 4th edition. USA: Blackwell Publishing Ltd; 2003.
2. Oakland JS. Total Quality Management and Operational Excellence: Text with Cases, 4th edition. London: Routledge; 2014.
3. Malhotra J, Malhotra K, Talwar P, Kannan P, Singh P, et al. ISAR Consensus Guidelines on Safety and Ethical Practices in In vitro Fertilization Clinics. J Hum Reprod Sci. 2021;14:S48-S68.
4. Pyzdek T, Keller PA. The Six Sigma Handbook, 4th edition. New York: McGraw-Hill Education; 2014.
5. Alpha Scientists in Reproductive Medicine and ESHRE Special Interest Group of Embryology. The Istanbul consensus workshop on embryo assessment: proceedings of an expert meeting. Hum Reprod. 2011; 26(6):1270-83.
6. Spriggs M. IVF mixup: white couple have black babies. J Med Ethics. 2003;29(2):65.
7. Parry R. (2011). An IVF mix-up meant I had to give birth to someone else's child–and give him away.
8. Brison D, Hooper M, Critchlow J, Hunter H, Arnesen R, Lloyd A, et al. Reducing risk in the IVF laboratory: implementation of a double witnessing system. Clin Risk. 2004;10(5):176-80.
9. Magli MC, Van den Abbeel E, Lundin K, Royere D, Van der Elst J, Gianaroli L, et al. Revised guidelines for good practice in IVF laboratories. Hum Reprod. 2008;23(6): 1253-62.
10. Novo S, Mora-Espí I, Gómez-Martínez R, Barrios L, Ibáñez E, Such X, et al. Traceability of human sperm samples by direct tagging with polysilicon microbarcodes. Reprod Biomed Online. 2015;31(2):162-70.
11. Perez O, Adriaanse HH, Navarrete G, Lay L, Tilley B, Kozlowski J, et al. A non-commercial witnessing system a journey to create a bar code system from dish labels to microscopic bar codes next to the embryo. Fertil Steril. 2022;118(4): p.e153.
12. Holmes R, Wirka KA, Catherino AB, Hayward B, Swain JE. Comparison of electronic versus manual witnessing of procedures within the in vitro fertilization laboratory: impact on timing and efficiency. F S Rep. 2021;2(2): 181-8.
13. Gupta S, Fauzdar A, Singh VJ, Srivastava A, Sharma K, Singh S. A Preliminary Experience of Integration of an Electronic Witness System, its Validation, Efficacy on Lab Performance, and Staff Satisfaction Assessment in a Busy Indian in vitro Fertilization Laboratory. J Hum Reprod Sci. 2020;13(4):333-9.
14. Alper M, Brinsden P, Wikland M, Fischer R. International standard for IVF centres. Hum Reprod. 2003;18(2):460-1.
15. OQRI. (2021). Guest editorial: Corruption rampant in India's ISO Certification Market.

16. Bento FC, Esteves S. Establishing a quality management system in a fertility center: experience with ISO 9001. Med Express (São Paulo, online). 2016;3(3).
17. Iso.org. (2022). ISO 15189:2022: Medical laboratories-Requirements for quality and competence.
18. Malhotra N, Shah D, Pai R, Pai HD, Bankar M. Assisted reproductive technology in India: a 3 year retrospective data analysis. J Hum Reprod Sci. 2013;6(4):235-40.
19. Nair TS, Memon P, Tripathi S, Srivastava A, Sunny Kujur M, Singh D, et al. Implementing a quality improvement initiative for private healthcare facilities to achieve accreditation: experience from India. BMC Health Serv Res. 2023;23(1):802.
20. McCall SJ, Branton PA, Blanc VM, Dry SM, Gastier-Foster JM, Harrison JH, et al. The College of American Pathologists Biorepository Accreditation Program: Results from the First 5 Years. Biopreserv Biobank. 2018;16(1):16-22.
21. Catt J. Australia: QMS in IVF Centres. In: Bento F, Esteves S, Agarwal A (Eds). Quality Management in ART Clinics: A Practical Guide. Boston, MA: Springer; 2013.
22. Prsindia.org. Issues for Consideration: Assisted Reproductive Technology (Regulation) Bill, 2021.

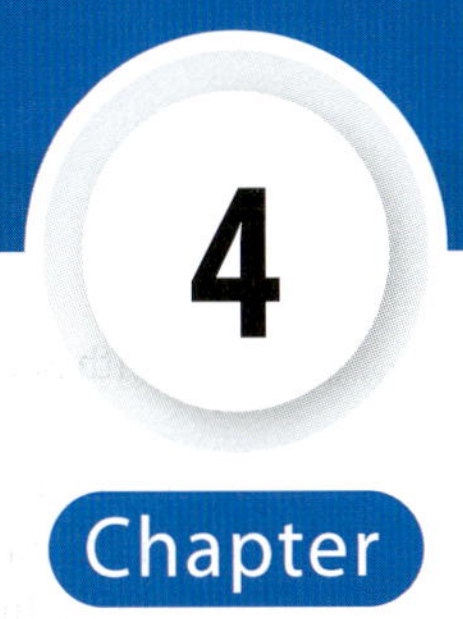

Chapter

Stem Cells: Will they Revolutionize Infertility Management?

Pankaj Kaingade, Gorakh G Mandrupkar

INTRODUCTION

The field of infertility management has made remarkable strides in recent years, offering hope to millions of couples facing reproductive challenges. However, there remain numerous cases where conventional treatments fall short of providing viable solutions. Stem cells is a groundbreaking area of research with the potential to revolutionize infertility management. This chapter explores the current state of stem cell research in the context of infertility, highlighting its promises, challenges, and future prospects.

UNDERSTANDING THE STEM CELLS

Stem cells are unique cells in the body that have the remarkable ability to develop into various different types of cells with specialized functions. They play a crucial role in growth, development, tissue repair, and maintaining the body's overall function. There are two main types of stem cells: (1) embryonic stem cells (ES cells) and (2) adult (or somatic) stem cells.

Embryonic stem cells are stem cells derived from the inner cell mass of an early-stage embryo known as a blastocyst. They are said to be pluripotent because of their plasticity and potentially unlimited capacity for self-renewal. To date, no approved medical treatments have been derived from ES cell research, due to its disadvantages such as ethical issues, immune rejections, and teratoma formation.

Adult stem cells are found in various tissues throughout the body including bone marrow, blood, skin, and organs. They are multipotent, meaning they have a more limited differentiation potential compared to ES cells. Adult stem cells primarily contribute to the repair and regeneration of the specific tissue they reside in. For example, hematopoietic stem cells in the bone marrow can give rise to different types of blood cells, while neural stem cells in the brain can generate neurons and glial cells **(Fig. 1)**.

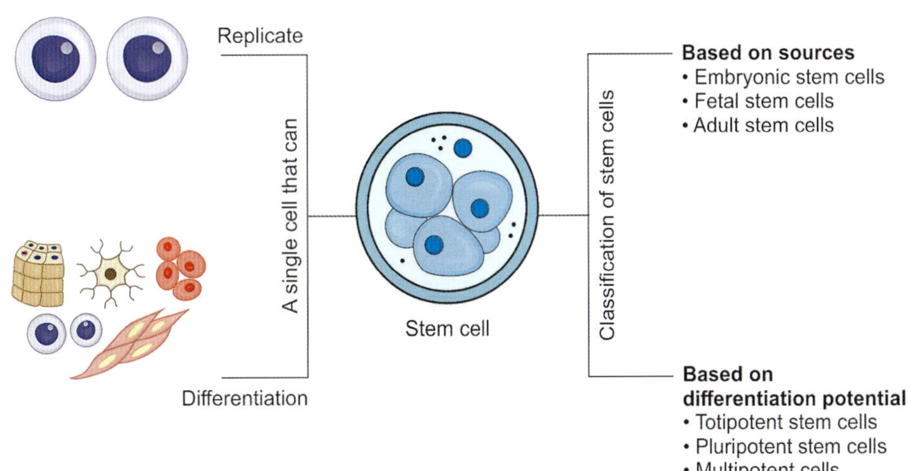

Fig. 1: Understanding the stem cells.

Stem cells have a wide range of potential applications across various fields of medicine, research, and beyond. Their unique ability to differentiate into different cell types and promote tissue regeneration has led to numerous possibilities.[1]

CONTRIBUTING FACTORS TO INFERTILITY

Infertility is indeed a complex issue influenced by a combination of genetic, medical, lifestyle, and environmental factors. Also, infertility is a complex issue that affects many individuals and couples. Medical conditions and hormonal imbalances can contribute to infertility in both men and women. In men, abnormal sperm production or function due to genetic defects, health problems such as diabetes or infections can lead to infertility.[2] Women may experience infertility due to alterations in ovarian, uterine tube, and uterine functioning, as well as disruptions in hormone levels.[3] In addition, genetic factors have been found to be responsible for nearly 50% of infertility cases.[2] Lifestyle factors such as smoking and alcohol consumption can also contribute to infertility. In women, smoking and alcohol consumption have been found to negatively influence fertility.[3] In men, lifestyle factors such as cigarette smoking, illicit drug use, and alcohol consumption can negatively affect fertility. Additionally, exposure to certain environmental factors, such as pesticides and other chemicals and radiation, can also contribute to infertility.[3]

Age is another important factor that contributes to infertility. In women, infertility in older women is likely due to the lower number and quality of eggs, and can also be due to health problems that affect fertility. In men, infertility can also be age-related, as the quality and quantity of sperm can decrease with age.[4-6]

ROLE OF STEM CELLS IN INFERTILITY

Stem cells have gained attention as a promising treatment option for infertility due to their unique properties and potential. Research on the use of stem cells in treating infertility has shown promising results. Studies have demonstrated the potential of stem cell therapy for both male and female infertility.[7] For example, bone marrow-derived mesenchymal stem cells (MSCs) have been found to improve injured tissue or form germ cells, making them a potential treatment option for infertility in both males and females.[8] Additionally, stem cell therapy using a patient's own stem cells has been found to be a safe and effective treatment option for diminished ovarian reserve.[9] However, more research is needed to fully understand the potential of stem cell therapy for infertility treatment. Stem cells have the potential to play a significant role in addressing certain causes of infertility. While the field is still in its early stages of research and clinical application, there are several ways in which stem cells could potentially contribute to infertility treatment. **Figure 2** enlists the potential applications of stem cells in infertility.

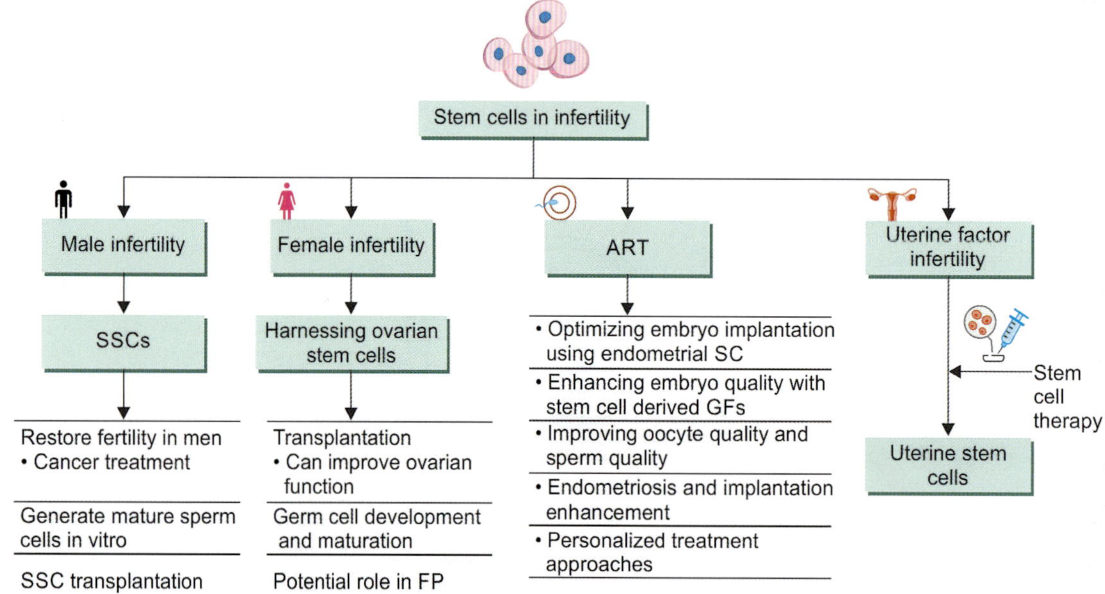

Fig. 2: Stem cell applications in infertility. (ART: assisted reproductive technology; FP: family planning; GFs: growth factors; SSCs: spermatogonial stem cells)

Male Infertility: Promise of Spermatogonial Stem Cells

Spermatogonial stem cells (SSCs) offer promising solutions for male infertility. SSCs are the foundation for spermatogenesis, the process by which sperm cells are produced, and thus play a crucial role in male fertility. Dysfunction of SSCs can lead to male infertility, making it important to understand the regulatory network of these cells. SSCs are unique in that they have the ability to self-renew and differentiate into mature sperm cells, making them a valuable resource for treating male infertility.[10]

There are numerous potential applications of SSCs in treating male infertility. One approach involves using SSCs to restore fertility in men who have undergone cancer treatment, which can damage or destroy the SSC population.[11] Another approach involves using SSCs to generate mature sperm cells in vitro, which can then be used for in vitro fertilization (IVF).[10] Additionally, SSC transplantation may be a viable option for treating male infertility caused by other sperm function defects. These potential applications of SSCs offer hope for men struggling with infertility.

Current research and clinical trials are exploring the use of SSCs for treating male infertility. These studies are investigating the safety and efficacy of SSC transplantation and in vitro differentiation of SSCs into mature sperm cells.[10-12] A recent breakthrough in the field involved the successful in vitro differentiation of human SSCs into mature sperm cells.[13] While there is still much to learn about the use of SSCs for treating male infertility, the promising results of these studies suggest that SSCs may offer a valuable solution for men struggling with infertility.

Female Infertility: Harnessing Ovarian Stem Cells

Ovarian stem cells are a unique cell population that have the potential to revolutionize the treatment of female infertility. While the existence of ovarian germline stem cells (GSCs) has been demonstrated in nonmammalian species, it was long believed that women have a finite ovarian reserve, which is fixed from birth. However, recent research has challenged this belief, with evidence suggesting that the ovary may contain a population of stem cells capable of generating new oocytes.[14] These ovarian stem cells have the potential to be harnessed for regenerative medicine including the treatment of female infertility.

Ovarian stem cells have been the focus of much research in the field of regenerative medicine. Recent preclinical studies have shown that stem cell transplantation can improve ovarian function by increasing the expression of related hormones and by promoting follicle growth.[15] Moreover, stem cells may provide a valuable model for germ cell development and maturation as well as a potential role in fertility preservation. In particular, MSCs have shown promise in restoring ovarian function and treating infertility.[14] These studies suggest that stem cell-based therapies may hold great potential for the treatment of female infertility.

While the use of ovarian stem cells for the treatment of female infertility is still in its early stages, the future prospects for this therapy are promising. Stem cell-based therapies offer a new hope for infertility treatment and may provide an alternative to current treatments such as IVF. However, further research is needed to fully understand the potential of ovarian stem cells in treating female infertility. Nonetheless, the potential of these cells offers a glimmer of hope for women struggling with infertility, and may lead to a breakthrough in the field of reproductive medicine.

STEM CELLS AND ASSISTED REPRODUCTIVE TECHNOLOGIES

Indeed, assisted reproductive technologies (ARTs) have significantly transformed infertility management, but there is always room for improvement in enhancing success rates and addressing challenges associated with these procedures. The integration of stem cells into existing ART procedures holds promise for improving various aspects of fertility treatments. Here are some potential ways stem cells could be integrated into ART to optimize outcomes:

- *Optimizing embryo implantation using endometrial stem cells:* Endometrial stem cells could play a role in enhancing the receptivity of the uterine lining for embryo implantation. By introducing stem cells or factors derived from them, it might be possible to improve the quality of the endometrium and create a more favorable environment for successful embryo attachment. This approach could benefit women with recurrent implantation failure or those with thin endometrial linings.[16,17]
- *Enhancing embryo quality with stem cell-derived growth factors:* Stem cells have the ability to secrete various growth factors and cytokines that support cell growth,

differentiation, and tissue repair. Incorporating stem cell-derived growth factors into culture media during IVF or embryo culture could potentially enhance embryo development and quality.[18,19] This approach might lead to higher rates of viable embryos available for transfer, improving the chances of successful pregnancy.

- *Improving oocyte and sperm quality:* Stem cells might offer insights into improving the quality of oocytes (eggs) and sperm. By studying the differentiation pathways of stem cells, researchers could identify factors or conditions that promote healthier gametes, potentially leading to improved success rates in IVF and other fertility treatments.[20]
- *Endometriosis and implantation enhancement:* For women with endometriosis, a condition where endometrial-like tissue grows outside the uterus, stem cells could contribute to developing innovative treatments. By targeting the underlying causes of implantation failure in endometriosis cases, stem cell therapies might improve the chances of successful pregnancies.[21]
- *Personalized treatment approaches:* Stem cells could allow for personalized treatment approaches in fertility care. By utilizing a patient's own stem cells, it might be possible to create customized therapies that are more compatible with their unique biology, potentially leading to improved outcomes.

UTERINE FACTOR INFERTILITY: PROMISE OF UTERINE STEM CELLS

Uterine factor infertility (UFI) is a condition that affects individuals who are unable to get pregnant due to either a complete lack of a uterus or a nonfunctioning uterus. UFI can also be caused by defective endometrial mesenchymal fibroblasts, which contribute to endometriosis and endometrial cancer.[22] This condition can be emotionally and psychologically challenging for those who experience it. However, recent research has shown promising results in the use of uterine stem cells for treating UFI.

Uterine stem cells are a type of adult stem cell that reside in the uterine endometrium.[23-25] These cells have the potential to differentiate into various cell types including endometrial and myometrial cells. Research and clinical trials have shown that uterine stem cell therapy can improve fertility in individuals with UFI. A study conducted by Santamaria X et al. in 2018 demonstrated that bone marrow-derived mesenchymal stem cells (BMDSCs) improved fertility in mice with induced Asherman syndrome.[26] Additionally, a 2021 study by Abuwala N et al. suggested that uterine endometrial stem cells and BMDSCs have the potential to become treatment targets for reproductive success and failure.[27]

While the use of uterine stem cells for treating UFI is still in the early stages of research, it shows great promise for improving fertility in individuals with this condition. Stem cell therapy has also been proposed as a potential therapeutic strategy for treating infertility associated with ovarian dysfunction. Furthermore, studies have revealed that intrauterine adhesion therapy can improve pregnancy outcomes and promote endometrial regeneration. Clinical trials using umbilical cord stem cells have also been successful in treating infertility due to intrauterine adhesions. With further research and development, uterine stem cell therapy may become a viable option for treating UFI and improving reproductive health.

POTENTIAL BENEFITS AND RISKS OF ENDOMETRIAL STEM CELLS

It is evident that in highly regenerative human endometrium, remodeling occurs during each menstrual cycle, after resection, parturition, and in postmenopausal women using hormone replacement therapy. It has been suggested that endometrial stem cells must play a role in endometrial remodeling and regeneration during menstrual cycle and pregnancy. Besides, bone marrow-derived stem/progenitor cells are also able to incorporate themselves into the endometrium, contributing to the vascular remodeling or transdifferentiating into endometrial cells.[23-25] Thus, the uniqueness of endometrial stem cells is known widely. In parallel, emerging research results suggest that irregular function of these stem cells may contribute to the abnormalities substantially contributing to endometrial disorders including endometriosis, causing dysmenorrhea, adenomyosis, subfertility, endometrial hyperplasia, and endometrial carcinoma. Such stem cells may also contribute to the pathogenetic process, because their high proliferation promotes rapid clonal expansion.

Thus, we call endometrial stem cells a "double-edged sword", wherein, on one side, they play a dynamic role in normal physiology and development throughout women's life as well on the other side; they contribute to the pathogenesis of various endometrial disorders through their abnormal proliferation and differentiation.

ETHICAL AND REGULATORY CONSIDERATION

Stem cell research for infertility treatment raises a number of ethical concerns, particularly surrounding the use of ES cells. ES cell research is controversial because it involves the destruction of human embryos, which some believe is morally unacceptable. Regulatory frameworks for stem cell research and treatment vary across different countries and regions. The International Society for Stem Cell Research (ISSCR) has developed guidelines that address the cultural, political, legal, and ethical issues associated with stem cell research.[28] In the United States, the Food and Drug Administration (FDA) considers stem cell-based products to be somatic cellular therapies that do not warrant a distinct regulatory approach. The moral status of embryos is also a critical consideration in determining the ethical position of each country and the national legislative decisions for stem cell research.

When considering stem cell research in infertility, it is important to balance the potential benefits and risks. While stem cells offer promise for new therapies in regenerative medicine, there are also risks associated with stem cell clinical trials.[29] Additionally, physical and mental health issues, as well as hormonal imbalances, are often associated with infertility and reproductive disorders. As such, it is important to carefully consider the ethical and regulatory frameworks surrounding stem cell research and treatment, while also balancing the potential benefits and risks for patients seeking infertility treatment.

FUTURE PROSPECTS AND CHALLENGES

Stem cell research has the potential to revolutionize infertility treatment, but it also presents several challenges. One of the current challenges in stem cell research for infertility is the difficulty in producing fully functional gametes from stem cells. Additionally, the safety and efficacy of using stem cells for fertility treatment are still being investigated. These challenges must be addressed before stem cell therapy can become a widely accepted treatment option for infertility.

Despite the current challenges, there are promising future applications of stem cells in infertility treatment. Stem cell-based strategies for ovarian regeneration and oocyte production have been proposed as potential clinical therapies for treating infertility in women.[30] Furthermore, stem cells have shown promise in overcoming issues related to infertility through cell-based therapies in various animal models. As research continues, stem cell therapy may become a viable option for individuals struggling with infertility.

REFERENCES

1. Rajabzadeh N, Fathi E, Farahzadi R. Stem cell-based regenerative medicine. Stem Cell Investig. 2019;6:19.
2. Coutton C, Fissore RA, Palermo GD, Stouffs K, Touré A. Male infertility: genetics, mechanism, and therapies. Biomed Res Int. 2016;2016:7372362.
3. Sharma R, Biedenharn KR, Fedor JM, Agarwal A. Lifestyle factors and reproductive health: taking control of your fertility. Reprod Biol Endocrinol. 2013;11:66.
4. Ubaldi FM, Cimadomo D, Vaiarelli A, Fabozzi G, Venturella R, Maggiulli R, et al. Advanced Maternal Age in IVF: Still a Challenge? The Present and the Future of Its Treatment. Front Endocrinol (Lausanne). 2019;10:94.
5. Brandt JS, Cruz Ithier MA, Rosen T, Ashkinadze E. Advanced paternal age, infertility, and reproductive risks: a review of the literature. Prenat Diagn. 2019;39(2):81-7.
6. Kulkarni V, Kaingade P, Kulkarni N, Bhalerao T, Nikam A. Assessment of semen parameters in consecutive ejaculates with short abstinence period in oligospermic males. JBRA Assist Reprod. 2022;26(2):310-14.
7. Saha S, Roy P, Corbitt C, Kakar SS. Application of stem cell therapy for infertility. Cells. 2021;10(7):1613.
8. Kemp KC, Hows J, Donaldson C. Bone marrow-derived mesenchymal stem cells. Leuk Lymphoma. 2005;46(11):1531-44.
9. Fàbregues F, Ferreri J, Méndez M, Calafell JM, Otero J, Farré R. In vitro follicular activation and stem cell therapy as a novel treatment strategies in diminished ovarian reserve and primary ovarian insufficiency. Front Endocrinol (Lausanne). 2020;11:617704.
10. Diao L, Turek PJ, John CM, Fang F, Reijo Pera RA. Roles of spermatogonial stem cells in spermatogenesis and fertility restoration. Front Endocrinol (Lausanne). 2022;13:895528.
11. Ebata KT, Yeh JR, Zhang X, Nagano MC. The application of biomarkers of spermatogonial stem cells for restoring male fertility. Dis Markers. 2008;24(4-5):267-76.
12. Azizi H, Niazi Tabar A, Skutella T. Successful transplantation of spermatogonial stem cells into the seminiferous tubules of busulfan-treated mice. Reprod Health. 2021;18(1):189.
13. Ibtisham F, Honaramooz A. Spermatogonial stem cells for in vitro spermatogenesis and in vivo restoration of fertility. Cells. 2020;9(3):745.
14. Ozakpinar OB, Maurer AM, Ozsavci D. Ovarian stem cells: From basic to clinical applications. World J Stem Cells. 2015;7(4):757-68.
15. Jiao W, Mi X, Qin Y, Zhao S. Stem cell transplantation improves ovarian function through paracrine mechanisms. Curr Gene Ther. 2020;20(5):347-55.

16. Nagori CB, Panchal SY, Patel H. Endometrial regeneration using autologous adult stem cells followed by conception by in vitro fertilization in a patient of severe Asherman's syndrome. J Hum Reprod Sci. 2011;4(1):43-8.
17. Ojosnegros S, Seriola A, Godeau AL, Veiga A. Embryo implantation in the laboratory: an update on current techniques. Hum Reprod Update. 2021;27(3):501-30.
18. Liu HC, He ZY, Mele CA, Veeck LL, Davis O, Rosenwaks Z. Human endometrial stromal cells improve embryo quality by enhancing the expression of insulin-like growth factors and their receptors in cocultured human preimplantation embryos. Fertil Steril. 1999;71(2):361-7.
19. Kaingade PM, Somasundaram I, Nikam AB, Sarang SA, Patel JS. Assessment of growth factors secreted by human breastmilk mesenchymal stem cells. Breastfeed Med. 2016; 11(1):26-31.
20. Kehler J, Hübner K, Garrett S, Schöler HR. Generating oocytes and sperm from embryonic stem cells. Semin Reprod Med. 2005;23(3):222-33.
21. Kong Y, Shao Y, Ren C, Yang G. Endometrial stem/progenitor cells and their roles in immunity, clinical application, and endometriosis. Stem Cell Res Ther. 2021;12(1):474.
22. Hur C, Rehmer J, Flyckt R, Falcone T. Uterine factor infertility: a clinical review. Clin Obstet Gynecol. 2019;62(2):257-70.
23. Gargett CE, Schwab KE, Zillwood RM, Nguyen HPT, Wu D. Isolation and culture of epithelial progenitors and mesenchymal stem cells from human endometrium. Biol Reprod. 2009;80(6):1136-45.
24. Masuda H, Matsuzaki Y, Hiratsu E, Ono M, Nagashima T, Kajitani T, et al. Stem cell-like properties of the endometrial side population: implication in endometrial regeneration. PLoS One. 2010;5(4):e10387.
25. Kaingade P, Nikam A, Kulkarni S, Somasundaram I. Marker profiles of human endometrial stem cells at various passages cultured in-vitro. J Stem Cell Res Ther. 2017;2(1):5-10.
26. Santamaria X, Cabanillas S, Cervelló I, Arbona C, Raga F, Ferro J, et al. Autologous cell therapy with CD133+ bone marrow-derived stem cells for refractory Asherman's syndrome and endometrial atrophy: a pilot cohort study. Hum Reprod. 2016;31(5):1087-96.
27. Abuwala N, Tal R. Endometrial stem cells: origin, biological function, and therapeutic applications for reproductive disorders. Curr Opin Obstet Gynecol. 2021;33(3):232-40.
28. Lovell-Badge R, Anthony E, Barker RA, Bubela T, Brivanlou AH, Carpenter M, et al. ISSCR Guidelines for Stem Cell Research and Clinical Translation: The 2021 update. Stem Cell Reports. 2021;16(6):1398-408.
29. Jarrige M, Frank E, Herardot E, Martineau S, Darle A, Benabides M, et al. The Future of Regenerative Medicine: Cell Therapy Using Pluripotent Stem Cells and Acellular Therapies Based on Extracellular Vesicles. Cells. 2021; 10(2):240.
30. Ali I, Padhiar AA, Wang T, He L, Chen M, Wu S, et al. Stem Cell-Based Therapeutic Strategies for Premature Ovarian Insufficiency and Infertility: A Focus on Aging. Cells. 2022;11(23):3713.

Chapter

Uterine Transplantation

Manisha Takhtani Kundnani

INTRODUCTION

One in 500 women of childbearing age are affected by absolute uterine factor infertility (AUFI).[1] It has been estimated that up to 1.5 million women worldwide cannot bear a child because of absolute uterine factor where either the uterus is absent or is unable to maintain a pregnancy.[2] Traditional motherhood choices available for such women include adoption and surrogacy. Where adoption allows for legal motherhood, surrogacy agreement bestows genetic and legal motherhood, but none of these treatments allows the women to experience childbearing herself. Uterine transplantation (UTx) is a new treatment modality which has recently emerged as a ray of hope for such women and offers them opportunity to become pregnant and give birth to genetically related offspring themselves. This technique helps bridge the discrepancies between procreative capability and reproductive desires in women with AUFI.

Although the procedure is relatively new, it has rapidly progressed from an experimental trial in animals to successful human procedures. More than 80 UTx procedures have been performed worldwide and >40 live births had been achieved by 2022.[3,4] Uterus transplantation is now becoming established as a clinical treatment. An International Society of Uterus Transplantation (ISUTx) was launched in 2020, and the first report from the registry was published in 2023.[4]

EVOLUTION OF UTERINE TRANSPLANTATION

The first uterine transplant was reported in the year 2000 in Saudi Arabia in a 26-year-old woman who underwent a postpartum hysterectomy because of postpartum hemorrhage. She received a uterus transplant from a 46-year-old woman who underwent hysterectomy for benign indication. This transplant however lasted only for 99 days and was removed because of complications such as thrombosis and necrosis.[5]

Following this, the second attempt to human uterus transplantation was done by a Turkish team in 2011, wherein a 21-year-old woman with Mayer-Rokitansky-Küster-Hauser (MRKH) syndrome received uterus from a brain-dead woman.[6,7] Though, the transplant was a success, the attempts at embryo transfer failed and did not result in successful pregnancy.

The first successful live birth after uterus transplant was reported by a Swedish team in the year 2014. The Swedish Uterine Transplant trial included nine women with AUFI of which eight were MRKH.[8] Of the nine transplants, seven were successful and two women became pregnant after the first embryo transfer. The first baby after transplant—baby Vincent was born preterm at 31 weeks due to obstetrical complications.[9,10] Following this live birth, uterus transplant has been attempted all over the world and has emerged as a new hope for women with AUFI.

INDICATIONS FOR UTERINE TRANSPLANT—POTENTIAL RECIPIENTS

Uterine transplant can be offered to women with absent uterus or those with uterus which is anatomically or physiologically dysfunctional. **Table 1** enlists the potential recipients of UTx.

POTENTIAL DONORS

The donors for uterine transplant can either be living or deceased donors. Most uterine transplants (approximately 80%) across the world so far have been performed using live donors, while only 20% have used deceased donors.[11-13]

TABLE 1: Potential indications of uterine transplant.

Uterus absent	*Uterus present*
• *Congenital:* – Mayer–Rokitansky–Küster–Hauser (MRKH) syndrome – Complete androgen insensitivity – Male-to-female transgender • *Posthysterectomy:* – Obstetric hemorrhage – Benign cause – Cancer	• Asherman syndrome • Severe adenomyosis • Multiple fibroids • Uterine malformation • Pelvic irradiation

TABLE 2: Live versus deceased donor—pros and cons.

Living donor	*Deceased donor*
Advantages: • Detailed history can be taken • Surgery can be well planned with multidisciplinary team • Any structural abnormality in the uterus can be detected and corrected • Better histocompatibility • Low risk of rejection • Less cold ischemia time	*Advantages:* • No surgical risk to the donor • Possibility of removal of longer vascular pedicles • May get potentially younger donors • Short surgical time
Disadvantages: • Higher surgical risk to donor • Longer surgical time • May not be able to obtain sufficient graft pedicle length • Higher age of donors • Psychological risks	*Disadvantages:* • Comprehensive assessment of donor not possible • Increased ischemia time • Higher chances of graft rejection • Systemic inflammatory changes after brain death can affect graft survival • Less convenient scheduling of procedure • Difficult to obtain consent from kin

As the procedure involves multidisciplinary expertise, an elective surgery using living donor is more convenient than an emergency procedure in case of deceased donor. The donors undergo all the investigations required for solid organ transplant including microbiological screening for human immunodeficiency virus (HIV), hepatitis B virus (HBV), hepatitis C virus (HCV), venereal disease research laboratory (VDRL), *Cytomegalovirus*, Epstein-Barr virus, *Toxoplasma*, and human T-cell lymphotropic virus. Tests specific for uterine transplant including Pap smear, sexually transmitted diseases (STDs), and vaginal culture to exclude *Candida* and bacterial vaginosis are also conducted. Any structural abnormalities in the uterus are ruled out by doing a transvaginal ultrasound. Magnetic resonance or computed tomography angiography provides necessary information about the vessels.

Many living donors across the world have been first-degree relatives to the recipients. While having a related donor provides immunological benefit,[14] the use of old donors is associated with arterial inflammation and atherosclerotic changes in the pelvic arteries which can result in organ of insufficient quality.[15] So far, 20 live births have been reported after uterine transplant from living donor. The procedure however carries a significant surgical risk to the donor.

Compared to the living donor, the use of deceased donor has advantage of more radical dissection, which enables taking out large caliber vessels thereby reducing the risk of graft thrombosis.[16] The deceased donor however is associated with systemic brain death inflammation that may affect organ quality and the cold ischemia time is longer in deceased donors.[17] The first successful live birth after uterine transplant from deceased donor happened in Brazil in 2017.[12] However, more cases and long-term follow-up is required to effectively compare uterine transplant from live and deceased donors. **Table 2** summarizes the difference between living and deceased donors.

SURGICAL CONSIDERATIONS OF UTERUS TRANSPLANT

The procedure of uterus transplantation is long and complex and involves multiple major surgeries and exposure to immunosuppressant drugs. It entails transplant of uterus including the cervix, vaginal cuff, surrounding ligaments and connective tissue, and major blood vessels. The common postoperative complications are graft thrombosis requiring emergency hysterectomy, graft ischemia, and postoperative hemorrhage.[5,11,18]

POSSIBLE COMPLICATIONS OF UTERUS TRANSPLANTATION

No surgery is without risks. UTx involves many major surgeries and therefore pose significant risk to the donor and recipient. **Table 3** summarizes the possible complication of uterus transplantation surgery.

TABLE 3: Reported complications in uterus transplantation procedures.

Possible complications to donor	*Possible complications to recipient*
• Major intra-/postoperative bleeding • Injury to ureter • Ureterovaginal fistula • Vaginal cuff dehiscence • Fecal impaction • Leg pain • Depression	• Major intra-/postoperative bleeding • Intra-abdominal hematoma/hemoperitoneum • Vascular thrombosis • Intrauterine abscess • Uterine prolapse • Vaginal stenosis • Vesicovaginal fistula • Urinary tract infections • Fungal infections • Viral infections • Graft rejection

FERTILITY AFTER UTERINE TRANSPLANT

Planning fertility with uterine transplant is a multifaceted process with several steps. The steps involved include the following **(Fig. 1)**:

- *Selection and medical evaluation of donor and recipient:* The donor and recipient selection is of utmost importance before planning and performing any uterus transplant. The Montreal criteria for the ethical feasibility of UTx has laid down a set criteria that must be fulfilled before enrolling a woman for uterus transplant, both donor and recipient.[19] **Box 1** enlists the Montreal criteria for ethical feasibility of UTx. A local multidisciplinary committee should be established including transplant surgeons, gynecologist, and reproductive medicine specialist, anesthetists, psychiatrist, infectious diseases specialists, nephrologists, immunologists, and counselors.
- *In vitro fertilization (IVF) procedure and embryo freezing:* This is done prior to the transplant procedure. The egg retrieval after the transplant may be difficult as the anatomy is distorted. Additionally, the risk of infections is higher as patient will be on immunosuppressant.
- *Uterus transplantation and administration of immunosuppressant:* Tacrolimus and azathioprine have been shown to be safe during pregnancy with no increased risk of congenital abnormalities.[20]
- Embryo transfer after successful transplantation is usually planned after few months to years after transplant surgery. Single embryo transfer is recommended to avoid the risks associated with multiple pregnancies. Pregnancy is considered a high risk and is closely monitored with frequent prenatal and antenatal visits.

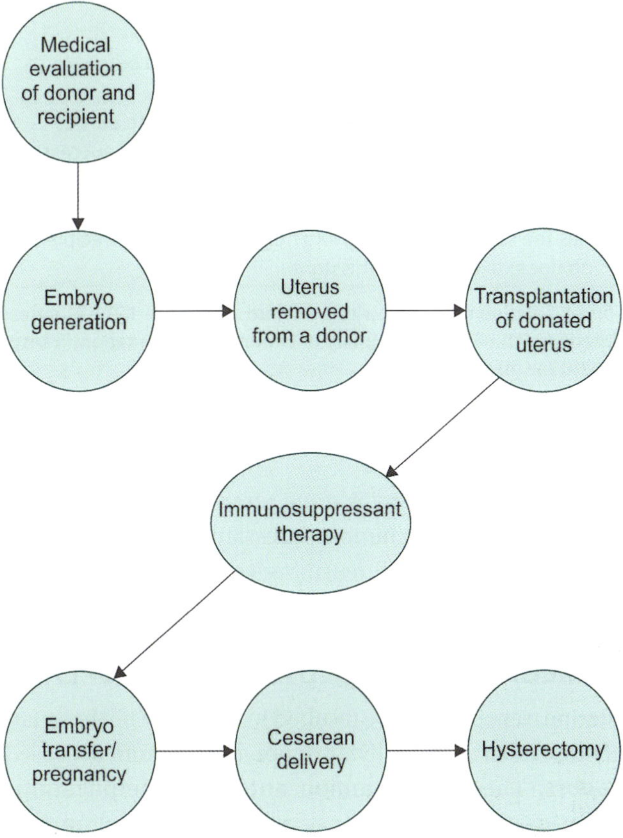

Fig. 1: Fertility after uterus transplantation.

BOX 1: Montreal criteria for ethical feasibility of uterine transplantation (UTx).[19]

The recipient:
- Is a genetic female of reproductive age with no medical contraindications to transplantation
- Has documented congenital or acquired uterine factor infertility (UFI) which has failed all current gold standard and conservative therapy.
- (c1) has a personal or legal contraindication to surrogacy and adoption measures, or (c2) seeks the UTx solely as a measure to experience gestation, with an understanding of the limitations provided by the UTx in this respect
- Has not had her decision to undergo UTx deemed as irrational by expert psychological evaluation
- Does not exhibit frank unsuitability for motherhood
- Is responsible enough to consent, informed enough to make a responsible decision, and not under coercion

The donor:
- Is a female of reproductive age with no medical contraindications to donation
- (h1) has repeatedly attested to her conclusion of parity, or (h2) has signed an advanced directive for post-mortem organ donation
- Has no history of uterine damage or disease
- Is responsible enough to consent, informed enough to make a responsible decision, and not under coercion

The healthcare team:
- Is part of an institution that meets Moore's third criteria as it pertains to institutional stability
- Has provided adequate informed consent to both parties regarding risks, potential sequelae, and chances of success and failure
- Has no conflict of interest independently or with either party
- Has the duty to preserve anonymity if the donor or recipient do not explicitly waive this right

Source: Adapted from Lefkowitz A, Edwards M, Balayla J. The Montreal Criteria for the Ethical Feasibility of Uterine Transplantation. Transpl Int. 2012;25(4):439-47.

- The baby is born by cesarean section as close to term as possible.
- Graft hysterectomy is done after the childbearing is complete and immunosuppressant is stopped.

The whole procedure length varies from patient to patient but can take as long as 2–5 years for many participants.

PREGNANCY AFTER UTERINE TRANSPLANT

Uterine transplants have resulted in many live births so far; of these most are from living donor and few from deceased donors. The most common antenatal complications experienced in recipients included preeclampsia, cholestasis, and preterm rupture of membranes.[21,22]

BOX 2: Ethical issues with uterine transplant.
- Nonessential organ transplant
- Risk to healthy live donor and recipient
- Prolonged immunosuppression
- Risk of teratogenicity
- Psychological risks

Delivery has been done by lower section cesarean section in all cases. Few cases had to undergo peripartum hysterectomy because of extensive hemorrhage.[23] No incidences of congenital abnormalities have been reported.

ETHICAL AND SOCIAL ISSUES WITH UTERUS TRANSPLANT

Uterine transplant is a nonvital organ transplant. A lot of medical, ethical, and social issues surround the topic. The transplant process is complex requiring multiple surgeries in otherwise healthy people; and involves multiple parties—the donor, the recipient, and the child. A detailed risk benefit analysis is thus required before planning the procedure. Alternative options for childbearing like adoption and surrogacy should be considered and discussed. **Box 2** summarizes the various ethical issues with uterine transplant.

CONCLUSION

Uterine transplant is a ray of hope for women with AUFI and allows them to bear a child themselves and experience motherhood. The procedure however is long and complex and is associated with significant morbidity involving 3–4 surgeries (transplant, cesarean section, and subsequent hysterectomy) and the risk associated with immunosuppression. Though the procedure is promising and approximately 20 babies have been born worldwide following it, it is still in its novel stages and the long-term outcome following is not available. The use of deceased donors is still a research concept and more cases and extensive follow-ups are required to compare the efficacy of each donor type.

REFERENCES

1. Johannesson L, Dahm-Kahler P, Eklind S, Brannstrom M. The future of human uterus transplantation. Womens Health Lond. 2014;10:455-67.
2. Flyckt R, Kotlyar A, Arian S, Eghtesad B, Falcone T, Tzakis A. Deceased donor uterine transplantation. Fertil Steril. 2017;107:e13.
3. Johannesson L, Richards E, Reddy V, Walter J, Olthoff K, Quintini C, et al. The first 5 years of uterus transplant in

the US: a report from the United States Uterus Transplant Consortium. JAMA Surg. 2022;157:790-7.

4. Brannstrom M, Tullius SG, Brucker S, Dahm-Kahler P, Flyckt R, Kisu I, et al. Registry of the International Society of uterus transplantation: first report. Transplantation 2023; 107:10-7.
5. Fageeh W, Raffa H, Jabbad H, Marzouki A. Transplantation of the human uterus. Int J Gynaecol Obstet. 2002;76:245-51.
6. Ozkan O, Akar M, Ozkan O, Erdogan O, Hadimioglu N, Yilmaz M, et al. Preliminary results of the first human uterus transplantation from a multiorgan donor. Fertil Steril. 2013; 99:470-6.
7. Erman Akar M, Ozkan O, Uraz BA, Dirican K, Cincik M, Mendilcioglu I. Clinical pregnancy following uterus transplantation. Fertil Steril. 2013;100(3):S142.
8. Akouri R, Brannstrom M. Human uterus transplantation with live births; outcome of first clinical trials. Geburtshilfe Frauenheilkd. 2016;76:43-51.
9. Brännström M, Johannesson L, Dahm-Kähler P, Enskog A, Mölne J, Kvarnström N, et al. First clinical uterus transplantation trial: a six-month report. Fertil Steril. 2014;101(5): 1228-36.
10. Johannesson L, Kvarnström N, Mölne J, Dahm-Kähler P, Enskog A, Diaz-Garcia C, et al. Uterus transplantation trial: 1-year outcome. Fertil Steril. 2015;103(1):199-204.
11. Chmel R, Novackova M, Janousek L, Matecha J, Pastor Z, Maluskova J, et al. Revaluation and lessons learned from the first 9 cases of a Czech uterus transplantation trial: Four deceased donor and 5 living donor uterus transplantations. Am J Transplant. 2019;19(3):855-64.
12. Ejzenberg D, Andraus W, Baratelli Carelli Mendes LR, Ducatti L, Song A, Tanigawa R, et al. Livebirth after uterus transplantation from a deceased donor in a recipient with uterine infertility. Lancet. 2019;392(10165):2697-704.
13. Flyckt RL, Farrell RM, Perni UC, Tzakis AG, Falcone T. Deceased donor uterine transplantation: innovation and adaptation. Obstet Gynecol. 2016;128:837-42.
14. Matter YE, Nagib AM, Lotfy OE, Alsayed AM, Donia AF, Refaie AF, et al. Impact of Donor Source on the Outcome of Live Donor Kidney Transplantation: A Single Center Experience. Nephrourol Mon. 2016;8(3):e34770.
15. Brucker SY, Brännström M, Taran FA, Nadalin S, Königsrainer A, Rall K, et al. Selecting living donors for uterus transplantation: lessons learned from two transplantations resulting in menstrual functionality and another attempt, aborted after organ retrieval. Arch Gynecol Obstet. 2018;297(3):675-84.
16. Sieunarine K, Zakaria FB, Boyle DC, Corless DJ, Noakes DE, Lindsay I, et al. Possibilities for fertility restoration: a new surgical technique. Int Surg. 2005;90(5):249-56.
17. Pratschke J, Neuhaus P, Tullius SG. What can be learned from brain-death models? Transpl Int 2005;18:15-21.
18. Wei L, Xue T, Tao KS, Zhang G, Zhao GY, Yu SQ, et al. Modified human uterus transplantation using ovarian veins for venous drainage: the first report of surgically successful robotic-assisted uterus procurement and follow-up for 12 months. Fertil Steril. 2017;108(2):346-356.e1.
19. Lefkowitz A, Edwards M, Balayla J. The Montreal Criteria for the Ethical Feasibility of Uterine Transplantation. Transpl Int. 2012;25(4):439-47.
20. Wiles KS, Tillett AL, Harding KR. Solid organ transplantation in pregnancy. Obstet Gynaecol. 2016;18:189-97.
21. Castellón LAR, Amador MIG, González RED, Eduardo MSJ, Díaz-García C, Kvarnström N, et al. The history behind successful uterine transplantation in humans. JBRA Assist Reprod. 2017;21(2):126-34.
22. Jackson RA, Gibson KA, Wu YW, Croughan MS. Perinatal outcomes in singletons following in vitro fertilization: a meta-analysis. Obstet Gynecol. 2004;103:551-63.
23. Jones BP, Kasaven L, Vali S, Saso S, Jalmbrant M, Bracewell-Milnes T, et al. Uterine Transplantation: Review of Livebirths and Reproductive Implications. Transplantation. 2021;105(8):1695-707.

Chapter

Ovarian Rejuvenation

Sunita Arora, Suyesha Khanijao

INTRODUCTION

A recent trend has come up to postpone the pregnancy due to modernization where one is more concerned about one's career than about knowing the downside of the concept of ovarian aging. With evolution in society in perceiving the gender inequality and developments of women's right comes a darker side of not knowing the negative part of delaying conception. The ovarian reserve declines with age from a peak of 6–7 million oogonia in utero to below 500,000 by onset of puberty. There is exponential decrease from age 37 years onward. In tandem, not just the quantity but quality also decreases.

With advent in recent technologies, a concept which has gain popularity is ovarian rejuvenation. A breakthrough research has helped us in understanding that approximately 1,000 quiescent residual primordial follicles remain in the ovaries at menopause. This is contrary to the earlier knowledge that human ovaries are born with a fixed number of ova, that determined her reproductive lifespan, the number depleting entirely during menopause.

Concept of ovarian rejuvenation comes from a long history of medical efforts of varied efficacy that gained notice more than a century ago. Ovarian rejuvenation is an innovative procedure that has intended to restore ovarian fertility and development during theperimenopausal and menopausal period. It has been used to enhance fertility in women with premature ovarian insufficiency (POI). The ovarian response to ovarian stimulation (OS) reflected by the number of oocytes retrieved is a keystone in in vitro fertilization (IVF) cycles and an independent factor in the success of treatment. Although the ideal number of oocytes needed might be a matter of debate, 10–15 follicles are considered to be the optimal response after OS.[1]

STRATEGIES AND METHODS FOR OVARIAN REJUVENATION

Multiple strategies have been proposed to rejuvenate the aging ovaries including dietary supplements, platelet-rich plasma (PRP), platelet-activated growth factors, stem cells, and so on.

Supplement with Diet

Coenzyme Q10, melatonin, and fish oil (omega 3) provide antioxidants to boost egg quality, support ovarian function, and help one sleep better. Omega 3 supplements preserve fertility and boost egg quality while Q10 provides antioxidants that support the mitochondria.[2] But all these antioxidants and nutrients can help only if taken for a duration of 3–6 months, and robust data to support this is still lacking.

Ovarian Rejuvenation with Platelet-rich Plasma

Platelet-rich plasma is a term used to describe a fraction of the blood after processing. It is typically isolated from autologous whole blood retrieved by phlebotomy into a citrate-based anticoagulant. This is then subjected to differential centrifugation, resulting in the removal of red blood and immune cells, leaving behind a high concentration of platelets within plasma. As per Government of India guidelines, medically we can only use autologous PRP derived from own blood cells with no or minimal manipulation in vitro.

The use of PRP for ovarian rejuvenation was first outlined a few years ago in Greece when a group of poor-prognosis infertility patients received an intraovarian injection of PRP followed by IVF with their own oocytes.[3]

Platelet-rich Plasma Preparation

Different workers have described PRP preparation with slight variations. A well-accepted PRP preparation for ovarian rejuvenation is as follows:

13.5 mL of peripheral blood sample mixed with 1.5 mL of anticoagulant (provided in PRP kit) is taken in two different conical tubes making a total of around 30 mL. After mixing well, both tubes are centrifuged at 1,500 rpm for 15 minutes. The blood separates into three layers—(1) an upper layer that contains platelets and white cells an intermediate thin layer (the buffy coat) that is rich in white blood cells and bottom layer that contains red bold cells (RBCs). The upper and intermediate layers are transferred to an empty sterile tube and plasma is centrifuged again at 3,200 rpm for 6 minutes with formation of soft pellet (erythrocytes and platelets) at the base. The upper two-thirds plasma which is platelet poor is discarded and the pellet is homogenized in the lower third (5 mL) of plasma to create the PRP. Around 30–50 mL of blood can yield 3–5 mL of PRP **(Fig. 1)**.

Indications of Platelet-rich Plasma in Reproductive Medicine

- Diminished ovarian reserve (DOR) is defined as a decrease in the number and/or quality of oocytes in the ovary, accompanied by decline in the level of anti-Müllerian hormone (AMH), a decrease in the number of antral follicles and an increase in the level of follicle-stimulating hormone (FSH). The American Society for Reproductive Medicine (ASRM) put forward an expert consensus in 2020 that DOR has no diagnostic criteria, but it is mainly manifested in the decline in the quality and quantity of oocytes and the decline in reproductive potential.

  Platelet-rich plasma is believed to rejuvenate the ovarian environment, possibly enhancing the quality of available eggs and improving the chances of successful conception.
- *Poor ovarian response (POR):* POR is when a woman's ovaries do not respond as expected to fertility medications. PRP might boost the ovaries responsiveness to these medications, potentially leading to a more successful IVF cycle.
- *Previous unsuccessful IVF cycles:* In cases of recurrent implantation failure, PRP can potentially improve ovarian function and egg quality, increasing the chances of a successful IVF cycle.
- *Menopause or perimenopause:* Menopause marks the end of a woman's reproductive years, while perimenopause is the transition phase leading up to it. In such cases, PRP has shown potential in rejuvenating the ovaries, possibly extending a woman's reproductive capabilities even during these phases.
- *Age-related infertility:*
  - As women age, the quality and quantity of their eggs often decline.
  - PRP can potentially stimulate the ovaries, enhancing the quality of the eggs and offsetting some age-related challenges.
- *Premature ovarian failure (POF):* POF is an early onset of menopause, occurring before age of 40 years.

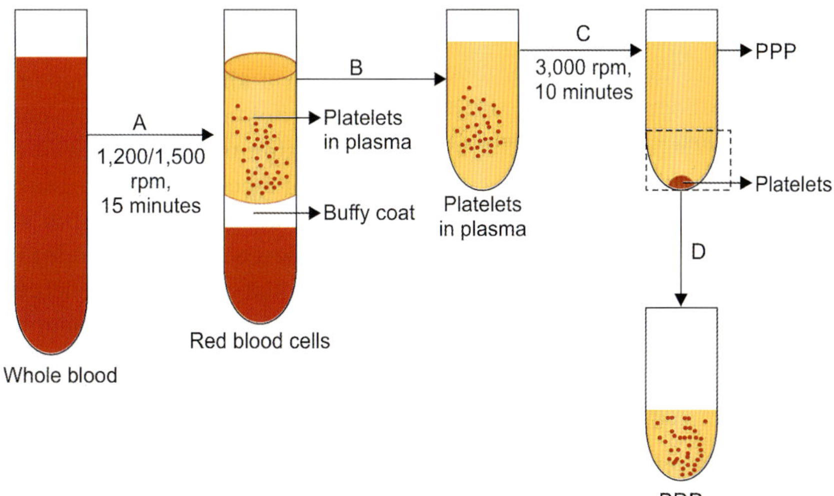

Fig. 1: Steps of preparation for platelet-rich plasma (PRP). (PPP: platelet-poor plasma)

Though not a cure, PRP can offer a glimmer of hope potentially reviving ovarian function to some extent.

- *Thin endometrial lining:* A thin endometrial lining can hinder embryo implantation, making pregnancy difficult. Subendometrial injection of PRP can help in regeneration of damaged endometrium.
- *Recurrent miscarriage:* Women who experience multiple miscarriages might have underlying ovarian function issues. There is a hypothesis that by rejuvenating the ovaries and potentially enhancing egg quality, PRP might reduce the risk of miscarriages.
- Unexplained infertility.

Timing of Procedure

It is preferable to do the procedure immediate post-menstrual before the follicles begin to grow, but in case of amenorrheic women, it can be done any time after excluding the pregnancy.

Advantages of Using Platelet-rich Plasma

- Therapeutic effect
- Cost-effective
- Ease of preparation
- Autologous nature

Mechanism of Action of Platelet-rich Plasma

The activation of platelets induces the release of variety of biologically active protein molecules which promote cell proliferation, growth, and differentiation. Biologically active mediation includes platelet-derived growth factors (PDGFs), transforming growth factor-β, epidermal growth factor, fibroblast growth factor, and hepatocyte growth factors. PRP induces accelerated angiogenesis and anabolism, inflammation and controls cell migration, differentiation, and proliferation. Some studies do suggest increase in AMH and antral follicle counts in 6 weeks to 3 months time post procedure.[4]

Routes of Insertion

- Laparoscopic route is preferred as most of the times these ovaries are small and PRP can be injected under vision. Around 2.5–3 mL prepared PRP is injected in each ovary either with single puncture or 2–3 punctures at different site.
- *Ultrasound route:* The insertion of PRP into the ovaries is administered with a nonsurgical and transvaginal ultrasound-guided injection performed under sedation or short general anesthesia. This can also be done immediately after ovum pick up in the same sitting. Though this route is less invasive with shorter recovery but may be less accurate for smaller ovaries.

Enriched Platelet Factors

With enriched platelet factors (EnPLAF), the ultrasound-guided/laparoscopic ovarian injection technique is identical to PRP. But, what is inserted into ovarian tissue is highly enriched (and platelet-free) autologous growth factors instead.

Studies indicate that the concentration of growth factors may be as much as 10–15 times higher than with PRP alone.

Advantage of the EnPLAF is that it can be refrigerated or even frozen for future use. It is an advanced PRP method with direct injection of proteins and growth factors into the ovaries after special treatment and centrifugation of platelets.[5] The most important benefit of the EnPLAF is that it contains a higher concentration of growth factors.

Stem Cell Ovarian Rejuvenation

It is a new innovation that works against premature menopause, thus can even help in POI. The knowledge and invention of ovarian stem cells was taken as the soil below the concept of ovarian rejuvenation by stem cells.

Many theories have been postulated behind the concept of using stem cell for rejuvenation:

- Recent research suggests that diminished ovarian reserve is a result of the aging of the niche rather than a defect in the germ cells. Stem cell niches are located in specific anatomic microenvironment that allows for stem cells self-renewal and maintenance of their undifferentiated potential. Stem cells have a rapid proliferation ability, achieving a thousandfold expansion of cell number in a 2-to-3-week period. Several mechanisms have been proposed to achieve tissue regeneration by adult stem cell therapy. The possible mechanisms include promoting angiogenesis, differentiating into functional cells, anti-inflammation, immunomodulation, antiapoptosis, antifibrosis, and a paracrine mechanism.[6]
- Many other theories have been proposed about tissue regeneration. One of the theories is the homing phenomenon where bone marrow-derived stem cells (BMDSCs) directly and impulsively migrate to the defective microenvironment and repair under the

stimulation of multiple factors, which facilitates ovarian recovery. BMDSCs differentiate into a variety of cells, such as theca cells, granulosa cells, corona radiata cells, and vascular endothelial cells.[7]

- Paracrine effects of stem cells have been evaluated for their ability to activate the preexisting quiescent follicles. BMDSCs secrete chemokines, growth factors, and hormones to influence adjacent cells (the paracrine effect). Paracrine signaling is important in anti-inflammation, immunoregulation, antiapoptosis, antifibrosis, and controlling oxidative stress, thus improving the microenvironment to promote the recovery of damaged tissues.[8]

Ovarian rejuvenation with stem cells is also called autologous stem cell transplant in the ovary (ASCOT). Bone marrow stromal cells were initially described by Owen and Friedenstein in 1988. They not only commit to osteoblasts, adipocytes, and chondroblasts, but also differentiate into granulosa, endometrial, and endothelial cells. Adult stem cells are often isolated from bone marrow, blood, adipose tissue, liver, and skin. However, as a natural consequence of aging, their quantity and quality decreases with the age affecting their regenerative potential, growth, and divisions.[9]

Pluripotent stem cells can differentiate into any cells derived from the endoderm, mesoderm, and ectoderm. Embryonic stem cells (ESCs) are the most pluripotent of all stem cells; they are derived from the inner cell mass of the blastocyst and possess unlimited ability to differentiate into various cell types.

They are widely used in research and therapeutics because of their ability to differentiate down multiple lineages of tissues/cells, such as chondrocytes, osteocytes, adipocytes, hepatocytes, and even neurons.

Procedure for Intraovarian Autologous Stem Cell Instillation

It is advisable to know base line AMH and antral follicle count and size of ovaries.

A detailed informed consent is mandatory before the procedure explaining its advantages, disadvantages, success rates, and risks involved. The hospital should be an approved center for stem cell work and should have taken ethical committee clearance from local body.

Bone marrow aspiration: Bone marrow aspiration is usually done from posterior iliac crest or long bone like femur under local/general anesthesia maintaining strict asepsis. Aspiration is done using Jamshidi needle (13G) and 20 mL syringe prewashed with heparin. Around 60 mL of bone marrow is aspirated. 16 mL BMDSCs were separated using the sepax (fully automated closed capability system) which uses optical sensor technology and simultaneous application of centrifugation and sedimentation.

Instillation of stem cells into the ovaries: Laparoscopic route is preferred than ultrasound-guided transvaginal route as most of the times these patients have small size ovaries; and hence, transvaginal route becomes less accurate. The patient is given general anesthesia. Three- to four-puncture laparoscopy is performed with 5-mm telescope. Ovaries are held at the cranial and caudal position with grasper and intraovarian instillation of about 1–2 mL of autologous bone marrow-derived stem cells (ABMDSCs) is done at 3–4 sites bilaterally **(Figs. 2A and B)**.

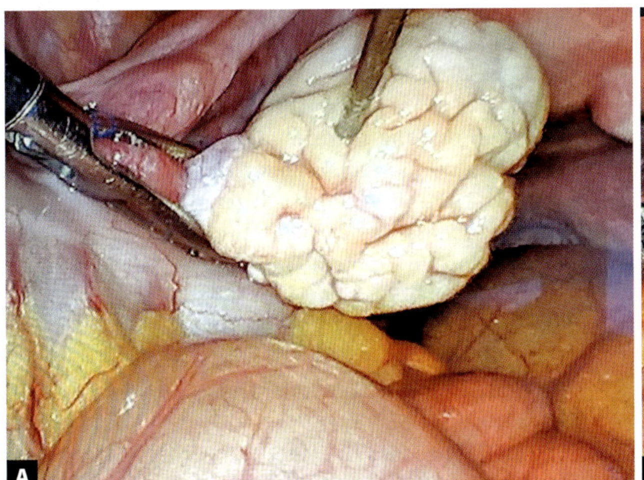

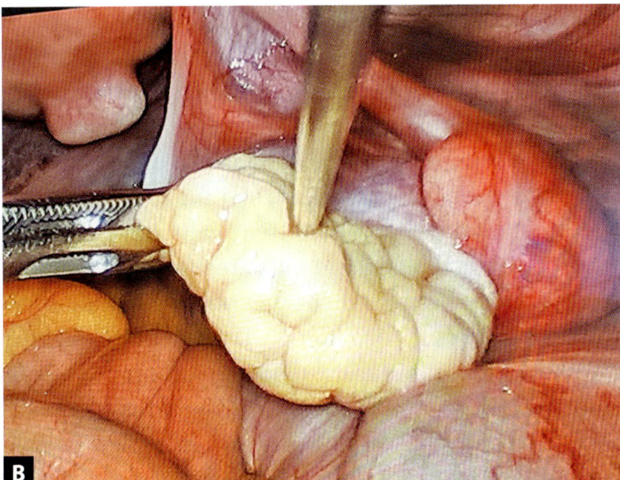

Figs. 2A and B: Laparoscopic intraovarian platelet-rich plasma (PRP) injection.

Follow-up of Patient

Patient should be followed up weekly for any side effects for 2–3 weeks. After 6 weeks of procedure antral follicle count and AMH can be reevaluated and patient can be subjected to OS drugs.

Complications of Stem Cells Procedure

Local site pain and infection at site of puncture for bone marrow aspiration is reported in rare cases. There are no long-term studies about potential risk of malignancy in the ovaries after stem cell injection and needs more data to reach at conclusions. However, use of stem cells in other degenerative disorders in medicine seems convincing and hence its growing interest for aging ovaries is on rise.

Drug-free In Vitro Activation of Ovarian Tissue for Premature Ovarian Insufficiency

This includes in vitro activation of ovarian fragments and orthotopic autotransplantation in same sitting. This is based on the concept that ovarian fragmentation disrupted ovarian hippo signaling that lead to follicular growth.[10] There are reports of natural pregnancy after in vitro drug-free activation of ovarian tissue.

CONCLUSION

Ovarian rejuvenation though seems very lucrative option but it gives improvement in 10% cases only. It is very important to counsel the patient undergoing the procedure about the success rates, steps involved, and pros and cons of the procedure. There are no long-term studies on safety profile of stem cells procedures as it has become more popular over last one decade only.

Administration of PRP for ovarian rejuvenation for infertility has attracted a lot of attention due to its potential in improving the ovarian reserve, its major advantages being ease of preparation and administration, no immunogenic or infection risk, and autologous nature.

With the knowledge that stem cells have unique property of regeneration and thus, treating degenerative illnesses, it serves as a game changer, offering solutions for scores of women suffering from POF, poor oocyte quality, endometrial degeneration/damage, or menopausal symptoms. Although the ovary as a target for stem cell therapy is relatively new, it has shown favorable results when applied to other organs which assure its safety and validity. ABMDSCs transplantation would prove a new paradigm in its role in ovarian rejuvenation. Stem cell therapy has become popular for treating POI. Oocyte and granulosa cell regeneration along with the reestablishment of hormone or cytokine profiles supporting stem cell follicular development may be involved in the improvement of both the damaged ovary function and fertility recovery. Increased understanding of its mechanism will help in promoting its wide clinical application and would give a ray of hope to the infertile couples who do not wish to opt for donor-assisted reproductive techniques.

REFERENCES

1. Abu-Musa A, Haahr T, Humaidan P. Novel Physiology and Definition of Poor Ovarian Response; Clinical Recommendations. Int J Mol Sci. 2020;21(6):2110.
2. Yang L, Chen Y, Liu Y, Xing Y, Miao C, Zhao Y, et al. The role of oxidative stress and natural antioxidants in ovarian aging. Front Pharmacol. 2021;11:617843.
3. Pantos K, Nitsos N, Kokkali G, Vaxevanoglou T, Markomichali C, Pantou A, et al. Ovarian rejuvenation and folliculogenesis reactivation in peri-menopausal women after autologous platelet-rich plasma treatment. Helsinki, Finland: ESHRE 32nd Annual Meeting; 2016. pp. 3-6.
4. Cakiroglu Y, Saltik A, Yuceturk A, Karaosmanoglu O, Kopuk SY, Scott RT, et al. Effects of intraovarian injection of autologous platelet rich plasma on ovarian reserve and IVF outcome parameters in women with primary ovarian insufficiency. Aging. 2020;12(11): 10211-22.
5. Tinjić S, Abazović Dž, Ljubić D, Vujović S, Vojvodić D, Božanović T, et al. Ovarian rejuvenation. Donald School J Ultrasound Obste Gynecol. 2019;13(2):64-8.
6. Anagani M, Agrawal P, Reddy BV, Mishra PC. Role of autologous bone marrow derived stem cells and platelet rich plasma for endometrial regeneration and repair and ovarian rejuvenation. Int J Reprod Contracept Obstet Gynecol. 2021;10(2):597-604.
7. He Y, Chen D, Yang L, Hou Q, Ma H, Xu X. The therapeutic potential of bone marrow mesenchymal stem cells in premature ovarian failure. Stem Cell Res Ther. 2018;9:263.
8. Tilly JL, Johnson AL. Modulation of hen granulosa cell steroidogenesis and plasminogen activator activity hy transforming growth factor alpha. Growth Factors. 1990;3:247-55.
9. Zhao YX, Chen SR, Su PP, Huang FH, Shi YC, Shi QY, et al. Using Mesenchymal Stem Cells to Treat Female Infertility: An Update on Female Reproductive Diseases. Stem Cells Int. 2019;2019:9071720.
10. Patel NH, Bhadarka HK, Patel NH, Patel MN. Drug-free In vitro Activation for Primary Ovarian Insufficiency. J Hum Reprod Sci. 2021;14(4):443-5.

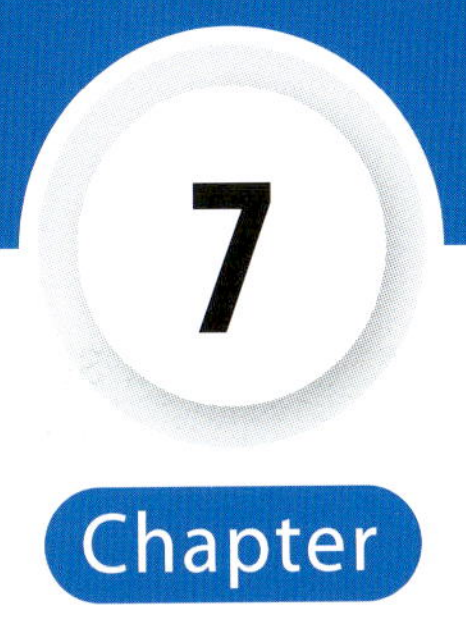

Chapter

Fertility Preservation in Cancer Patients and Pregnancy after Fertility Preservation

Puneet Rana Arora, Avantika Sharma, Jyoti Pandey

INTRODUCTION

With the advancement in cancer therapy, most patients have a improved life span and live longer. It is thus important to know the consequences of cancer treatments and quality of life after cancer. One of the long-term sequelae of cancer treatment infertility. Infertility can occur due to gonadotoxic effects of chemotherapy agents used in treatment of oncological conditions. American Society of Clinical Oncology recommends that oncologists should address the possibility of infertility to all patients and refer them to a reproductive specialist at the earliest possible opportunity.[1,2]

Occurrence of cancer between the ages of 15 and 30 years is 2.7 times more common than during the first 15 years of life, is much less common than cancer in older age-groups, and accounts for 2% of all invasive cancers.[3] In India, about 5.8% of all cancer cases registered are in age-group of 15–29 years in most urban cancer registries.[4,5]

With recent advances in treatment and improved cancer care, almost 80% of children and adolescents become long-term survivors of cancer.[6] The impact of cancer therapy on future fertility is closely related to the age of the women at the time of treatment and it also depends on the duration, dose intensity, and type of treatment.

A recent study has shown that women who received specialized counseling about future reproductive outcomes reported less regret and greater quality of life.[7] The grief associated with infertility may affect quality of life even 10 years after treatment of cancer. Cancer-related infertility has shown to cause long-term distress and impaired quality of life in cancer survivors, especially for women who did not receive sufficient information on fertility preservation options before starting their treatment.

IMPACT OF CANCER TREATMENT ON FERTILITY

Effect of Chemotherapy

Follicular depletion is physiologically age-dependent. Rapid depletion occurs around the age of 38 years when the reserve is just about 10% of the number present at menarche. The gonadotoxic effect is dependent on type and dosage of the cytotoxic drug administered as well as on the age of the woman. Effects of various chemotherapy agents are enlisted in **Table 1**.

The extent of gonadal failure is dependent on age at diagnosis and the cumulative dose of chemotherapy agents. Young women treated with adjuvant chemotherapy for breast cancer have higher risk of chemotherapy-related amenorrhea and premature ovarian insufficiency compared to those who receive chemotherapy after the age of 35 years for newly diagnosed breast cancer.[8]

Effect of Radiotherapy

Radiotherapy effects on the fertility potential of female are dependent on the dose. A dose of 6 Gy to the ovary of a woman below 30 years of age is usually reversible, but it will lead to premature ovarian insufficiency. In a woman over 30 years of age, doses of 14.3 Gy radiation will usually lead to irreversible infertility.[9,10] Thus, radiotherapy affects fertility as well as hormone production.[9]

Uterus is a relatively resistant organ to radiotherapy as compared with ovaries. Uterine irradiation may lead to poor implantation.[9-11] The reason could be many factors, which may include decreased uterine volume and blood flow that results in increased midtrimester losses, preterm labor, and intrauterine growth retardation.[12] Irradiation to the vagina can lead to less lubrication and stenosis causing

TABLE 1: Classes of chemotherapy agents and their infertility effects.

Class of agents	*Example*	*Mechanism of action*	*Infertility risk*
Alkylating agents	• Cyclophosphamide • Mechlorethamine • Chlorambucil • Busulfan • Melphalan	The active metabolites form cross-links with DNA with resultant inhibition of DNA synthesis and function. DNA double-strand breaks, with resultant p63-mediated apoptotic death in human primordial follicles	High risk
Platinum-based compounds	• Cisplatin • Carboplatin	Covalently bind to DNA to form intra- and interstrand DNA cross-links, leading to DNA breakage during replication. This inhibits DNA transcription, synthesis, and function. Specific toxicity has not been shown in human primordial follicles	Intermediate risk
Antimetabolites	• Methotrexate • 5-Fluorouracil • Cytarabine	Inhibition of DNA, RNA, thymidylate, and purine synthesis; no DNA damage in human follicles, hence not gonadotoxic	Low risk
Vinca alkaloids	• Vincristine • Vinblastine	Inhibition of tubulin polymerization and disruption of microtubule assembly during mitosis; this arrests mitosis during metaphase and leads to cell death. No DNA damage in human follicles, hence not gonadotoxic	Low risk
Anthracycline antibiotics	• Daunorubicin • Bleomycin • Adriamycin (doxorubicin)	Inhibition of DNA synthesis and function; it interferes with DNA transcription; it inhibits topoisomerase II, which leads to DNA breaks; it also forms toxic oxygen-free radicals, which induce DNA strand breaks, thereby inhibiting DNA synthesis and function; doxorubicin induces DNA double-strand breaks causing p63-mediated apoptotic death in human primordial follicles	Low risk except adriamycin (intermediate risk)

physical impairments and vaginismus leading to infertility as well as major psychosexual issues.[9,13]

FERTILITY PRESERVATION METHODS IN FEMALES

Fertility preservation techniques are now evolving and have provided opportunities to women in reproductive age-group to have their eggs or embryos preserved. Oocyte freezing is also a very widely practised method by women who wish to delay their childbearing due to social or medical cause. Medical causes in which fertility preservation is indicated are as follows:

- Cancer treatments
- *Hematologic conditions:* Thalassemia major, aplastic anemia, Fanconi's anemia
- *Autoimmune diseases:* Systemic lupus erythematosus (SLE), scleroderma
- Severe endometriosis
- *Genetic disorders*: Turner's syndrome, galactosemia
- Transgender individuals

Medical

- *Oocyte/embryo cryopreservation:* Embryo cryopreservation is a widely practised fertility preservation strategy. It can be used when a delay of 10–12 days is acceptable before starting the treatment. Women are given at least 10–12 days of injections before the oocytes are retrieved. A male partner or donor sperm is needed for formation of embryos. Embryo cryopreservation is a safe technique. Compared to embryo cryopreservation, oocyte freezing is associated with lower pregnancy rates (4.6–12% vs. 30–40%).[14,15]
- *In vitro maturation:* Oocytes from unstimulated ovaries can be used for fertility preservation for women in whom gonadotropin administration is contraindicated due to estrogen-sensitive disease. This method also avoids risk of delaying the cancer treatment.[16]
- *Preantral or primordial follicle culture:* The culture of primordial follicles involves a combination of inhibitory, stimulatory, and maintenance factors.[17,18] Primordial follicles can be activated or can be put to dormant state within ovarian cortical tissue by following steps: (1) Once activated preantral follicles are isolated, (2) they are grown individually till antral stages. (3) These are further grown to obtain full grown oocytes. (4) After this, they are tested for competence to undergo maturation and fertilization.
- *Ovarian suppression by gonadotropin-releasing hormone (GnRH) agonist therapy:* The use of GnRH

agonist suppresses the gonadotropin level and maintains the ovaries in an artificial dormant state.[19] Studies have shown that these agents reduce the organ damage and the local tissue ischemia caused by chemotherapeutic agents. For maximum benefit, GnRH agonist administration should be started 2–4 weeks before initiating chemotherapy. The menopausal symptoms associated with GnRH treatment is more frequent in older women compared to younger ones. The possible mechanisms by which these agents reduce the effect of chemotherapy are as follows:

- Simulation of prepubertal hypogonadotropic milieu
- Decrease in ovarian perfusion due to low estrogen levels
- Possible upregulation of antiapoptotic molecule such as sphingosine-1-phosphate
- Possible protection of ovarian germinative stem cells.[20-23]

Surgical

- *Ovarian tissue cryopreservation:* Ovarian cortex has abundant primordial follicles where oocytes are arrested in the diplotene state of prophase of the first meiotic division. This method can also be used as a method of fertility preservation in young prepubertal girls. Women below 40 years of age are ideal candidates for this method due to high ovarian reserve. This method does not require ovarian stimulation, male partner, or donor sperm, thus avoiding any delay in the treatment onset.[15] Laparoscopic surgery is a preferred approach to obtain cortical ovarian tissue of 0.5–2 cm and this tissue is then cryopreserved for either later reimplantation or in vitro maturation of eggs.[24] The main risk with this method is reintroduction of malignant cells. The risk is high for patients with leukemia, neuroblastoma, and Burkitt's lymphoma.[20,25] Hence, before autotransplantation thawed tissues should be checked for malignant cells.
- *Ovarian tissue autotransplantation:* This method is useful for women who need to have pelvic or peritoneal irradiation due to cancer. Ovaries or ovarian tissue are removed and transplanted in area away from the field of irradiation.
- *Uterus transplantation:* This is still considered experimental. This method may be useful in women who had to get hysterectomy done due to advanced or invasive disease of uterine cervix or body.

PREGNANCY FOLLOWING CANCER TREATMENT

Significant number of postpubertal women may not have completed their family at the time of diagnosis of cancer. These women may express a desire for pregnancy after treatment.[26] Studies have demonstrated a significantly lower pregnancy rate in cancer survivors compared to that of general population,[27-29] and the former more likely use ART (assisted reproductive techniques) for conception. Posttreatment pregnancy rate depends on the type of cancer, the lowest rates are reported for women with a history of breast or cervical cancer. While counseling the women or couple regarding fertility after the treatment of cancer factors related to disease, treatment as well as personal factors should be considered. These factors are mentioned in **Box 1**.

Adult cancer survivors who are not able conceive spontaneously and also did not have a chance of fertility preservation strategies due to lack of time or lack of accessibility at the time of diagnosis of cancer should be counseled regarding the safety of ART procedures.

Lower live birth rates have been reported with the use of autologous oocytes in cancer survivors compared with healthy women (24.7% vs. 47.7%).[30] A human live birth has been reported following the treatment of ovarian tissue for 48 hours in vitro with bpV(HOpic) and 740YP, an Akt stimulant, followed by replacement and in vitro fertilization (IVF).[31]

The time period between the disease and the start of pregnancy is an important aspect while planning pregnancy after treatment of breast cancer. The Royal College of Obstetricians and Gynaecologists (RCOG)

BOX 1: Factors to be considered before planning pregnancy after cancer treatment.

Personal factors	*Factors related to disease/ treatment*
• Age • Sex • BMI • Smoking • Presence of a partner • Prior medical condition • Prior fertility treatment • Prior fertility preservation treatment • Hereditary conditions	• Type of cancer (biology and prognosis) • Site of cancer • Type of treatment (surgery, chemotherapy, RT) • Dose and duration of treatment • Interval since completion of treatment • Follow-up after treatment

(BMI: body mass index; RT: radiotherapy)

recommends that premenopausal breast cancer women should wait for at least 2 years before attempting to conceive.[32] As young women have lower survival rates and an increased risk of local relapse and metastases, they should wait for 3 years before planning pregnancy.[32] The possible explanation for this could be that duration of 2–3 years helps to differentiate patients with better prognosis from those with more aggressive disease. There is a statistically nonsignificant increase in mortality risk in women who become pregnant <6 months after diagnosis. However, risk reduces significantly if pregnancy occurs 2–5 years after diagnosis. In between, there is a nonsignificant reduction in the risk of mortality.[33,34]

The POSITIVE trial showed no clear worsening of breast cancer outcomes in the short term after temporary interruption of endocrine therapy to allow for pregnancy in selected women with a history of hormone receptor-positive breast cancer. Longer-term follow-up is needed to further inform the safety of this strategy.[35]

Studies have shown that there is an increased risk of obstetric and birth complications in female cancer survivors in terms of increased risk of prematurity [relative risk (RR): 1.56; 95% confidence interval (CI): 1.37–1.77], low birth weight (RR: 1.47; 95% CI: 1.24–1.73), elective (RR: 1.38; 95% CI: 1.13–1.70) and emergency cesarean section (RR: 1.22; 95% CI: 1.15–1.30), assisted vaginal delivery (RR: 1.10; 95% CI: 1.02–1.18), and postpartum hemorrhage (RR: 1.18; 95% CI: 1.02–1.36).[36,37] The risk of these complications appears to be higher when the interval between the end of cancer treatment and conception is short.[38]

CONCLUSION

- Fertility preservation should preferably be offered to women at the time of diagnosis before initiating the cancer treatment.
- Oocytes or embryo cryopreservation can be safely and efficiently done before the initiation of anticancer therapy if a delay of 2 weeks is possible for starting the anticancer treatment without compromising the safety of women.
- Women should be managed by a multidisciplinary team consisting of reproductive medicine and cancer treatment facility for timely referral for counseling and access to oocyte and embryo cryopreservation.
- Women should be counseled regarding the importance of age for achieving a successful pregnancy.
- Pregnant women after treatment of cancer should be monitored more closely due to the increased chances of developing obstetric and perinatal complications.
- With adequate treatment and follow-up, women should not be discouraged from having a pregnancy for safety reasons, even with a prior history of hormone receptor-positive breast cancer.

REFERENCES

1. Lee SJ, Schover LR, Partridge AH, Patrizio P, Wallace WH, Hagerty K, et al.; American Society of Clinical Oncology. American Society of Clinical Oncology recommendations on fertility preservation in cancer patients. J Clin Oncol. 2006;24:2917-31.
2. Loren AW, Mangu PB, Beck LN, Brennan L, Magdalinski AJ, Partridge AH, et al.; American Society of Clinical Oncology. Fertility preservation for patients with cancer: American Society of Clinical Oncology clinical practice guideline update. J Clin Oncol. 2013;31:2500-10.
3. Bleyer A, Viny A, Barr R. Cancer in 15- to 29-year-olds by primary site. Oncologist. 2006;11:590-601.
4. Arora RS, Alston RD, Eden TO, Moran A, Geraci M, O'Hara C, et al. Cancer at ages 15-29 years: the contrasting incidence in India and England. Pediatr Blood Cancer. 2012;58:55-60.
5. Kalyani R, Das S, Kumar ML. Pattern of cancer in adolescent and young adults—a ten year study in India. Asian Pac J Cancer Prev. 2010;11:655-9.
6. Revel A, Revel-Vilk S. Fertility preservation in young cancer patients. J Hum Reprod Sci. 2010;3:2-7.
7. Vadaparampil ST, Quinn GP. Improving communication between oncologists and reproductive specialists to promote timely referral of patients with cancer. J Oncol Pract. 2013;9:300-21.
8. Turnbull AK, Patel S, Martinez-Perez C, Rigg A, Oikonomidou O. Risk of chemotherapy-related amenorrhoea (CRA) in premenopausal women undergoing chemotherapy for early stage breast cancer. Breast Cancer Res Treat. 2021; 186(1):237-45.
9. Ajala T, Rafi J, Larsen-Disney P, Howell R. Fertility preservation for cancer patients: a review. Obstet Gynecol Int. 2010;2010:160386.
10. Wallace WH, Thomson AB, Saran F, Kelsey TW. Predicting age of ovarian failure after radiation to a field that includes the ovaries. Int J Radiat Oncol Biol Phys. 2005;62:738-44.
11. Critchley HO, Wallace WH. Impact of cancer treatment on uterine function. J Natl Cancer Inst Monogr. 2005;34:64-8.
12. Chhabra S, Kutchi I. Fertility preservation in gynecological cancers. Clin Med Insights Reprod Health. 2013;7:49-59.
13. Liao L, Doyle J, Crouch NS, Creighton SM. Dilation as treatment for vaginal agenesis and hypoplasia: a pilot exploration of benefits and barriers as perceived by patients. J Obstet Gynaecol. 2006;26:144-8.

14. Chan JL, Wang ET. Oncofertility for women with gynecologic malignancies. Gynecol Oncol. 2017;144(3):631-6.
15. Levine JM, Kelvin JF, Quinn GP, Gracia CR. Infertility in reproductive-age female cancer survivors. Cancer. 2015; 121(10):1532-9.
16. Huang JY, Buckett WM, Gilbert L, Tan SL, Chian RC. Retrieval of immature oocytes followed by in vitro maturation and vitrification: a case report on a new strategy of fertility preservation in women with borderline ovarian malignancy. Gynecol Oncol. 2007;105:542-4.
17. Nelson SM, Telfer EE, Anderson RA. The ageing ovary and uterus: new biological insights. Hum Reprod Update. 2013; 19:67-83.
18. Hsueh AJ, Kawamura K, Cheng Y, Fauser BC. Intraovarian control of early folliculogenesis. Endocr Rev. 2015;36:1-24.
19. Hickman LC, Valentine LN, Falcone T. Preservation of gonadal function in women undergoing chemotherapy: a review of the potential role for gonadotropin-releasing hormone agonists. Am J Obstet Gynecol. 2016;215(4):415-22.
20. Blumenfeld Z, Katz G, Evron A. 'An ounce of prevention is worth a pound of cure': the case for and against GnRH-agonist for fertility preservation. Ann Oncol. 2014;25(9): 1719-28.
21. Blumenfeld Z. How to preserve fertility in young women exposed to chemotherapy? The role of GnRH agonist in addition to cryopreservation of embryos, oocytes, or ovaries. Oncologist. 2007;12:1044-54.
22. Blumenfeld Z, von Wolff M. GnRH-analogues and oral contraceptives for fertility preservation in women during chemotherapy. Hum Reprod Update. 2008;14:543-52.
23. Blumenfeld Z. GnRH-agonists in fertility preservation. Curr Opin Endocrinol Diabetes Obes. 2008;15:523-8.
24. Loren AW, Mangu PB, Beck LN, Brennan L, Magdalinski AJ, Partridge AH, et al. Fertility preservation for patients with cancer: American society of clinical oncology clinical practice guideline update. J Clin Oncol. 2013;31(19):2500-10.
25. Donnez J, Dolmans MM. Transplantation of ovarian tissue. Best Pract Res Clin Obstet Gynaecol. 2014;28:1188-97.
26. Letourneau JM, Ebbel EE, Katz PP, Katz A, Ai WZ, Chien AJ, et al. Pretreatment fertility counseling and fertility preservation improve quality of life in reproductive age women with cancer. Cancer. 2012;118(6):1710-7.
27. Cvancarova M, Samuelsen SO, Magelssen H, Fosså SD. Reproduction rates after cancer treatment: experience from the Norwegian radium hospital. J Clin Oncol. 2009; 27:334-43.
28. Green DM, Whitton JA, Stovall M, Mertens AC, Donaldson SS, Ruymann FB, et al. Pregnancy outcome of female survivors of childhood cancer: a report from the Childhood Cancer Survivor Study. Am J Obstet Gynecol. 2002; 187:1070-80.
29. Stensheim H, Cvancarova M, Møller B, Fosså SD. Pregnancy after adolescent and adult cancer: a population-based matched cohort study. Int J Cancer. 2011;129:1225-36.
30. Luke B, Brown MB, Missmer SA, Spector LG, Leach RE, Williams M, et al. Assisted reproductive technology use and outcomes among women with a history of cancer. Hum Reprod. 2016;31(1):183-9.
31. Kawamura K, Cheng Y, Suzuki N, Deguchi M, Sato Y, Takae S, et al. Hippo signaling disruption and Akt stimulation of ovarian follicles for infertility treatment. Proc Natl Acad Sci USA. 2013;110:17474-9.
32. Royal College of Obstetricians and Gynaecologists. (2011). Pregnancy and Breast Cancer. Green-top Guideline No. 12.
33. Ives A, Saunders C, Bulsara M, Semmens J. Pregnancy after breast cancer: Population based study. BMJ. 2007; 334:194.
34. Mueller BA, Simon MS, Deapen D, Kamineni A, Malone KE, Daling JR. Childbearing and survival after breast carcinoma in young women. Cancer. 2003;98:1131-40.
35. Partridge AH, Niman SM, Ruggeri M, Peccatori FA, Azim HA Jr, Colleoni M, et al.; International Breast Cancer Study Group; POSITIVE Trial Collaborators. Interrupting Endocrine Therapy to Attempt Pregnancy after Breast Cancer. N Engl J Med. 2023;388(18):1645-56.
36. Stensheim H, Klungsøyr K, Skjaerven R, Grotmol T, Fosså SD. Birth outcomes among offspring of adult cancer survivors: a population-based study. Int J Cancer. 2013;133(11):2696-705.
37. van der Kooi ALF, Kelsey TW, van den Heuvel-Eibrink MM, Laven JSE, Wallace WHB, Anderson RA. Perinatal complications in female survivors of cancer: a systematic review and meta-analysis. Eur J Cancer. 2019;111: 126-37.
38. Hartnett KP, Mertens AC, Kramer MR, Lash TL, Spencer JB, Ward KC, et al. Pregnancy after cancer: does timing of conception affect infant health? Cancer. 2018;124(22): 4401-7.

Chapter

Oocyte and Sperm Vitrification

Navin Desai, Rishina Bansal, Kavya MP, S Lavanya

INTRODUCTION

The procedure of cryopreservation involves preservation of sperm, oocytes, or an embryo at subzero temperatures through a process of solidification in order to preserve them for a prolonged period of time in liquid nitrogen at temperatures under –196°C.

Cryopreservation is one of the keystones in clinical infertility treatment.

HISTORICAL BACKGROUND OF CRYOPRESERVATION

More than two centuries ago, in 1776, Spallanzani was the first to report the maintenance of motility of human spermatozoa after exposure to low temperatures. Mantegazza in 1866 suggested sperm banks for frozen human sperm. In 1949, Polge et al. discovered the effectiveness of glycerol as a cryoprotective agent for fowl spermatozoa.[1] Freezing of human spermatozoa was reported shortly afterward by Bunge and Sherman, observing that human spermatozoa, after freezing were viable when thawed to fertilize and to produce normal embryonic development and offspring.[2] The first birth after freezing human spermatozoa with glycerol in liquid nitrogen vapor was described by the same group. The development of human sperm cryobanks in the 1970s gave rise to a growing need for standardization. The first association of human sperm banks was set up in France, the Center d'Etude et de Conservation du Sperme, in 1973, followed by the creation of the American Association of Tissue Banks in 1976, which also covered cryopreservation of gametes.

The growing use of cryopreserved human semen led to the First International Meeting on Human Semen Cryopreservation, held in Paris in 1978. The pioneers of oocyte cryopreservation set out their goals almost 50 years ago. In 1957, Lin, Sherman, and Willet demonstrated that the mouse oocyte can survive cooling to –5°C in a 5% glycerol-containing medium.[3] In 1958, Sherman and Lin reported the birth of live young following in vitro fertilization (IVF) of mouse oocytes that had been "frozen" at –10°C in a 5% glycerol-containing medium.[4] However, no oocytes survived exposure to a temperature of –20°C. The question with regard to these experiments is whether the oocytes were really frozen at –10°C, or whether they were reduced to a "super cooled" state.

In 1972, Whittingham and coworkers applied mathematically based cryopreservation protocols to mouse embryos, leading to the first report of birth after storage of mouse embryos at –196°C in liquid nitrogen.[5] The protocols that they had been using for freezing the mouse embryos were largely copied for the human embryo, and in 1983, the first paper on a pregnancy from a cryopreserved human embryo was published by Trounson and Mohr.[6]

It was again Wittingham who reported on the first successful cryopreservation of the mouse oocyte at –196°C in liquid nitrogen followed by the birth of live young.[7] But oocyte cryopreservation was not very successful as it did not find widespread clinical application due to low survival rates, and also questions about the genetic safety appeared in the literature. It was found that the degree of polyploidy increased significantly after cryopreservation of mouse and human oocytes. Almost all clinical teams stopped oocyte cryopreservation around 1987; and only a few research teams continued to investigate the effects of cryopreservation on the oocyte before considering moving oocyte cryopreservation back to the clinic again.[8]

Cryoprotectants are chemical compounds that prevent cells or tissues from damage due to freezing. They are used in both slow freezing and vitrification methods, but the concentration of cryoprotectant is much higher in vitrification.[9] Ethylene glycol has been widely used as cryoprotectant in both slow freezing and vitrification methods due to its high permeable nature and low toxicity.[10]

Cryoprotectants can be categorized into two types:

1. Cryoprotectants that permeate cell membranes include dimethyl sulfoxide (DMSO), glycerol, and 1,2-propanediol.
2. Membrane-impermeable cryoprotectants include polymers such as polyvinylpyrrolidone, hydroxyethyl starch, 2-methyl-2,4-pentanediol, and other sugars.

METHODS OF SPERM CRYOPRESERVATION

Cryopreservation can be done using either conventional slow freezing technique or vitrification.

Conventional Slow Freezing Technique

Basic principle of conventional slow freezing technique is dehydration of cells[11] using low concentration of cryoprotectant to achieve equilibrium. After liquefaction, freezing must be performed within 1 hour for better post-thaw results. In this method, ice crystals are formed at a certain temperature due to gradual decreasing in temperature. The slow cooling is achieved either by using a programmable freezer or by lowering the samples into liquid nitrogen vapor manually. After initial equilibration with cryoprotectant for 5–10 minutes at 20°–25°C, freezing starts with keeping the sample at –20°C for 15–20 minutes and then at –86°C for 60 minutes and finally samples are stored in liquid nitrogen under –196°C using cryovials **(Fig. 1)**.[12]

Slow freezing can be performed for fresh ejaculated sample or washed samples, surgically retrieved samples, and also for testicular tissue.

Vitrification

Basic principle of vitrification is based on extremely high cooling rate, which prevents ice crystals formation. The processed semen sample is loaded in straws or cryoloops and then rapidly cooled by direct contact with liquid nitrogen (–196°C).[13] Sperm vitrification method can be used with patients with severe oligospermia or azoospermia, who have undergone testicular sperm extraction (TESE)/micro-TESE procedure.

It is now regarded as the potential alternative to the conventional slow freezing technique. Two conditions required to allow vitrification are an increase in viscosity and a depression of the freezing temperature. These conditions are achieved by addition of cryoprotectants which act like antifreeze.

This method of cryopreservation is more commonly used for oocytes and embryos, whereas vitrification of spermatozoa is still a challenge due to their specific characteristics.[14]

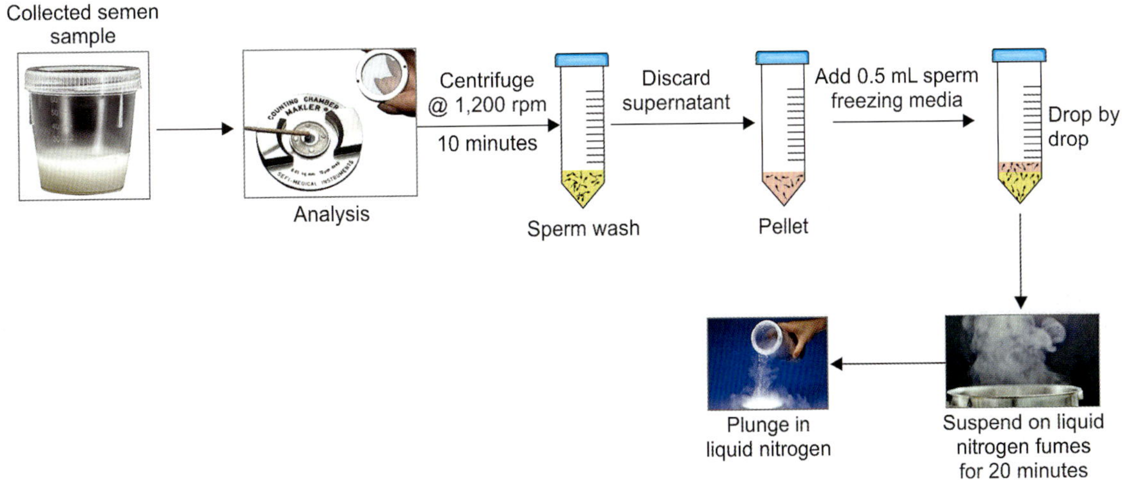

Fig. 1: Semen freezing.

OPEN AND CLOSED SYSTEMS OF VITRIFICATION

Vitrification techniques differ from each other in many technical details including equilibration of the solutions, dilution parameters, storage, etc. One other aspect which varies is the open and closed type of vitrification.

Closed system: In the closed system, the samples are physically separated from liquid or vapor phase nitrogen during the entire cooling, storage, and warming procedure.

Open vitrification: In the open system, the samples are physically allowed for possible direct contact to liquid- or vapor-phase nitrogen to improve the overall efficiency of vitrification by increased cooling rate.

OOCYTE CRYOPRESERVATION

Human oocyte cryopreservation is a technology where oocytes are extracted, frozen, and stored. Later, when the patient is ready to become pregnant, the eggs can be thawed, fertilized, and transferred to the uterus as embryos. In1999, the birth of the first baby from an embryo derived from vitrified-warmed oocytes was reported by Kuleshova and coworkers in the journal of Human Reproduction.[15]

The technique of oocyte vitrification is used for three main indications; they are:

1. In the case of female fertility preservation to preserve fertility in women diagnosed with cancer and seeking oncological treatment that may affect their fertility
2. Social egg freezing for women delaying parenthood due to competing priorities such as education or career or not having found a suitable partner yet
3. Oocyte vitrification allows better planning of IVF cycles, as this procedure offers the possibility of collecting oocytes in low responders and vitrifying the oocytes from several ovarian stimulations to perform intracytoplasmic sperm injection (ICSI) procedure. In addition, oocyte vitrification also allows the use of vitrified donor oocyte without having synchronization with recipient treatment cycle **(Fig. 2)**.

EMBRYO CRYOPRESERVATION

Vitrification of human embryos allows us to maximize the potential for conception from any one IVF cycle and prevents wastage of embryos. Vitrification has become a well-established and widely used procedure that allows expansion of therapeutic strategies when IVF/ICSI is used to treat infertility. As a result of the increasing use of embryo vitrification, more than a million children have been born worldwide after transfer of cryopreserved embryos.[16]

Embryo vitrification provides a solution in situations such as:

- Canceling of embryo transfer in the same cycle as stimulation for ICSI/IVF due to reasons such as

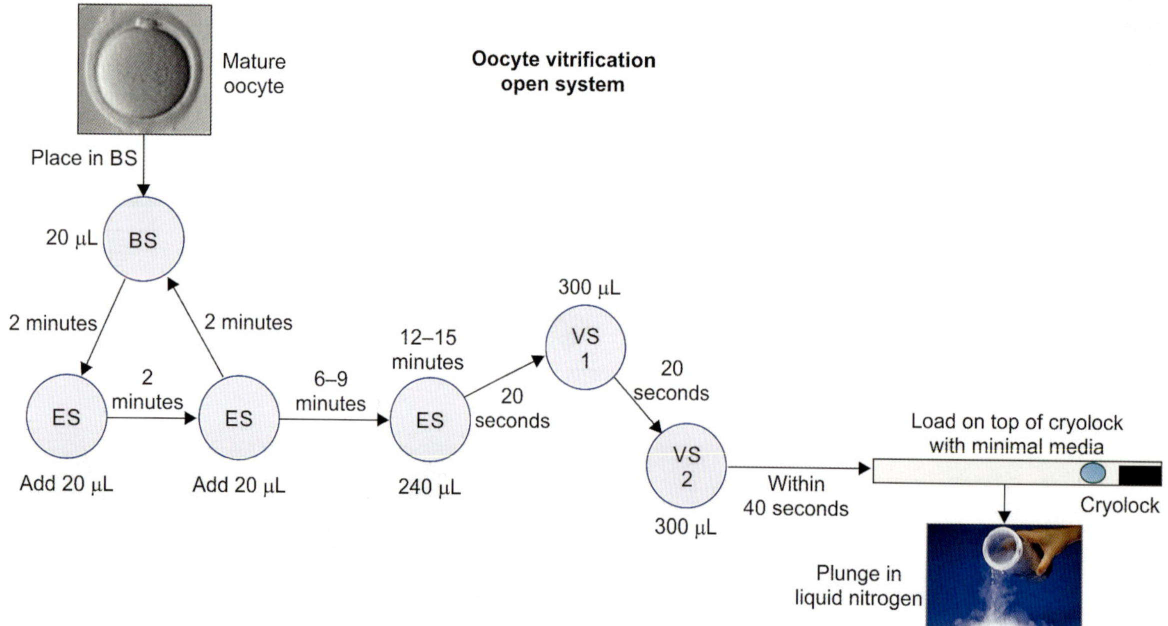

Fig. 2: Oocyte vitrification. (BS: basic solution; ES: equilibrium solution; VS: vitrification solution)

risk of ovarian hyperstimulation syndrome (OHSS), inadequate endometrial preparation, or emergency management.

- When the embryo transfer done in the same cycle as stimulation for ICSI/IVF, and there are one or more good-quality embryos that can be used for subsequent cycles in case of negative result or because the patient wants to plan for another child in future.
- When couple decides to cryopreserve embryos instead of oocytes and sperm separately, for their fertility preservation.
- When embryo(s) are biopsied for the preimplantation genetic testing (PGT) procedure such as to rule out genetic abnormalities, the result is not expected for several days.
- Vitrification allows for the preservation of either donor eggs or the embryos when there is no synchronization of donor treatment cycle with recipient treatment cycle.

Note: Vitrification has better post-thaw survival rates when compared to conventional slow freezing methods. Research has found an approximately 85% survival rate with vitrification and 70% rate for conventional slow freezing.

Method

The basic method is as follows: Cleavage stage embryos or blastocyst stage embryos are pre-equilibrated in 7.5% DMSO and 7.5% ethylene glycol, followed by a short incubation in 15% DMSO and 15% ethylene glycol, and then immediately loaded into a straw and submerged into liquid nitrogen **(Fig. 3)**.

OVARIAN TISSUE CRYOPRESERVATION

Ovarian tissue cryopreservation is still an experimental technique. This method allows fertility preservation in prepubertal girls or unmarried women diagnosed with cancer. Ovarian tissue for cryopreservation can be extracted either by laparoscopy or by minilaparotomy, and these surgeries can be performed at any point of women's menstrual cycle.[17]

The procedure involves removing small pieces of the ovarian cortex from the patient's ovaries.

The ovarian cortex contains the egg precursor cells. The extracted immature tissues are dissected into thin 1-mm strips and stored under liquid nitrogen using slow freezing technique. Later, once it is confirmed that patient is cured from cancer, these strips are transplanted into the ovary.

SINGLE-SPERM VITRIFICATION

The development of ICSI technology has extended the therapeutic capacity of assisted reproductive technology for men with azoospermia via the surgical isolation of sperm from the testis/epididymis. Thus, cryopreservation of their sperm is performed to avoid repeated surgical retrievals and to preserve their sperm from any side effects. The conventional cryopreservation techniques are inadequate for preserving individually selected sperm. The technique for freezing single sperm was first developed in 1997 and has been explored from the perspective of frozen carriers, freezing programs, and cryoprotectant formulations.

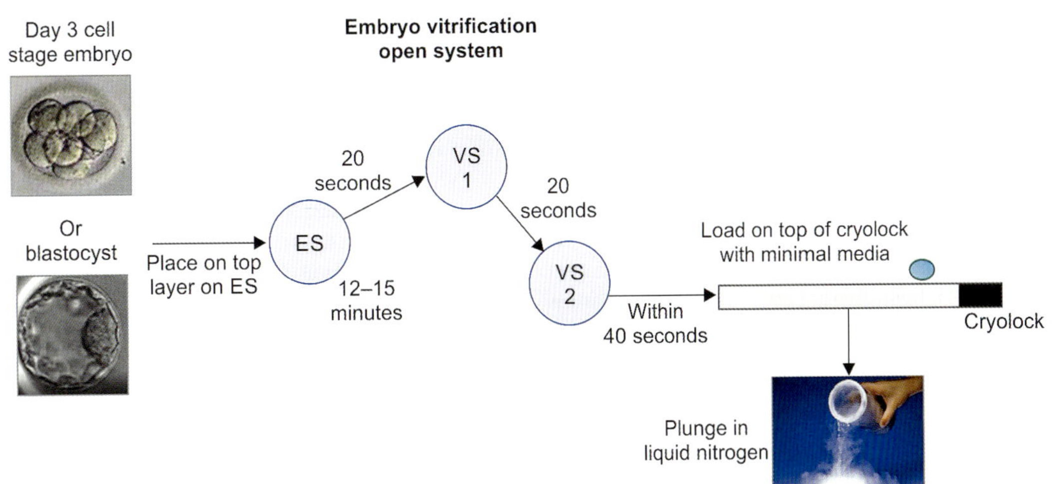

Fig. 3: Embryo vitrification. (ES: equilibrium solution; VS: vitrification solution)

Among these methods, advances in frozen carriers have directly improved single-sperm freezing technology.

Methods

Samples are evaluated for the presence of motile sperm before cryopreservation. Motile or twitching sperm are isolated with an ICSI needle for single-sperm cryopreservation. Selected sperm are loaded on the High Security Straw in ~0.5 μL of fluid to facilitate recovery. Test-yolk buffer–glycerol (Irvine) is used as the cryoprotectant.[18]

CONCLUSION

There are many factors that can affect the outcome of a cryopreservation procedure, from sperm quality, egg quality, and embryo quality, to patient demographics, stimulation protocols, quality of drug administration, culture conditions, laboratory quality, vitrification and warming procedures, and uterine preparation. All of these variables must be carefully observed and managed in order to achieve successful cryopreservation outcomes.

It is important to remember that there are no guarantees for success. Not every cryopreserved sperm, egg, or embryo will survive the warming process. Not every thawed egg will become fertilized and develop as a potent blastocyst. Not every embryo that will develop may be healthy enough to transfer. Freezing sperm, eggs, or embryos may help patient become pregnant later, but there is no method or process that offers guaranteed success. When cells do not survive, we assume it is from intracellular ice formation or osmotic effects or toxicity or handling technique, but we really are just guessing. We have no way of seeing what is happening inside the cell and can only make assumptions, many of which are incorrect. These unknowns and the continued push to find simpler, more effective methods of embryo storage keep us looking to the future for a deeper understanding of the complexities of human gamete and embryo vitrification.

REFERENCES

1. Polge C, Smith AU, Parkes AS. Revival of Spermatozoa after Vitrification and Dehydration at Low Temperatures. Nature. 1949;164:666.
2. Bunge RG, Sherman JK. Fertilizing capacity of frozen human spermatozoa. Nature. 1953;172:767-8.
3. Lin TP, Sherman JK, Willett EL. Survival of unfertilized mouse eggs in media containing glycerol and glycine. J Exp Zool. 1957;134(2):275-91.
4. Sherman JK, Lin TP. Survival of Unfertilized Mouse Eggs During Freezing and Thawing. Proc Soc Exp Biol Med. 1958;98(4):902-5.
5. Whittingham DG, Leibo SP, Mazur P. Survival of mouse embryos frozen to –196 degrees and –269 degrees C. Science. 1972;178(4059):411-4.
6. Trounson A, Mohr L. Human pregnancy following cryopreservation, thawing and transfer of an eight-cell embryo. Nature. 1983;305(5936):707-9.
7. Whittingham DG. Fertilization in vitro and development to term of unfertilized mouse oocytes previously stored at –196 degrees C. J Reprod Fertil. 1977;49(1):89-94.
8. Van der Elst J, Verheyen G, Van Steirtegehem A. Cryoconservation: Sperms and oocytes. In: Rabe T, Diedrich K, Runnebaum B (Eds). Manual on Assisted Reproduction. Germany: Springer-Verlag Berlin Heidelberg; 1997. pp. 223-51.
9. Elder K, Brian D. Cryopreservation. In Vitro Fertilization, 2nd edition. Cambridge: Cambridge University Press; 2000. pp. 192-228.
10. Emiliani S, Van den Bergh M, Vannin AS, Biramane J, Englert Y. Comparison of ethylene glycol, 1,2-propanediol and glycerol for cryopreservation of slow-cooled mouse zygotes, 4-cell embryos and blastocysts. Hum Reprod. 2000; 15:905-10.
11. Gupta SAA, Sharma R, Ahmady A. Sperm banking via cryopreservation. In: RMB RB, Nabil A, Agarwal A, Sabanegh E (Eds). Medical and Surgical Management of Male Infertility. New Delhi: Jaypee Brothers Medical Publishers; 2014.
12. World Health Organization. WHO laboratory manual for the examination and processing of human semen, 6th edition. Geneva: World Health Organization; 2021.
13. Gao F. Human Sperm Vitrification: Review of Recent Progress. Embryology Update. IntechOpen; 2023.
14. Sharma R, Kattoor AJ, Ghulmiyyah J, Agarwal A. Effect of sperm storage and selection techniques on sperm parameters. Syst Biol Reprod Med. 2015;61(1):1-12.
15. Kuleshova LL, Wang XW, Wu YN, Zhou Y, Yu H. Vitrification of encapsulated hepatocytes with reduced cooling and warming rates. Cryo Letters. 2004;25(4):241-54.
16. Fahy GM, MacFarlane DR, Angell CA, Meryman HT. Vitrification as an approach to cryopreservation. Cryobiology. 1984;21:407-26.
17. Mayerhofer K, Ott J, Nouri K, Stoegbauer L, Fischer EM, Lipovac M, et al. Laparoscopic Ovarian Tissue Harvesting for cryopreservation: an effective and safe procedure for fertility preservation. Eur J Obstet Gynecol Reprod Biol. 2010;152(1):68-72.
18. Desai N, Goldberg J, Austin C, Sabanegh E, Falcone T. Cryopreservation of individually selected sperm: methodology and case report of a clinical pregnancy. J Assist Reprod Genet. 2012;29(5):375-9.

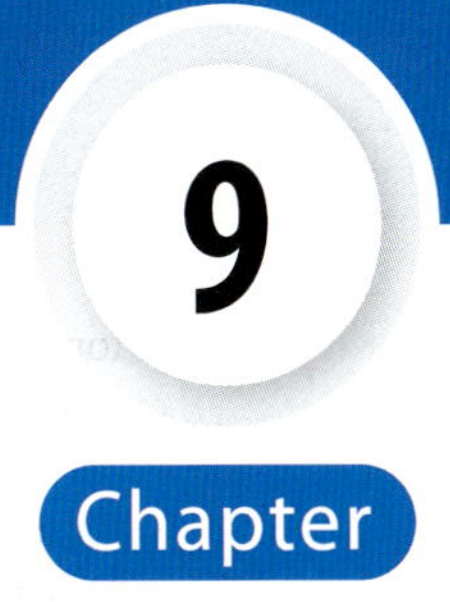

Chapter

Current Practices in In Vitro Maturation

Durga G Rao, Krishna Chaitanya Mantravadi

INTRODUCTION

In vitro maturation (IVM) refers to the growth of oocytes progressing from prophase 1 stage, i.e., from germinal vesicle (GV) through meiosis I to reach metaphase II (MII) stage after recovery from follicles that have not been exposed to preovulatory trigger.[1]

Pincus and Enzmann introduced IVM using immature rabbit oocytes in 1935. Cha et al. demonstrated the use of IVM in humans in 1991.[2] Trounson et al. are credited with the creation of the first IVM baby in 1994 using oocytes from a patient (unstimulated ovaries) with polycystic ovaries.[3]

The original idea behind the retrieval of immature oocytes followed by maturation (in vitro) was to mitigate ovarian hyperstimulation syndrome (OHSS) risk in the case of women with polycystic ovary syndrome (PCOS), thereby intending to reduce the financial burden, number of injections, and duration of treatment.[4]

In vitro maturation is a relatively recent development in the field of assisted reproduction and as it has evolved over the years. This chapter gives an overview of the current practices in IVM **(Fig. 1)**.

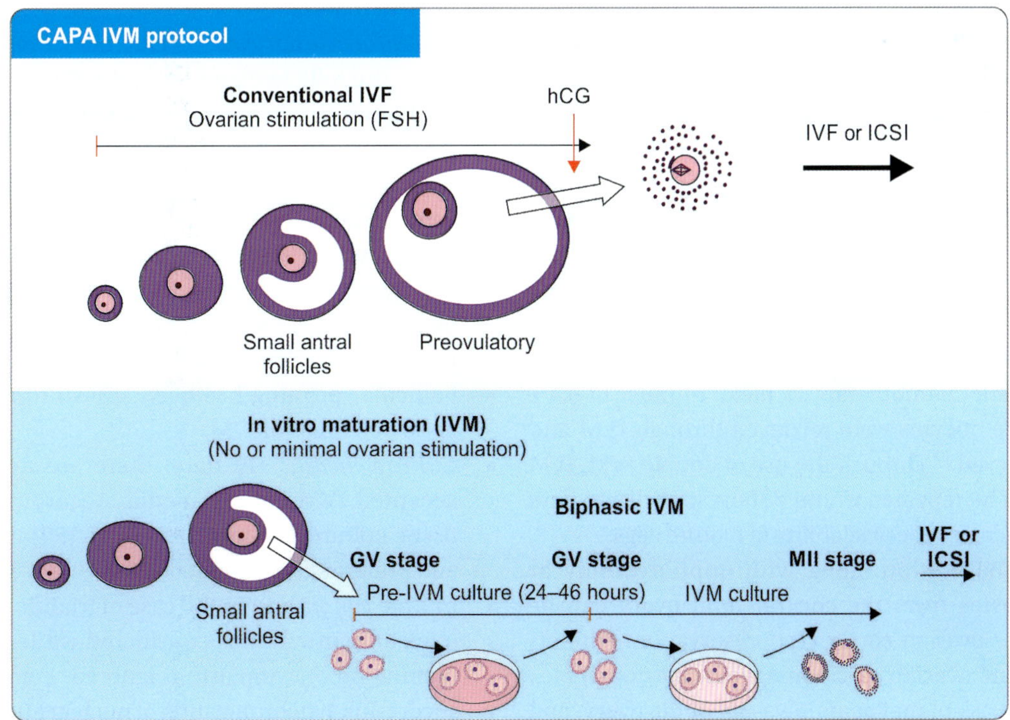

Fig. 1: Pictorial depiction of conventional in vitro fertilization (IVF) with human chorionic gonadotropin (hCG) trigger and overview of in vitro maturation (IVM). (CAPA IVM: capacitation IVM; FSH: follicle-stimulating hormone; GV: germinal vesicle; ICSI: intracytoplasmic sperm injection; MII: metaphase II)

INDICATIONS OF IN VITRO MATURATION

- *Polycystic ovary syndrome:* IVM is very helpful in the case of PCOS and results in 32–44% pregnancy rate and 22–29% delivery rates.[5]
- *History of OHSS:* Application of antagonist protocol and agonist trigger with freeze-all policy does not totally eliminate the risk of OHSS. However, IVM has been shown to eliminate the risk of OHSS.[6]
- *Women with ovulatory cycles:* IVM helps normo-ovulatory women by eliminating the side effects of stimulation, resulting in a pregnancy rate of approximately 30%.[1]
- *Recurrent fertilization failure-poor oocyte or embryo quality:* IVM has shown better results in women with recurrent fertilization failures, poor oocyte, or embryo quality.[7,8]
- *Resistant ovary syndrome (ROS):* For women with ROS, IVM is an excellent alternative to egg donation and several live births have also been reported.[7] These women have primary or secondary amenorrhea and have high levels of FSH and luteinizing hormone (LH) though their anti-Müllerian hormone (AMH) level and antral follicle counts are normal.
- *Fertility preservation in cancer:* In case of patients with cancer, for whom hormonal treatment might not be suitable and chemotherapy needs to be started immediately, IVM is the best option to preserve fertility.[9] There is reduced use of expensive drugs and limited monitoring in IVM. In prepubertal girls and women who have estrogen receptor-positive breast cancer, wherein oocyte cryopreservation is necessary, IVM of oocytes can be done through transvaginal follicular aspiration or oocytes can be taken from extracorporeal ovarian tissue. In 248 breast cancer patients with a mean age of 31.5 ± 0.3 years, before neoadjuvant chemotherapy, a mean number of 6.4 ± 0.3 mature oocytes were retrieved through IVM and cryopreserved.[10] Through the use of double IVM, IVM cycles can be repeated within a short span of <10 days so as to increase the availability of mature eggs.

In vitro maturation along with oophorectomy or ovarian biopsies from the contralateral ovary can be performed for ovarian cortex cryopreservation. Patients with borderline ovarian carcinoma, neuroblastoma, etc., have a higher risk of malignant invasion of the ovary, and IVM of oocytes from excised ovarian tissue oocyte-IVM (OTO-IVM) may be the best choice of treatment for these women. Ovarian tissue transplantation may reintroduce tumors. Hence, OTO-IVM remains experimental even today.[7]

- *IVM for rescuing IVF cycles:* Sometimes oocytes retrieved after ovarian stimulation (OS) and the trigger may be immature and in these cases, rescue IVM is proposed as it can result in good-quality oocytes.

FACTORS AFFECTING IN VITRO MATURATION (FIG. 2)

- *Woman's age:* A study on the effect of IVM conducted on 133 patients (aged 1–35 years) who took up fertility preservation via ovarian tissue cryopreservation indicated that the highest IVM rates were observed in the patients between menarche to 25 years and the lowest IVM rates (<10%) were reported in women ≥30 years and premenarche girls (<6 years).[11]
- *Time of in vitro culture:* The IVM culture time of human oocytes is around 24–30 hours, which can result in IVM rates of 40–60%. Longer culture time may be needed to increase the maturation rate, but at the same time, it may affect embryo quality and embryo utilization rate. A shorter culture time may lead to cytoplasmic immaturity as cytoplasmic maturation lags behind nuclear maturation.[8]
- *Time of oocyte retrieval:* Usually, oocyte retrieval is done when the follicle diameter of the dominant follicle is 10–12 mm or when the thickness of the endometrium is 5–6 mm in the case of women with PCOS who do not have leading follicles. Although there is no common agreement on the timing of oocyte retrieval in the IVM process, oocyte retrieval is preferred when the dominant follicle is ≤14 mm as sibling immature oocytes may be affected adversely if a dominant follicle >14 mm is present at the time of oocyte retrieval.
- Follicular priming has been shown to influence the cycle outcomes of IVM.
- *Culture media:* Till date, there are no universally accepted IVM culture media. According to studies, tissue culture medium 199 (TCM-199) is widely used and preferred for human oocytes.[8]
- *Culture conditions:* In the case of traditional IVM, only nuclear maturation is considered while synchronous maturation of cytoplasm is ignored. For an IVM to be successful, synchronization of nuclear and cytoplasmic maturation is a must. To prevent the resumption of meiosis, the biphasic IVM has an additional step of

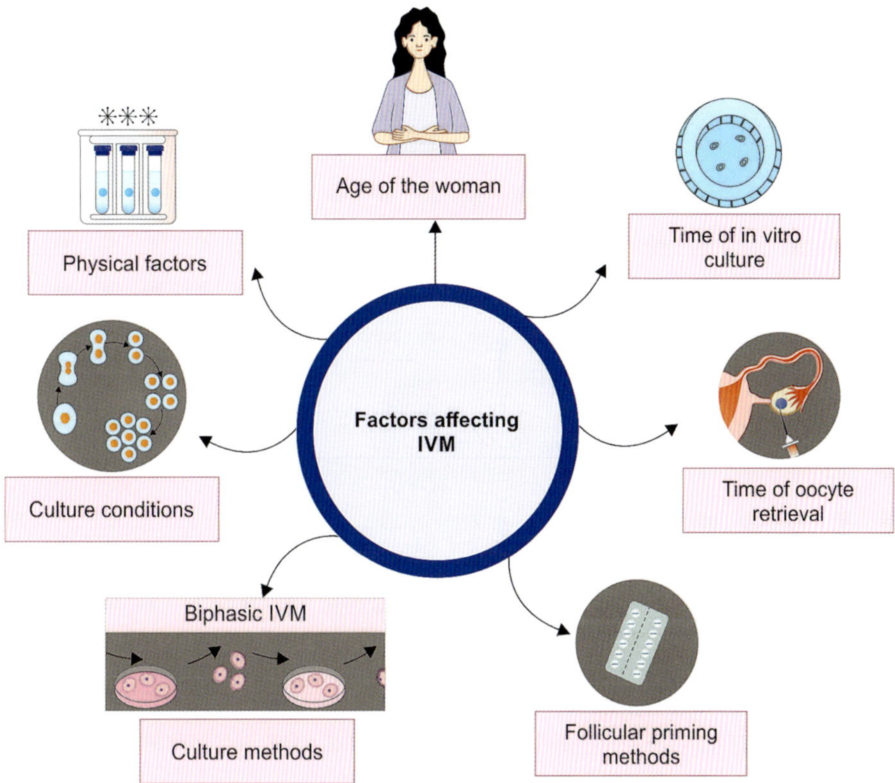

Fig. 2: Pictorial depiction of factors affecting the outcomes of an in vitro maturation (IVM) cycle.

pre-IVM culturing period for 24 hours before IVM culturing. This extra step promotes the synchronization of nuclear and cytoplasmic maturation.[8]

- Physical factors such as aspiration pressure, needles used, and temperature also play a vital role.[8]

TYPES OF IVM AND STIMULATION PROTOCOLS IN IVM (FIG. 3)

- *Unstimulated/standard IVM cycles:* FSH stimulation is not done and immature oocytes are collected and IVM is performed followed by ICSI (intracytoplasmic sperm injection). Standard IVM cycle includes only one-step culture and oocytes remain in the immature meiotic stage.
- *FSH priming IVM cycle:* Gonadotropins 150–300 IU are given from day 3 to day 5 with oocyte retrieval on day 7 without hCG trigger. It has the advantage of easy follicular preparation. The major disadvantage in this type is that the growth of dominant follicles may lead to apoptosis of smaller follicles, which may have a negative impact on the quality of the oocyte.[7]
- Human chorionic gonadotropin (hCG) priming with 10,000 IU to prime intermediate-sized follicles 36 hours before oocyte retrieval; the advantage here is improved oocyte maturation and implantation potential. There is no indisputable evidence that suggests the use of hCG trigger before oocyte retrieval and IVM has a considerable impact on clinical pregnancy or live birth rates.[7]
- *FSH and hCG priming IVM cycles, combing the above protocols:* This is called truncated IVF wherein FSH injections and hCG trigger are given.[7,12]
- *Random-start IVM:* Cycle-independent start especially for women with cancer and who do not have time for a conventional IVF and for those women who can tolerate only minimal hormonal stimulation; hCG trigger is also not given in this protocol.[7]
- *Rescue IVM:* IVM cycle converted after a full-blown gonadotropin stimulation and an hCG trigger due to the retrieval of a larger number of immature oocytes; these oocytes do not have cumulus cells and are cultured in vitro from immature GV to MII stage. However, this procedure has not been beneficial.[7]

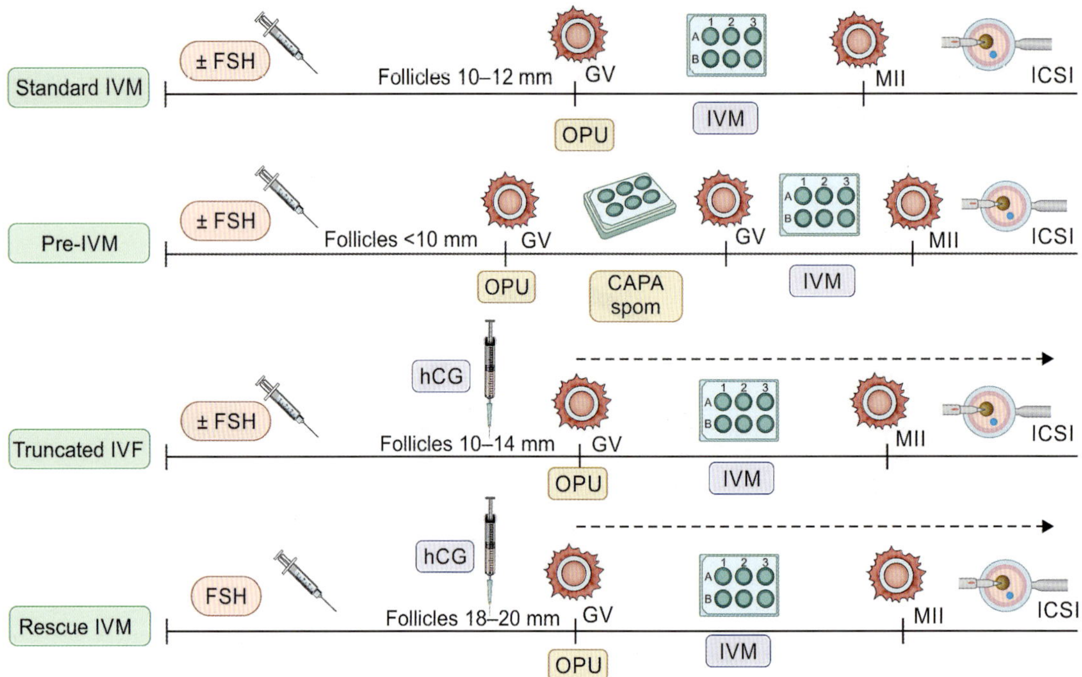

Fig. 3: Pictorial depiction of various in vitro maturation (IVM) protocols reported in the literature. (FSH: follicle-stimulating hormone; GV: germinal vesicle; hCG: human chorionic gonadotropin; ICSI: intracytoplasmic sperm injection; MII: metaphase II; OPU: ovum pickup)

- *Aromatase inhibitor use (letrozole 2.5 mg twice daily for 5 days starting from day 3 of the cycle) for OS:* Letrozole results in an increase in FSH levels, and an increased androgenic microenvironment leads to the development of primordial follicles. Therefore, letrozole may help women with hormone-sensitive tumors without exposing them to sustained elevated estrogen levels, for OS.[13]
- Estrogen suppression is a new protocol that uses oral estradiol valerate on day 3 of the cycle to suppress the dominant follicle development and ovulation while maintaining a uniform cohort of small follicles. Early-onset estrogen supplementation may improve the quality of retrieved immature oocytes and help in the maturation of oocytes in stimulated IVM cycles.[14]

CAPACITATION IN VITRO MATURATION

Capacitation IVM (CAPA IVM) is the recent and most significant development in clinical IVM in the recent times. Conventional IVM results in relatively low MII rates (50%), while the CAPA procedure gives high MII rates (70%).[15]

The first step of CAPA IVM is the pre-IVM step wherein immature oocytes are exposed to C-type natriuretic peptide (CNP) followed by the IVM step which is initiated 22–24 hours post oocyte retrieval. Oocytes are examined at 30 hours post retrieval and subjected to ICSI. After ICSI, a freeze-all strategy is preferred and a frozen embryo replacement cycle is planned as the endometrium may not be adequately thick. The culture media include CNP, estrogen, insulin, FSH, and amphiregulin **(Figs. 4A to F)**.[7]

ADVANTAGES OF BIPHASIC IN VITRO MATURATION CULTURE

- Maintenance of oocytes in a meiotically arrested stage
- Retaining the physical contact and paracrine signaling system of communication
- Maintenance of an environment that enables the oocytes to acquire developmental competence over 24 hours (pre-IVM step)
- Enabling meiosis to resume and progress under an environment similar to post-LH surge follicular environment.[7]

IN VITRO MATURATION VERSUS CONVENTIONAL IN VITRO FERTILIZATION

In vitro maturation is safe, inexpensive, and a better alternative when compared to IVF (hyperstimulation) in the case of women with PCOS.[16,17] One cycle of IVM

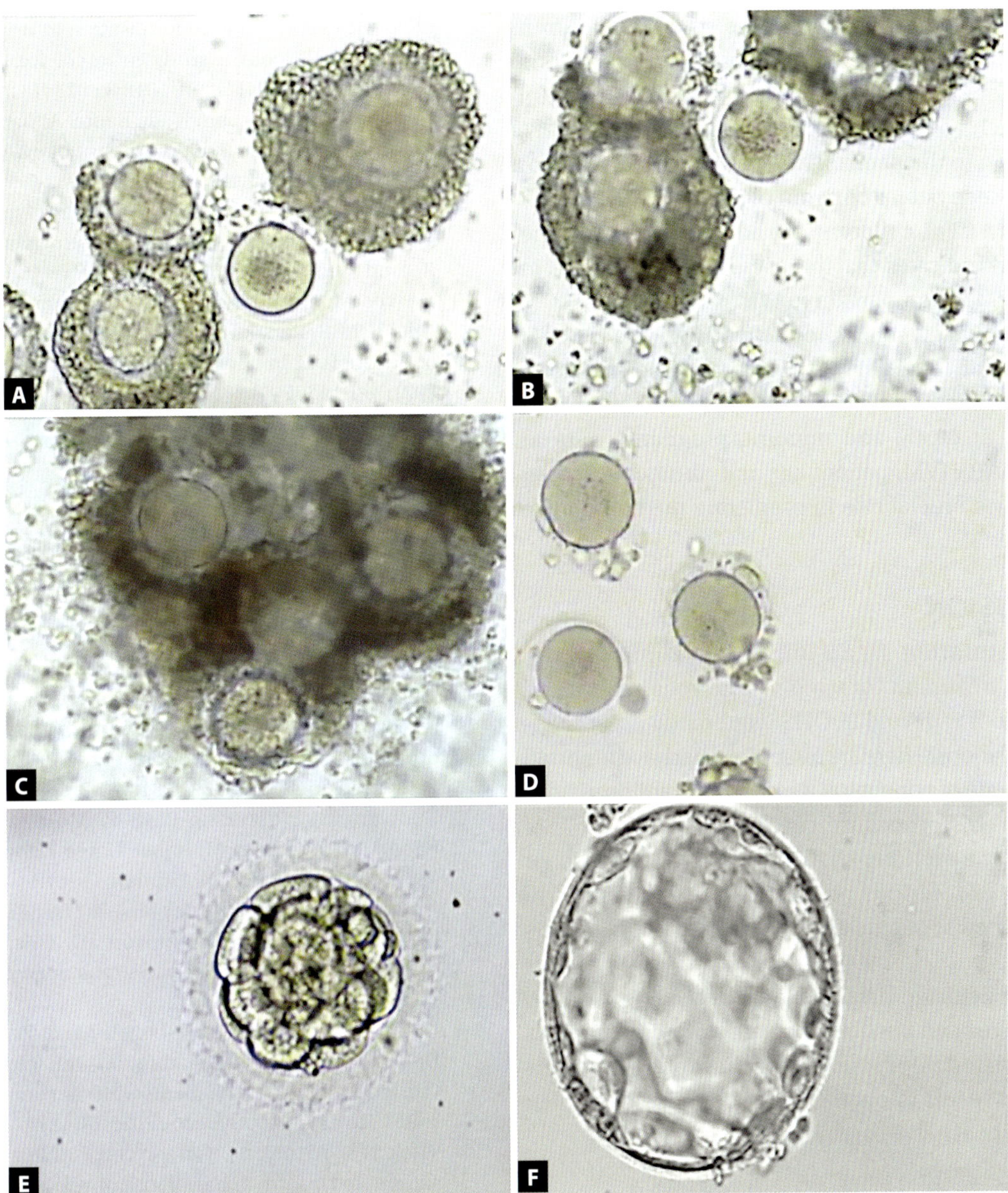

Figs. 4A to F: Oocytes and embryos from a biphasic capacitation in vitro maturation (CAPA IVM) cycle. (A) At oocyte retrieval; (B) 22 hours—post oocyte retrieval; (C) 30 hours—post oocyte retrieval; (D) Postdenudation; (E) Day 3—cleavage-stage embryo; (F) Day 5—blastocyst-stage embryo.

is considered to be inferior to one IVF cycle when the cumulative live birth rate is taken into consideration in case of single blastocyst transfer (freeze-all cycle).[18]

Safety Profile

In vitro maturation is recommended for women with PCOS as it is much safer in comparison to conventional OS and IVF and it is devoid of OHSS.[1,19] As the rates of miscarriage are high in the case of fresh embryo transfer IVM, the freeze-all strategy is preferred.[6,20] There is no significant difference in outcomes in the case of ectopic pregnancies, gestational diabetes, antepartum hemorrhage in both IVM and conventional IVF.[7,19-22] According to a study, there was an increase in hypertensive disorders in IVM pregnancies in comparison to IVF. However, this was not observed in the randomized controlled trial (RCT) of CAPA IVM vs traditional IVF.[7,21]

There are concerns regarding the risks the children born out of IVM may have, as oocyte meiosis occurs in vitro.[23] Recent studies have shown that neonatal outcomes such as congenital anomalies, preterm births, and admission to the neonatal intensive care unit are not different between babies born out of IVM and IVF.[24,25]

A study on IVM children and adolescents up to the age of 19 years indicated that there was no increased risk in the case of IVM in comparison to IVF.[26]

American Society for Reproductive Medicine (ASRM) in 2021 indicated that IVM was not merely experimental.[27]

Recent studies report the cumulative clinical pregnancy rate at 60.4% and ongoing pregnancy rate at 43.6%.[28] In CAPA IVM, patient age and number of frozen embryos play a crucial role in predicting the cumulative live birth rate.[29]

CONCLUSION

In vitro maturation is a simple, economical, and harmonious treatment for women who require assisted reproduction. It is devoid of OHSS and many other long-term complications. There are no studies that have reported an alarming rate of congenital anomalies in children born out of IVM. This procedure can be the best course of action not only for fertility-challenged couples but also for those who opt for fertility preservation. Patients need to be well informed about the advantages and disadvantages of IVM.

Without calculated risks and great decision-making, it would not have been possible to create wonderful families through assisted reproductive techniques. The new biphasic IVM seems to offer a new ray of hope to women who struggle to achieve parenthood.

REFERENCES

1. Ellenbogen A, Shavit T, Shalom-Paz E. IVM results are comparable and may have advantages over standard IVF. Facts Views Vis Obgyn. 2014;6(2):77-80.
2. Cha KY, Koo JJ, Ko JJ, Choi DH, Han SY, Yoon TK. Pregnancy after in vitro fertilization of human follicular oocytes collected from nonstimulated cycles, their culture in vitro and their transfer in a donor oocyte program. Fertil Steril. 1991;55(1):109-13.
3. Trounson A, Wood C, Kausche A. In vitro maturation and the fertilization and the developmental competence of oocytes recovered from untreated polycystic ovarian patients. Fertil Steril. 1994;62(2):353-62.
4. Vuong LN, Ho VNA, Ho TM, Dang VQ, Phung TH, Giang NH, et al. Effectiveness and safety of in vitro maturation of oocytes versus in vitro fertilisation in women with high antral follicle count: study protocol for a randomised controlled trial. BMJ Open. 2018;8:e023413.
5. Grynberg M, El Hachem H, de Bantel A, Benard J, le Parco S, Fanchin R. In vitro maturation of oocytes: uncommon indications. Fertil Steril. 2013;99(5):1182-8.
6. Huang JY, Chian RC, Tan SL. Ovarian hyperstimulation syndrome prevention strategies: in vitro maturation. Semin Reprod Med. 2010;28(6):519-31.
7. De Vos M, Grynberg M, Ho TM, Yuan Y, Albertini DF, Gilchrist RB. Perspectives on the development and future of oocyte IVM in clinical practice. J Assist Reprod Genet. 2021;38(6):1265-80.
8. Yang H, Kolben T, Meister S, Paul C, van Dorp J, Eren S, et al. Factors Influencing the In Vitro Maturation (IVM) of Human Oocyte. Biomedicines. 2021;9(12):1904.
9. Nogueira D, Fajau-Prevot C, Clouet M, Assouline P, Deslandres M, Montagut M. Outcomes of Different In Vitro Maturation Procedures for Oocyte Cryopreservation for Fertility Preservation and yet Another Live Birth in a Cancer Patient. Life (Basel). 2023;13(6):1355.
10. Grynberg M, Poulain M, le Parco S, Sifer C, Fanchin R, Frydman N. Similar in vitro maturation rates of oocytes retrieved during the follicular or luteal phase offer flexible options for urgent fertility preservation in breast cancer patients. Hum Reprod. 2016;31:623-9.
11. Karavani G, Wasserzug-Pash P, Mordechai-Daniel T, Bauman D, Klutstein M, Imbar T. Age-Dependent in vitro Maturation Efficacy of Human Oocytes—Is There an Optimal Age? Front Cell Dev Biol. 2021;9:667682.
12. De Vos M, Smitz J, Thompson JG, Gilchrist RB. The definition of IVM is clear-variations need defining. Hum Reprod. 2016;31(11):2411-5.
13. Hatırnaz Ş, Hatırnaz ES, Başbuğ A, Kanat Pektaş M, Erol O, Dahan M, et al. In vitro maturation with letrozole priming: Can it be a solution for patients with cancerophobia? A pilot study. Turk J Obstet Gynecol. 2020;17(4):247-52.
14. Vitek WS, Witmyer J, Carson SA, Robins JC. Estrogen-suppressed in vitro maturation: a novel approach to in vitro maturation. Fertil Steril. 2013;99(7):1886-90.
15. Sanchez F, Le AH, Ho VNA, Romero S, Van Ranst H, De Vos M, et al. Biphasic in vitro maturation (CAPA-IVM) specifically improves the developmental capacity of oocytes from small antral follicles. J Assist Reprod Genet. 2019;36(10):2135-44.
16. Xu Y, Qiao J. Comparison of in vitro maturation and in vitro fertilization for polycystic ovary syndrome patients: a systematic review and meta-analysis. Ann Transl Med. 2021;9(15):1235.
17. Zheng X, Guo W, Zeng L, Zheng D, Yang S, Xu Y, et al. In vitro maturation without gonadotropins versus in vitro fertilization with hyperstimulation in women with polycystic ovary syndrome: a non-inferiority randomized controlled trial. Hum Reprod. 2022;37(2):242-53.

18. Vuong LN, Nguyen LK, Le AH, Pham HH, Ho VN, Le HL, et al. Fresh embryo transfer versus freeze-only after in vitro maturation with a pre-maturation step in women with high antral follicle count: a randomized controlled pilot study. J Assist Reprod Genet. 2021;38(6):1293-302.
19. Vuong LN, Ho VNA, Ho TM, Dang VQ, Phung TH, Giang NH, et al. In-vitro maturation of oocytes versus conventional IVF in women with infertility and a high antral follicle count: a randomized non-inferiority controlled trial. Hum Reprod. 2020;35(11):2537-47.
20. Mackens S, Mostinckx L, Drakopoulos P, Segers I, Santos-Ribeiro S, Popovic-Todorovic B, et al. Early pregnancy loss in patients with polycystic ovary syndrome after IVM versus standard ovarian stimulation for IVF/ICSI. Hum Reprod. 2020;35(12):2763-73.
21. Strowitzki T, Bruckner T, Roesner S. Maternal and neonatal outcome and children's development after medically assisted reproduction with in-vitro matured oocytes-a systematic review and meta-analysis. Hum Reprod Update. 2021;27(3):460-73.
22. Söderström-Anttila V, Salokorpi T, Pihlaja M, Serenius-Sirve S, Suikkari AM. Obstetric and perinatal outcome and preliminary results of development of children born after in vitro maturation of oocytes. Hum Reprod. 2006; 21(6):1508-13.
23. Saenz-de-Juano MD, Ivanova E, Romero S, Lolicato F, Sánchez F, Van Ranst H, et al. DNA methylation and mRNA expression of imprinted genes in blastocysts derived from an improved in vitro maturation method for oocytes from small antral follicles in polycystic ovary syndrome patients. Hum Reprod. 2019;34(9):1640-9.
24. Roesner S, von Wolff M, Elsaesser M, Roesner K, Reuner G, Pietz J, et al. Two-year development of children conceived by IVM: a prospective controlled single-blinded study. Hum Reprod. 2017;32:1341-50.
25. Shu-Chi M, Jiann-Loung H, Yu-Hung L, Tseng-Chen S, Ming-I, Tsu-Fuh Y. Growth and development of children conceived by in-vitro maturation of human oocytes. Early Hum Dev. 2006;82:677-82.
26. Yu EJ, Yoon TK, Lee WS, Park EA, Heo JY, Ko YK, et al. Obstetrical, neonatal, and long-term outcomes of children conceived from in vitro matured oocytes. Fertil Steril. 2019; 112:691-69.
27. Practice Committees of the American Society for Reproductive Medicine and the Society for Assisted Reproductive Technology. In vitro maturation: a committee opinion. Fertil Steril. 2013;99(3):663-6.
28. Vuong LN, Pham TD, Ho TM, De Vos M. Outcomes of clinical in vitro maturation programs for treating infertility in hyper responders: a systematic review. Fertil Steril. 2023; 119(4):540-9.
29. Pham HH, Le AH, Nguyen AM, Ha UD, Nguyen TC, Pham TD, et al. Cumulative live birth rate after oocyte in vitro maturation with a pre-maturation step in women with polycystic ovary syndrome or high antral follicle count. J Assist Reprod Genet. 2023;40(4):827-35.

Chapter

Endometrial Microbiota

Anu Chawla, Manisha Nandi

INTRODUCTION

The microbiome was first defined as "an ecological community of symbiotics, commensals, and pathogens that share our body space". The Human Microbiome Project pioneered the profound understanding of the human microbiota; however, the exact bacterial growth that can be considered as normal still remains uncertain. The uterine cavity was initially described as a sterile environment till recently when culture-based techniques and traditional microscopy were the tools used for the assessment of the microbiome.[1] In the later years, with the arrival of techniques like *next-generation sequencing* (NGS), newer techniques like 16S rRNA gene sequencing helped authors to define the various commensals found inside the uterus. However, it is still not clear as to where these commensals originate from. For example, it is hypothesized that uterine colonization occurs from the bloodstream, oral cavity, gut, and vagina, and seeding into the uterine cavity can primarily take place via the placement of contraceptive devices and assisted reproductive technology (ART) procedures and also as an attachment of the microorganisms to the male spermatozoa during coitus.[2] Irrespective of its site of origin, recent studies consistently have demonstrated that the uterine microbiome is largely diverse but scarcely populated in comparison to the lower genital tract, and its primary composition is yet to be fully unraveled.[3]

CHARACTERISTICS OF THE HUMAN MICROBIOME FOUND IN THE HUMAN REPRODUCTIVE TRACT

In healthy women, the normal vaginal microbiome is in general dominated by the lactobacilli spp.; however variations with hormonal status and age are evident. For instance, the vaginal microbiota during the years of infancy is primarily a mixture of anaerobic and aerobic bacterial populations that includes enterobacteria, *Prevotella*, *Staphylococcus*, and *Streptococcus* species, with the onset of puberty, the estrogenic environment is brought on that causes the pH to fall and glycogen to rise, leading to the subsequent domination of the lactobacilli spp. For the categorization of the microbiota found in the vagina, it has been again subclassified into five primary communities. Over 70% of women usually have the flora primarily consisting of *Lactobacillus crispatus*, *Lactobacillus iners*, *Lactobacillus gasseri*, or *Lactobacillus jensenii* species, which corresponds to CST I, II, III, and V. However, a minor population also shows CST IV, which is marked by a lower population of lactobacilli species and the predominance of anaerobes that include *Gardnerella*, *Atopobium*, *Aerococcus*, *Dialister*, *Prevotella*, *Megasphaera*, and *Sneathia*.

Recent studies on the healthy upper genital tract commensals are not yet available. Although, the flora of the upper tract has been evaluated by means of quantitative polymerase chain reaction (qPCR) techniques in over 95% of endometrial biopsies from asymptomatic hysterectomized patients. To illustrate further, the upper tract flora is qualitatively and quantitatively contrasting from that found in the lower tract. Studies applying NGS of the 16S rRNA genes have recently been put into comparison with the endometrial and vaginal flora of fertile, nonpregnant patients. Mitchell and colleagues reported that the bacterial communities were found in the endometrial biopsies of the entire study population of women, with *Lactobacillus* species being dominant and the others were *Gardnerella*, *Atopobium*, *Prevotella*, and *Sneathia*. Approximately in 25% of the subjects, the bacteria detected in the endometrial samples were different in great terms from those found in the lower genital tract, which suggests that the upper and lower genital tract floras are mostly not identical.[4]

FACTORS PLAYING A ROLE IN DETERMINING THE MICROBIOTA OF THE HUMAN REPRODUCTIVE TRACT (FIG. 1)

- *Age:* Microbiome found in the reproductive tract alters along the lifespan of a woman, and the composition and diversity tend to decline in the later years of life.
- *Medical history:* Both extragenital and genital diseases, including a history of sexually transmitted infections (STIs) can also have an effect on the microbiome analysis.
- *Ethnicity:* Hispanics and African Americans show a trend to have more colonization of non-*Lactobacillus* species in the endometrium as compared to the Caucasians.

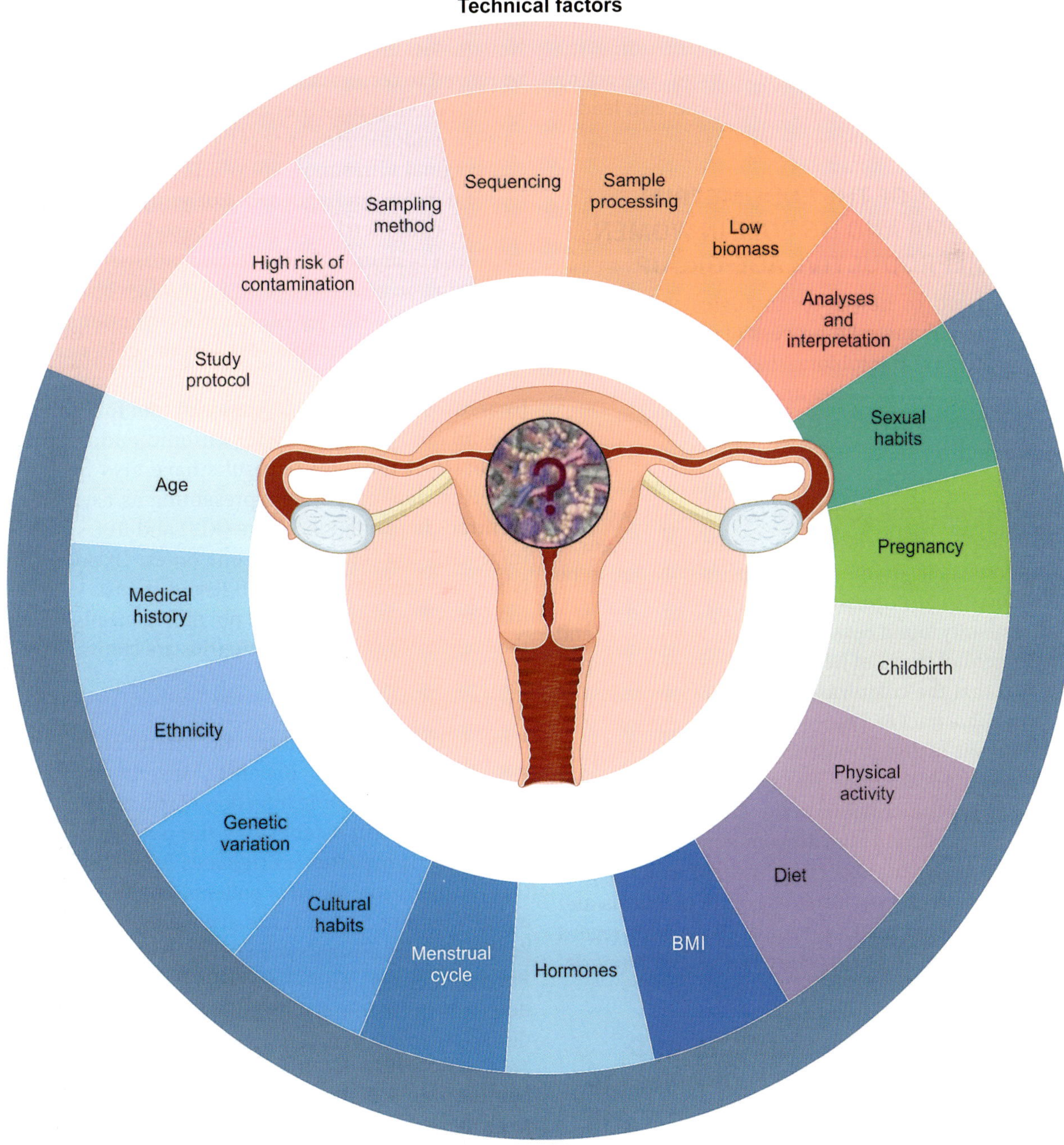

Fig. 1: Factors playing a role in determining the microbiota of the human reproductive tract. (BMI: body mass index)

- *Genetics:* The genetics of the host can have an effect on the microbiome composition and maintenance.
- *Hormones and the role of the menstrual cycle:* Hormonal fluctuations in the circulating progesterone and estrogen levels can have an influence on the endometrial microbiome.
- *Body mass index (BMI):* Obesity has been primarily associated with an altered intestinal and genital microbiome composition.
- *Physical activity:* Exercising has shown to impact microbial composition.
- *Study protocols:* Various protocols (including the collection techniques, sample storage, extraction methods, and the choice of primers) can also lead to the difference in results.

PHYSIOLOGY OF THE ENDOMETRIAL MICROBIOMA AND ITS ROLE IN WOMEN OF THE REPRODUCTIVE AGE-GROUP

With the advent of newer technologies that help in detection and enhance the process of characterization of the low biomass microbiota, the composition of the endometrial flora can be better understood.

- The uterine cavity of a healthy woman is mostly dominated by lactobacilli species. However, the lactobacilli-deficient communities of bacteria are also detected in the genital tract of a healthy woman, which implies that without any pathological signs, a non-lactobacilli-dominated community can also be considered to be normal.
- The similarity found between the flora in the lower and upper genital tracts of healthy women also supports the fact that the colonization process starts from the lower genital tract and ascends to the uterine cavity.
- In a subset of the population, other physiological and biochemical conditions present in the uterus can cause the microbiota in the uterine cavity to be significantly different from the communities of bacteria found in the vagina. For these women, endometrial sampling is necessary for an accurate diagnosis and to make a meaningful, clinical decision with regard to determining the characteristics of the bacterial communities.

GYNECOLOGICAL PATHOLOGIES AND ALTERATION OF UTERINE FLORA (FIG. 2)

Chronic Endometritis

Chronic endometritis is the primary pathology commonly due to alteration of the uterine flora. The disease is marked by chronic inflammation of the endometrial mucosa caused by the colonization of the endometrial cavity by the common bacterial population such as *Escherichia coli, Enterococcus faecalis, Proteus* spp., *Gardnerella vaginalis, Klebsiella pneumoniae, Staphylococcus, Streptococcus* spp., *Pseudomonas aeruginosa*, and pathogens of the genital tract such as *Ureaplasma* and *Mycoplasma* species, and also yeasts such as *Candida* species and *Saccharomyces cerevisiae*. The incidence of chronic endometritis generally has been established to be approximately 19%, and it is found to be around 45% in subfertile patients. Nonetheless, this higher prevalence is primarily found to be related to recurrent pregnancy loss (RPL) in IVF cycles as compared to the other causes of subfertility. Because chronic endometritis is mostly not detectable through transvaginal ultrasonography, it is rarely suspected and hence remains undiagnosed. Currently, the diagnosis of chronic endometritis is mainly based on identification by means of immunohistochemical analysis for CD138 in the stroma on taking samples and through histopathology of the plasma cells, by means of conventional staining techniques. Although this serves as the gold standard for the diagnosis, some researchers have recently reported hysteroscopy to be a gold standard tool for a diagnosis. The treatment protocols for chronic endometritis on the basis of the culture results have also been stated in recent data on patients presenting as asymptomatic recurrent implantation failure (RIF) and RPL subjects for improving the reproductive outcomes. Of note, culture is not performed routinely in terms of cost, with a long turnaround time period, and not all organisms which are the culprits for chronic endometritis are cultivable.

Endometriosis

Even with abundant data, the origin of the disease yet remains unclear. Recently, several studies have established the chronic infection of the uterine cavity as a potent cause in establishing the pathogenesis of the disease. This hypothesis originates from demonstrating that the menstrual blood of patients with the disease have a high count of *E. coli*. It has also been found that other pathogenic organisms, such as *Enterococcus, Gardnerella, Staphylococcus*, and *Streptococcus*, were primarily detected in endometrial samples of patients with the disease, followed by others such as *Actinomyces, Prevotella, Fusobacterium, Corynebacterium*, and *Propionibacterium*, in comparison to the *Lactobacillus* species, which was predominately found in the healthy group. Additionally, bacterial population from the *Staphylococcus* and Streptococcaceae spp. were substantially higher in

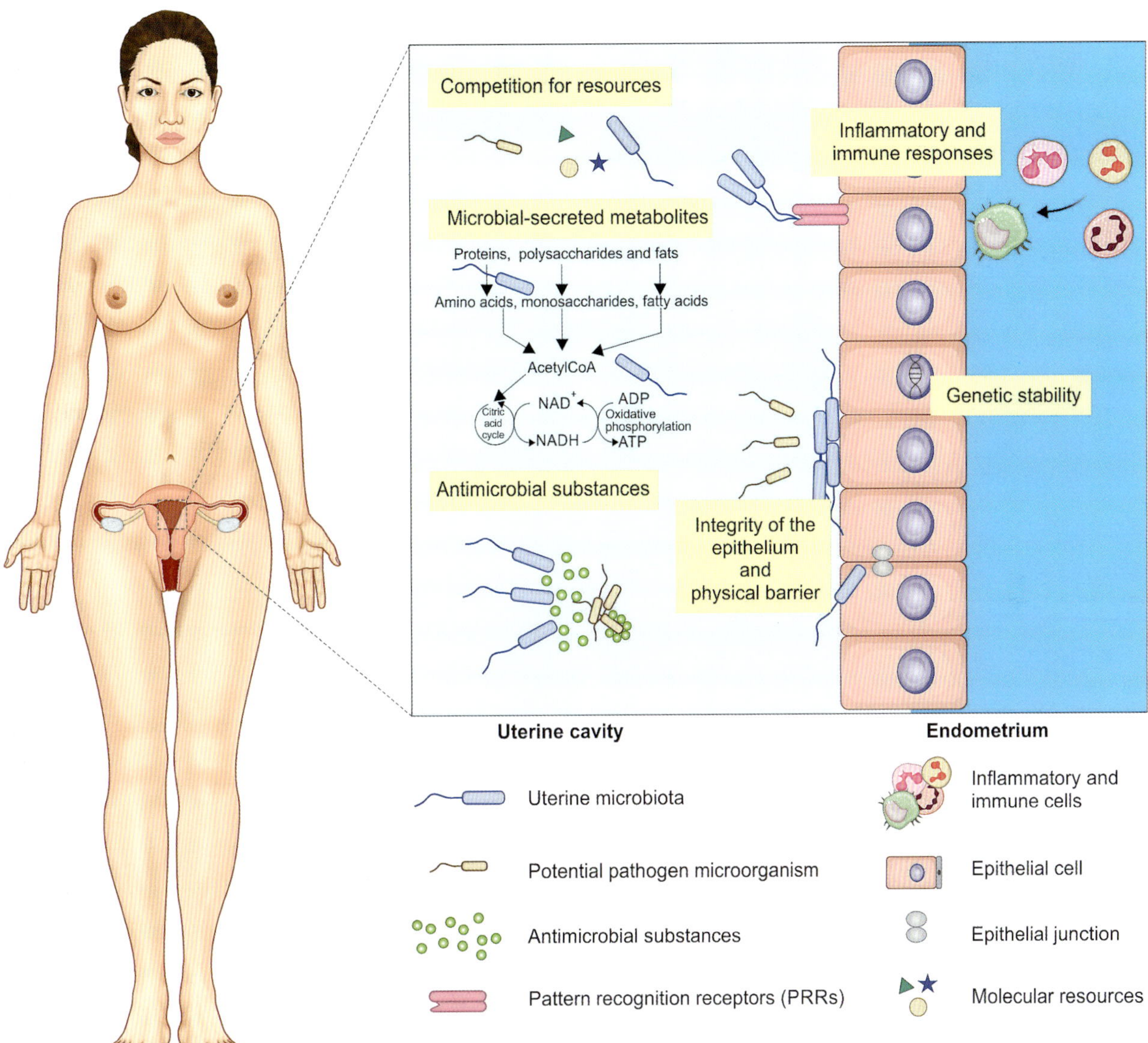

Fig. 2: Gynecological pathologies and alteration of uterine flora.

the cystic fluids of the patients with endometriomas in comparison to the control group of women. To sum up, these findings tend to be in favor of the positive correlation of chronic endometritis with endometriosis; this hypothesis could, however, be established by the theory of seeding of ectopic endometrial tissues owing to inflammation caused by impaired uterine contractility and dysperistalsis in women with endometriosis.

Other Gynecological Diseases

Bacterial infections are commonly found to be in association with colorectal infections with the pathogens: *Porphyromonas* and fusobacteria. Discussing the genital tract, bacterial vaginosis has been found to influence the prevalence of pelvic inflammatory disease (PID) and cervical intraepithelial neoplasia (CIN). In order to further investigate the role of the microbes in the emergence of the gynecological cancers, cervical, vaginal, ovarian, fallopian, peritoneal, and urinal samples from 32 patients who underwent hysteroscopy for endometrial hyperplasia, endometrial cancer, and other benign diseases were investigated with the study of the bacterial 16S rRNA genes. There was an abundance of many populations of microbes; for example, *Bacteroides, Anaerostipes, Dialister, Peptoniphilus, Anaerotruncus, Ruminococcus, Atopobium,* and *Porphyromonas* in the genital tract of women with uterine cancer and endometrial hyperplasia as compared to those with benign diseases, which suggests the role of inflammation and infection by the microbes for the onset of the diseases **(Fig. 3)**.

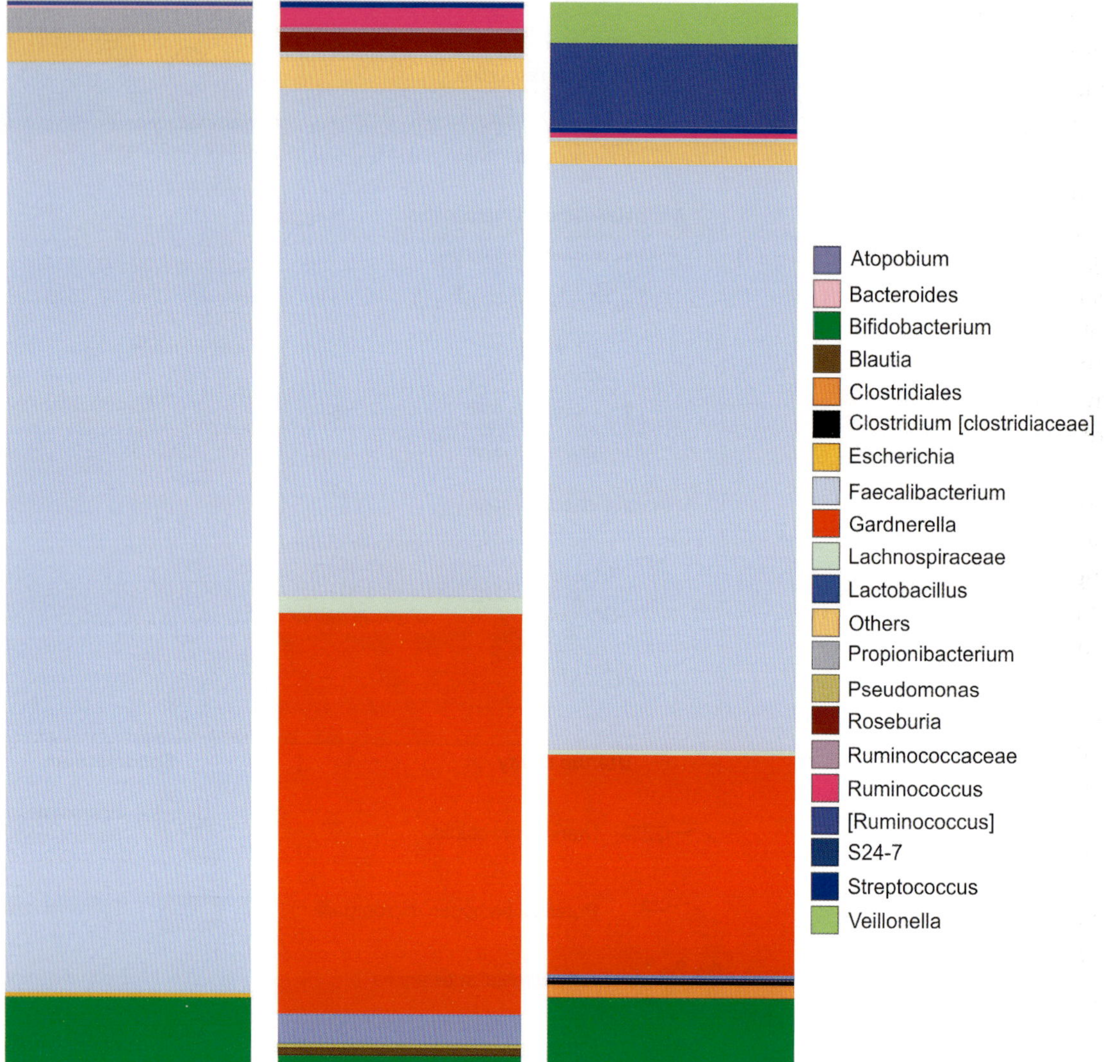

Fig. 3: Low abundance of endometrial *Lactobacillus* (MICA) is associated with poor reproductive outcome. Average abundance of the 20 most abundant taxa in endometrial fluid samples from in vitro fertilization (IVF) patients with receptive endometrium. Patients are grouped by their reproductive outcome. (MISC: biochemical or clinical miscarriage)

Source: Reprinted with permission from Elsevier: Moreno I, Codoñer FM, Vilella F, Valbuena D, Martinez-Blanch JF, Jimenez-Almazán J, et al. Evidence that the endometrial microbiota has an effect on implantation success or failure. Am J Obstet Gynecol. 2016;215:684-703.

ROLE OF MICROBIOTA: FERTILITY CONSIDERATIONS

Vaginal Flora and Its Role in Assisted Reproductive Technology

Recent studies have been promising with regard to determining the role of the vaginal flora in women of the reproductive age-group.

- The vagina has shown to exhibit the alpha and the lowest beta diversities when phylotypes were taken into consideration for classification and comparison with the other body sites such as the oral cavity and skin. This was mainly because lactobacilli species tend to dominate in the lower genital tract. Hence, in healthy women it is relatively simple to identify the normal flora and detect abnormalities.
- The vaginal flora has been exclusively studied with pertinence to ART by means of sequencing and culture methods. With culture, the presence of *Staphylococcus* and Enterobacteriaceae species

detected at the time of embryo transfer has been found to be associated with poor outcomes in terms of clinical pregnancy rates.

- Sequencing-based studies have demonstrated that a low diversity is associated with better outcomes with the dominance of lactobacilli species.
- During ovarian stimulation, the vaginal flora undergoes changes owing to the role of estrogen in the menstrual cycle. It is not recommended to study the endometrial microbiota during controlled ovarian hyperstimulation and this also supports frozen embryo transfer so as to have a better overview of the physiological status before planning embryo transfer.

Repeated Implantation Failure

The occurrence of RIF has also been found to be associated with changes in the endometrial microbiota. A recent study was conducted with 46 patients undergoing IVF cycles with RIF or women who were attempting ART treatment for the first time.[5] Women with low diversity of microbes and dominance of lactobacilli species had better outcomes. One group of researchers attempted to restore the lactobacilli dominance in women with RIF, and a decrease in the responsiveness to treatment protocols was reported on those patients with dominance of *Gardnerella* spp.

ENDOMETRIAL DYSBIOSIS MANAGEMENT PROTOCOLS (FIG. 4)

- *Antibiotics:* Secnidazole and amoxicillin for the treatment of gynecological pathologies; however, the administration of antibiotics as the first line to alter microbiota remains controversial.[6]
- *Probiotics:* Recolonization of the genital tract has been discussed as an additional approach. The administration of antibiotics along with probiotics has been tried in various clinical scenarios to improve the reproductive outcomes.

Reproductive Outcomes and Endometrial Flora Composition

- The concept of the human uterus being a nonsterile environment has led to the evolution of the theories regarding the role of the microbiota in reproductive health of a woman.
- The dominance of lactobacilli spp. has been suggested to represent the ideal environment for implantation and pregnancy. Nevertheless, the exact role of endometrial microbiota in terms of positive reproductive outcomes has not been delineated so far.[7]

ALTERATIONS OF THE MICROBIOME IN PREGNANCY

Originally proposed as relatively sterile, recent data have shown that various microbial agents tend to grow in the amniotic fluid and the fetomaternal compartments of healthy pregnant women. The identification of the organisms growing around the fetus has improved over the years with the advent of culture-independent techniques. Of note, three routes have been suggested for

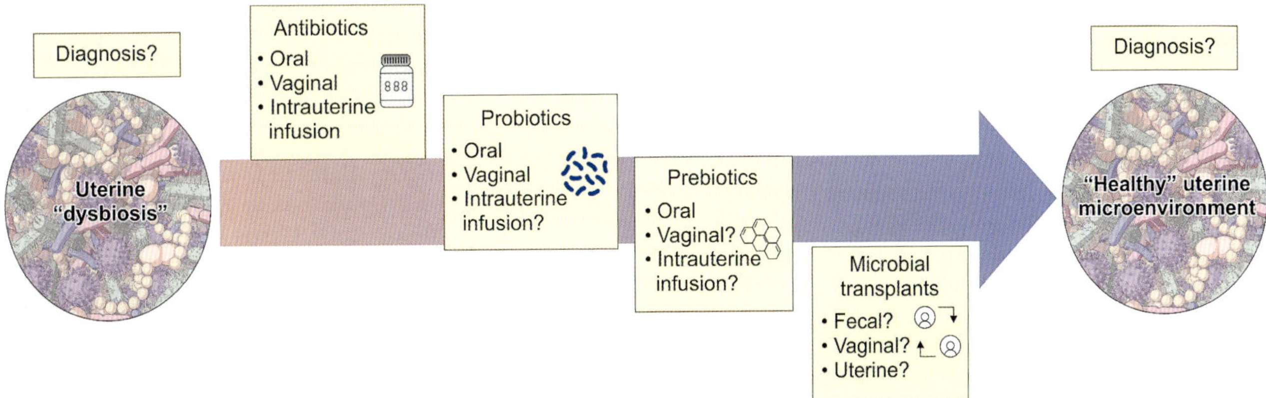

Fig. 4: Current and future strategies for modifying uterine microbial composition. Intrauterine drug delivery represents an attractive alternative to achieve local and systemic effects due to the high-contact surface exposed, the mucoadhesion of the epithelium, and the high absorption of drugs into the bloodstream. Several strategies for modifying endometrial microbial composition are being applied, nevertheless the core microbial composition is not established. The standard protocols for detecting uterine microbes and treatment protocols of dysbiosis are yet to be established.[7]

the colonization of the fetus. The first two are characterized mainly by the ascension from the lower genital tract to the uterine cavity or hematogenous route of spread from the placenta and the oral cavity. A third proposal from recent studies has linked the bacterial communities in both the vaginal and gastrointestinal microbiome. Irrespective of the route of colonization, transfer of bacteria from mother to fetus can have a pivotal role for sustenance of pregnancy, fetal development, or for the potential preparation of the fetal microbiota for planning postnatal healthcare. Hence, the maternal-fetal microbiome acts as the primary target for the assessment of the detrimental pregnancy outcomes and provides the treatment options for improving the chances of a healthy child birth.[8]

PLACENTAL MICROBIOME

The basal plate of placenta was demonstrated to have the presence of a diverse population of bacterial communities. The commensals might be involved in initiation of endotoxin tolerance for future bacterial exposure and preparation of the neonatal gut to receive nutrition.[9]

PRETERM BIRTHS

A shift from the healthy uterine microbiome characterized by increase of flora like *Ureaplasma parvum* and *Ureaplasma urealyticum, E. coli, Mycoplasma hominis, Bacteroides, G. vaginalis, Streptococcus* species, *Sneathia sanguinegens*, and *Fusobacterium nucleatum* associated with decrease in *L. crispatus* is associated with preterm birth. The mechanism of the bacterial infections causing preterm birth has the involvement of proinflammatory mediators such as tumor necrosis factor alpha (TNF-α), interleukin 1 beta (IL-1 β), IL6, IL8, monocyte chemoattractant protein 1 (MCP-1), and prostaglandins that initiate contractions, and with additional bacteria induced initiation of hyaluronidase and matrix metalloproteinases (MMPs) that cause breaks in the epithelium of the cervix and trigger the onset of preterm labor. To prevent bacteria-related preterm birth, various authors have studied the impact of prophylactic antibacterial agents during the late trimesters on the clinical outcomes. The results of recent publications demonstrated that prophylactic antimicrobial coverage reduces maternal infections but had no role in reducing the rate of preterm birth.

PREECLAMPSIA

The theory of linking preeclampsia with variations in vaginal flora is based on the concept of activation of the inflammation cascade and angiogenic pathways, which leads to impaired trophoblastic invasion, endothelial dysfunction, and increased blood pressure.[10]

CHALLENGES OF STUDYING THE ENDOMETRIAL MICROBIOTA

The following are the challenges of studying the endometrial microbiota:

- Lack of consensus on the taxonomic core due to limitations of studies
- Unstandardized methods and practices with differences in clinical approach
- Lack of research and larger studies to establish standard protocols

CONCLUSION

- Newer technologies and innovative thinking are paving the way toward a better clinical approach.
- The studies with time should characterize the relationship and transition from singular approach of focus from physiology to pathology and involve multidisciplinary actions.
- No substantial consensus is yet available to correlate the alteration of microbiome to the cause or effect of disease development.

REFERENCES

1. NIH HMP Working Group; Peterson J, Garges S, Giovanni M, McInnes P, Wang L, Schloss JA, et al. The NIH Human Microbiome Project. Genome Res. 2009;19(12):2317-23.
2. Moreno I, Codoñer FM, Vilella F, Valbuena D, Martinez-Blanch JF, Jimenez-Almazán J, et al. Evidence that the endometrial microbiota has an effect on implantation success or failure. Am J Obstet Gynecol. 2016;215(6):684-703.
3. Toson B, Simon C, Moreno I. The Endometrial Microbiome and Its Impact on Human Conception. Int J Mol Sci. 2022;23(1):485.
4. Moreno I, Franasiak JM. Endometrial microbiota—new player in town. Fertil Steril. 2017;108(1):32-9.
5. Ichiyama T, Kuroda K, Nagai Y, Urushiyama D, Ohno M, Yamaguchi T, et al. Analysis of vaginal and endometrial microbiota communities in infertile women with a history

of repeated implantation failure. Reprod Med Biol. 2021; 20(3):334-44.
6. Recine N, Palma E, Domenici L, Giorgini M, Imperiale L, Sassu C, et al. Restoring vaginal microbiota: biological control of bacterial vaginosis. A prospective case-control study using Lactobacillus rhamnosus BMX 54 as adjuvant treatment against bacterial vaginosis. Arch Gynecol Obstet. 2016;293(1):101-7.
7. Molina NM, Sola-Leyva A, Saez-Lara MJ, Plaza-Diaz J, Tubić-Pavlović A, Romero B, et al. New Opportunities for Endometrial Health by Modifying Uterine Microbial Composition: Present or Future? Biomolecules. 2020;10(4):593.
8. Leoni C, Ceci O, Manzari C, Fosso B, Volpicella M, Ferrari A, et al. Human Endometrial Microbiota at Term of Normal Pregnancies. Genes (Basel). 2019;10(12):971.
9. Panzer JJ, Romero R, Greenberg JM, Winters AD, Galaz J, Gomez-Lopez N, et al. Is there a placental microbiota? A critical review and re-analysis of published placental microbiota datasets. BMC Microbiol. 2023;23(1):76.
10. Theis KR, Romero R, Winters AD, Greenberg JM, Gomez-Lopez N, Alhousseini A, et al. Does the human placenta delivered at term have a microbiota? Results of cultivation, quantitative real-time PCR, 16S rRNA gene sequencing, and metagenomics. Am J Obstet Gynecol. 2019;220(3):267.e1-267.e39.

Metabolomics in Assisted Reproductive Technology

Kedar N Ganla, Priyanka H Vora

INTRODUCTION

Science has evolved from genomics to transcriptomics to proteomics and now metabolomics. Metabolomics is the science involving a systematic analysis of the inventory of metabolites representing the functional phenotype at a cellular level. It includes small molecules (<1 kDa), amino acids, lipids, nucleotides, adenosine triphosphate (ATP), and hormones.[1,2]

Metabolomics, a subdiscipline of systems biology, is concerned with the comprehensive profiling of small molecule metabolites in biological samples. When applied to assisted reproductive technology (ART), it provides profound insights into reproductive health, embryo viability, and potential pregnancy outcomes. This chapter explores the role of metabolomics in enhancing the success rates of ART procedures, primarily in vitro fertilization (IVF).

METABOLOMICS: A BRIEF OVERVIEW

Before delving into its application in ART, it is essential to understand the basics of metabolomics. Metabolomics investigates the unique chemical fingerprints left by cellular processes.[3] These fingerprints, or metabolites, offer unparalleled insights into an organism's physiological state and potential responses to various stimuli.

Two crucial pathways for ATP generation in embryonic cellular metabolism are (1) aerobic glycolysis/tricarboxylic acid (Krebs) cycle and (2) anaerobic glycolysis (Embden-Meyerhof) pathway.

Krebs cycle dominates up to cleaving embryonic development whereas pyruvate and lactate are predominant energy suppliers in the morula to blastocyst stage which requires minimal glucose.[4-6]

Quieter amino acid metabolism, viz., decreased glycine and leucine with increased asparagine levels is seen in the culture media with increased clinical pregnancy and live birth rates.[7]

APPLICATIONS IN ASSISTED REPRODUCTIVE TECHNOLOGY

Embryo Assessment

One of the primary challenges in IVF treatments is selecting the most viable embryos for transfer. Traditional methods, while effective, offer only a limited view of embryo health.[8] Metabolomic profiling of the culture medium can provide a holistic assessment of embryo viability, revolutionizing selection procedures.[9] Embryo culture media analysis is a noninvasive method, analyzing the culture media. It yields valuable information about embryo metabolism. Lactate production and amino acid turnover patterns are pivotal in assessing embryo vitality.[10] It is beneficial in assessing embryos giving an accurate and deep understanding of the embryonic phenotype which can produce improved pregnancy results.

Oocyte Quality

Oocyte quality plays a pivotal role in successful fertilization and subsequent embryo development. The metabolic profile of follicular fluid, the nurturing environment of the oocyte, can shed light on its quality and the likelihood of successful fertilization.

Follicular fluid profiling: The follicular fluid metabolome can potentially discern between competent and suboptimal oocytes.[11]

Biomarker discovery: Specific metabolites, when present in aberrant concentrations, might be indicative of oocyte health.[12]

Endometrial Receptivity

Successful implantation requires a receptive endometrium. By studying the metabolomic signature of the endometrial fluid, it is possible to determine the best time for embryo transfer, thereby increasing the chances of implantation.[13]

The metabolome of the endometrial fluid reveals the endometrial state. Perturbations in certain metabolites can indicate a nonreceptive endometrium.

Metabolomics and Male Fertility

Semen analysis provides basic insights, but metabolomics delves deeper.

Seminal plasma analysis: Variances in the metabolomic profiles of seminal plasma might elucidate underlying causes of male infertility, offering robust diagnostic markers.[14]

Metabolomics and Miscarriage

Recent advances spotlight the potential of metabolomics in predicting miscarriage risks.

Plasma metabolite profiles: Aberrant profiles could offer foresight into possible miscarriages, paving the path for proactive interventions.[15]

METABOLOMIC TECHNIQUES

Mass Spectrometry

Advanced mass spectrometry (MS) techniques allow for the identification of a vast array of metabolites, even in minute quantities.[16] It allows for the identification and quantification of metabolites based on their mass-to-charge ratio. Chromatography refers to a group of laboratory methods employed for mixture separation. This process entails passing a mixture, known as the "mobile phase," through a "stationary phase" fixed to columns and capillaries. The stationary phase separates the analytes into their individual components based on the analytes affinity for it. It is influenced by the physical (size) or chemical (polarity) properties of the analyte. Chromatographic-coupled MS needs detailed biological sample understanding beforehand along with sample preparation knowledge. Consequently, the application of chromatographic techniques may lead to the loss of metabolites due to discrimination between different metabolite classes.[2]

Nuclear Magnetic Resonance Spectroscopy

Recent advancements in nuclear magnetic resonance (NMR) provide more detailed data on metabolites, enabling better interpretation of metabolic activities.[17] It utilizes the magnetic properties of atomic nuclei to determine the physical and chemical properties of the molecules in the sample. In this, one is able to obtain information simultaneously at structural and quantitative level along with identification of even the most complex metabolite within the mixture not requiring any preparation of sample or of separating it.[18]

Gas Chromatography–Mass Spectrometry

Especially beneficial for metabolites that are volatile, thermally stable, and possess a low molecular weight (<350 Da). Gas chromatography-mass spectrometry (GC–MS) separates compounds before they are analyzed and quantified.[16]

Optical Spectroscopy

It evaluates the interaction between a species and electromagnetic radiation that is either absorbed, emitted, or scattered by the analyzed sample. This encompasses analytical techniques such as ultraviolet/visible absorption, luminescence, circular dichroism spectroscopies, and vibrational spectroscopies [including infrared (IR), near-infrared (NIR), and Raman spectroscopies]. Optical spectroscopy, in contrast to NMR or MS, is relatively uncomplicated and employs basic optical components, such as light sources, mirrors, lenses, gratings, and detectors. Moreover, these instruments exhibit exceptional stability over time, are easily maintainable, and can be operated by individuals with minimal training. Optical spectroscopic technologies generally facilitate swift measurements, viz., less than a second to a few minutes and nondestructive analyses across a broad spectrum.[19]

Fourier-transform Infrared Spectroscopy

A widely employed method for analyzing molecular species in biological samples, it is a vibrational spectroscopic technique.

Near-infrared Spectroscopy

This method is employed for tracking lactate levels in the blood[20] and assessing the metabolite content of culture media in IVF.[21] Primarily, it gauges the overtone and vibrational frequencies resulting from the combination of functional groups. Its application extends to conducting comprehensive spectral profile comparisons.

POTENTIAL BENEFITS AND BREAKTHROUGHS

Tailored Treatments

Metabolomics offers a personalized understanding of patient reproductive health, paving the way for treatments tailored to individual needs.[22]

Enhanced Success Rates

With deeper insights into embryo and oocyte health, ART procedures can be optimized for higher success rates.[23]

Reduced Multiple Pregnancies

With more accurate embryo selection, there is a decreased need to transfer multiple embryos, reducing the risks associated with multiple pregnancies.

CHALLENGES AND CONSIDERATIONS

While metabolomics holds tremendous potential in ART, it is essential to recognize the challenges.

Ethical and Moral Implications

Metabolomics, by offering clearer insights into embryo health, brings forth ethical considerations, especially in relation to embryo selection and potential genetic interventions.[24] The potential to select embryos based on certain metabolic markers might raise ethical questions, especially if used for nonmedical traits.

Data Interpretation

The vast amount of data generated through metabolomic analysis requires sophisticated tools and expertise for interpretation.[25]

Standardization

For consistent results and interpretations, standardized protocols across medical facilities are imperative.[26]

CONCLUSION

Metabolomics, with its ability to offer a window into the intricate metabolic activities of reproductive cells, has the potential to revolutionize the field of ART. By ensuring the selection of the most viable embryos, determining the optimal time for implantation, and offering insights into oocyte quality, metabolomics paves the way for more successful, efficient, and safe ART procedures. As with any advancing field, continued research, collaboration, and ethical considerations will be pivotal in harnessing its full potential.

REFERENCES

1. Posillico JT, the Metabolomics Study Group for Reproductive Technologies. Selection of viable embryos and gametes by rapid, non-invasive metabolomic profiling of oxidative stress biomarkers. In: Cohen J, Elder K (Eds). Human Preimplantation Embryo Selection. London, UK: Taylor and Francis; 2007. pp. 325-36.
2. Pasikanti KK, Ho PC, Chan EC. Gas chromatography/mass spectrometry in metabolic profiling of biological fluids. J Chromatogr B Analyt Technol Biomed Life Sci. 2008;871:202-11.
3. Zhang A, Sun H, Wang P, et al. Metabolomics in cell biology and medicine: past, present, and future. Biomed J. 2019;42(1):19-29.
4. Biggers JD, Whittingham DG, Donahue RP. The pattern of energy metabolism in the mouse oocyte and zygote. Proc Natl Acad Sci USA. 1967;58:560-7.
5. Conaghan J, Handyside AH, Winston RM, Leese HJ. Effects of pyruvate and glucose on the development of human preimplantation embryos in vitro. J Reprod Fertil. 1993;99: 87-95.
6. Devreker F. Uptake and release of metabolites in human preimplantation embryos. In: Cohen J, Elder K (Eds). Human Preimplantation Embryo Selection. London, UK: Taylor and Francis; 2007. pp. 325-36.
7. Sturmey RG, Hawkhead JA, Barker EA, Leese HJ. DNA damage and metabolic activity in the preimplantation embryo. Hum Reprod. 2009;24(1):81-91.
8. Gardner DK, Lane M, Stevens J, Schoolcraft WB. Noninvasive assessment of human embryo nutrient consumption as a measure of developmental potential. Fertil Steril. 2001;76(6):1175-80.
9. Vergouw CG, Heijnen EM, Meintjes M, et al. Metabolomic profiling by MS reveals embryo viability. Reprod Biomed Online. 2019;38(1):87-94.
10. Lee CI, Chen CH, Huang CC, Cheng EH, Chen HH, Ho ST, et al. Embryo morphokinetics is potentially associated with clinical outcomes of single-embryo transfers in preimplantation genetic testing for aneuploidy cycles. Reprod Biomed Online. 2019;39(4):569-79.
11. Sanchez MA, Cui J, Rojo D, et al. Follicular fluid metabolomics reveals altered metabolic pathways in polycystic ovary syndrome. J Clin Sci. 2019;133(21):2181-96.

12. Wu HX, Liu KX, Zhang YH, et al. Metabolomic signatures in oocytes of aged mice and its relevance in the decline of oocyte quality with age. Aging. 2020;12(8):7626-43.
13. Garrido-Gomez T, Castillo-Mayén MG, Salcedo-Amaya AM, Calle A, Cruz M, Ríos FJ, et al. Defining the window of implantation by metabolomic profiling of the endometrial microenvironment. J Clin Endocrinol Metab. 2020; 105(4):292.
14. Amaral A, Agarwal A, Roychoudhury S, Sharma R, Gupta S, Henkel R. Metabolomics in male reproductive health: a review. J Androl. 2020;8(4):927-45.
15. Kang B, Pirhaji M, Martin AT, Shariati P, Cavalleri G, Norman JM, et al. Metabolomic prediction of pregnancy outcomes in ART: a systematic review. J Mol Reprod Dev. 2021;88(2):104-16.
16. Thompson NJ, Rosati S, Rose R, Heck A. The impact of mass spectrometry on the study of intact antibodies: from post-translational modifications to structural analysis. Chem Commun (Comb). 2013:49(6):538-48.
17. Du X, Smith AB, Johnson CD, et al. Recent advances in high-resolution NMR spectroscopy. Anal Chem. 2018;90(1): 1104-10.
18. Lindon J, Holmes E, Nicholson JK. Metabonomics—Techniques and Applications. Metabometrix Ltd. Business Briefing: Future Drug Discovery. 2004;1-6.
19. Dunn WB, Ellis DI. Metabolomics: Current analytical platforms and methodologies. Trends Anal Chem. 2005;24: 285-94.
20. Lafrance D, Lands LC, Burns DH. In vivo lactate measurement in human tissue by near-infrared diffuse reflectance spectroscopy. Vib Spectrosc. 2004;36:195-202.
21. Seli E, Sakkas D, Scott R, Kwok JS, Rosendahl S, Burns DH. Non-invasive metabolomic profiling of human embryo culture media using Raman and near infrared spectroscopy correlates with reproductive potential of embryos in women undergoing in vitro fertilization. Fertil Steril. 2007; 88:1350-7.
22. Seli E, Robert C. Metabolomics and the quest for personalized assisted reproductive technology outcomes. J Biomol. 2019;9(9):448.
23. Agarwal A, Aponte-Mellado A, Premkumar BJ, Shaman A, Gupta S. The effects of oxidative stress on female reproduction: a review. Reprod Biol Endocrinol. 2012; 10:49.
24. Racowsky C, Stern JE, Gibbons WE, et al. The decision to cancel a cycle of IVF: ethical considerations. J Hum Reprod. 2018;33(3):411-5.
25. Zhang A, Sun H, Wang P, et al. Advanced techniques and tools in metabolomics analysis. Trends Anal Chem. 2019; 120:115323.
26. Teahan O, Gamble S, Holmes E, Waxman J, Nicholson JK, Bevan C, et al. Impact of analytical bias in metabonomic studies of human blood serum and plasma. Anal Chem. 2006;78(13):4307-18.

Chapter

Noninvasive Chromosomal Screening

Jyoti Tripathi, Aswati Nair

INTRODUCTION

Chromosomal errors can occur in embryos during the segregation phase or meiosis 1.[1] These chromosomal abnormalities could result in implantation failure or multiple or recurrent pregnancy losses.[2,3] The occurrence of chromosomal abnormalities is substantially higher in patients with advanced maternal and paternal age, resulting in issues like chromosomal translocations, monosomies, trisomies, and at times chromosomal deletions which may be detrimental to the healthy continuation of pregnancy.

BACKGROUND

One of the most common methods used to detect chromosomal abnormalities in the embryos is to perform preimplantation genetic testing on the embryos or preimplantation genetic testing for aneuploidy (PGT-A) and then subsequently transfer only the chromosomally normal embryo. PGT-A can utilize various methods for comprehensive chromosomal screening of the embryos. These methods include comparative genomic hybridization (array-CGH),[4,5] single-nucleotide polymorphism (SNP) arrays,[6-9] multiplex quantitative polymerase chain reaction (PCR),[10] and next-generation sequencing (NGS).[11,12] Many studies and clinical trials have established the role of PGT-A in detecting such chromosomal abnormalities and thus improving the pregnancy rates and lowering the miscarriage rates.[13-16] With the help of a laser, a small opening is created in the zona pellucida from where a few of the trophectoderm cells of the blastocyst are taken out and sent for analysis. The major drawback of trophectoderm biopsy for PGT-A is the invasive nature of this procedure. The technical possibility of laser associated embryo damage cannot be ruled out completely.

Noninvasive chromosomal screening (NICS) of the embryos is based on sequencing the genomic deoxyribonucleic acid (DNA) secreted into the culture medium from the embryo. It therefore avoids the need for an embryo biopsy and results in overall safety of the embryos. NICS is soon turning out to be a promising tool to detect chromosomal aneuploidies in the embryos.

HISTORY

Since long there were efforts made to develop a noninvasive method of chromosomal testing of the embryos, which could help testing the embryos for normalcy without causing any damage to the embryos.[17,18] Palini S et al. first through their work demonstrated the presence of DNA in the blastocele fluid.[19] Gianaroli L et al. performed a pilot study on chromosome screening using blastocentesis and then analyzing the blastocele fluid.[20] Soon, Stigliani S et al. observed genomic and mitochondria DNA contents in the culture medium, which when analyzed could correlate with the embryo quality.[20,21] Wu H et al. reported the PCR detection of the secreted genomic DNA in the culture medium for preimplantation genetic diagnosis (PGD) of α-thalassemia cases.[22] Although the mechanism of secretion is not known, it is most likely that the DNA in the media results from the apoptotic cells of the growing embryo. The genome-wide analysis of the secreted DNA in the culture medium has not been previously reported, and would provide the basis for PGT-A, assuming that the detected DNA arises from cells of the growing embryo. From the perspective of noninvasiveness and ease in handling the embryos, blastocyst culture medium would be an ideal source for chromosome screening. However, such an approach would require high sensitivity and reproducibility of the whole-genome amplification (WGA) of the DNA from the blastocyst culture medium so as to have a near accurate assessment of the chromosomal normalcy of the embryos.

Studies have reported the utilization of secreted genomic DNA in the culture medium for PGD of X-linked disorders and α-thalassemia cases.[17,22] Hammond ER et al. and Vera-Rodriguez M et al. reported a mixed origin of DNA in spent medium with varied proportions of maternal contamination.[23,24] Capalbo A et al. found that spent medium only produced a diagnosis concordance of 20.8% with trophectoderm biopsy for monogenetic disorder, making the feasibility of using spent medium for noninvasive genetic assessment more controversial.[25]

More recently, a noninvasive chromosome screening (NICS) assay that incorporates a multiple annealing and looping-based amplification cycle (MALBAC)-NGS strategy conducted on the spent medium of in vitro fertilization (IVF) embryos has been validated.[26]

METHODOLOGY

Preparation

It is pertinent to have a good preparation prior to the procedure. All the materials (except the embryos) should be exposed to ultraviolet (UV) light before the procedure if it is available. If it is not available, use extra care to avoid DNA contamination. All the materials employed for the culture of the embryos, like dishes, media aliquots, etc. for these embryos should always be manipulated with gloves. Label the PCR tubes prior to media collection. Keep the tubes in the freezer at –20°C. After the media collection, the tubes have to be placed inside the freezer again at –20°C until shipping.

Procedure

Oocytes should be thoroughly denuded to remove all cumulus cells prior to intracytoplasmic sperm injection (ICSI) to avoid any DNA contamination. After denudation extra washes should be performed at least 5–6 times, with 6 microdroplets, each containing 20 µL of the fresh medium to ensure that each oocyte enters the culture dish without any cumulus cells, thus minimizing contamination with maternal DNA which is crucial for an accurate report.

After that the oocytes can undergo the standard protocol for fertilization and embryo development by ICSI.

After day 4, the embryos should be subjected to extra washes and should be placed in a 10 µL of fresh medium in a new dish. It should be one embryo per dish. It will be wiser to use a fresh media bottle to prepare the dishes. Plus there has to be a negative control dish that will be exposed to the same culture conditions, but without previous contact with any embryo. There has to be mandatorily one negative control per patient. On day 6 and 7, embryos should be removed outside the culture drop for vitrification. Spent culture medium (SCM) should not be sent for embryos which have undergone vitrification, assisted hatching, or for a collapsed blastocyst.

Next, the SCM of each embryo should be collected in labeled PCR tubes along with the negative control medium. Immediately after collection, the tubes should be centrifuged for a few seconds. The tubes should then be placed in a cool rack at –20°C for 24 hours till they are shipped.

The complementary DNA (cDNA) from the SCM undergoes WGA followed by NGS. Whole-genome amplified products are sequenced using an Illumina HiSeq 2500 platform and the chromosome ploidy information is obtained.

Accuracy

The advent of NICS niPGT-A in ART has aroused interest of practitioners and research groups as an alternative to traditional trophectoderm biopsy for PGT-A testing. Various research groups are trying to compare the concordance rates of standard trophectoderm biopsy-based PGT-A versus niPGT-A.

Noninvasive PGT-A (niPGT-A) and minimally invasive PGT-A (miPGT-A) can be performed by:

- Genetic assessment of the embryonic spent blastocyst culture medium (SBM)[19]
- miPGT-A involves genetic assessment of the blastocele fluid that collects in the blastocoel cavity (BF)[19,20,27,28]
- Combination of the above two approaches.

Several studies have reported high cell-free fetal DNA (cfDNA) amplification rates in SBM ranging from 80 to 100%.[28] Although wide variation has been reported in the concordance rates between niPGT-A and trophectoderm PGT-A, ranging from as low as 3.5% being reported in a proof of concept study[29] to 30.4% in another study,[24] 65% in yet another one[30] and later studies stating as high as 85.7%.[26]

Similarly, variations in the concordance rates between BF and trophectoderm biopsy for PGT-A have been reported ranging from lack of concordance to remarkable correlation between the two methods. The highest reported concordance rate was of 97.4% by Gianaroli L et al.[20] In the report by Kuznyetsov V et al., they have shown a 97.8% concordance between this miPGT-A technique and trophectoderm biopsy.[31]

There are various explanations reported for these discrepancies in concordance values. These include the embryo culture technique, embryo handling technique, manipulation of blastocyst (assisted hatching and vitrification), and method used for DNA analysis. Maternal DNA contamination from the residual cumulus cells during embryo handling can lead to high rate of false-negative results.[23-25,30]

Advantages of Noninvasive Chromosomal Screening (NICS) Compared to Conventional PGT-A[26,32]

- Procedure for collection of SCM is easy to perform.
- Does not require special expertise and training compared to biopsy.
- Does not require any extra equipment in the IVF laboratory.
- Does not require invasive testing and micromanipulation of the embryos and reduces risk of any potential harm to the embryo development and forthcoming pregnancy.
- Cost-effective compared to trophectoderm biopsy.
- SCM-PGT can be offered to those embryos also where trophectoderm PGT-A cannot be done.

Disadvantages Compared to Conventional PGT-A

- Needs changes in IVF laboratory protocols
- Low amount of cfDNA is obtained in SCM affecting the genetic assessment and results
- Discordance in results due to maternal contamination of DNA leading to lower sensitivity and specificity.

CHALLENGES BEFORE IMPLEMENTATION

It is important to improve the results in order to provide consistent and reliable results in noninvasive preimplantation genetic testing-A (niPGT-A). This requires certain changes and adaptation in the IVF laboratory protocols on routine basis.

To improve the amount of cfDNA obtained during the procedure it is recommended to extend the time in the culture media, reduce the culture drop volume, and decrease maternal contamination. Genetic counseling and detailed discussion about the procedure, various options, and the outcome with the patients is very essential.

CONCLUSION

The advent of PGT has revolutionized the field of ART and has improved the clinical outcomes. Trophectoderm biopsy PGT-A is a well-established gold standard procedure and has the most reliable results.

Noninvasive PGT-A is an emerging technology which has promising future in the field of ART. The current stage of niPGT-A requires more well-defined research before implementation in routine clinical practice.

REFERENCES

1. Battaglia DE, Goodwin P, Klein NA, Soules MR. Influence of maternal age on meiotic spindle assembly in oocytes from naturally cycling women. Hum Reprod 1996;11(10): 2217-22.
2. Munné S. Chromosome abnormalities and their relationship to morphology and development of human embryos. Reprod Biomed Online. 2006;12(2):234-53.
3. Korenberg JR, Chen XN, Schipper R, Sun Z, Gonsky R, Gerwehr S, et al. Down syndrome phenotypes: the consequences of chromosomal imbalance. Proc Natl Acad Sci U S A. 1994;91(11):4997-5001.
4. Hellani A, Abu-Amero K, Azouri J, El-Akoum S. Successful pregnancies after application of array-comparative genomic hybridization in PGS-aneuploidy screening. Reprod Biomed Online. 2008;17(6):841-7.
5. Gutiérrez-Mateo C, Colls P, Sánchez-García J, Escudero T, Prates R, Ketterson K, et al. Validation of microarray comparative genomic hybridization for comprehensive chromosome analysis of embryos. Fertil Steril. 2011;95(3): 953-8.
6. Thornhill AR, Handyside AH, Ottolini C, Natesan SA, Taylor J, Sage K, et al. Karyomapping-a comprehensive means of simultaneous monogenic and cytogenetic PGD: comparison with standard approaches in real time for Marfan syndrome. J Assist Reprod Genet. 2015;32(3):347-56.
7. Natesan SA, Handyside AH, Thornhill AR, Ottolini CS, Sage K, Summers MC, et al. Live birth after PGD with confirmation by a comprehensive approach (karyomapping) for simultaneous detection of monogenic and chromosomal disorders. Reprod Biomed Online. 2014;29(5):600-5.
8. Treff NR, Northrop LE, Kasabwala K, Su J, Levy B, Scott RT Jr. Single nucleotide polymorphism microarray-based concurrent screening of 24-chromosome aneuploidy and unbalanced translocations in preimplantation human embryos. Fertil Steril. 2011;95(5):1606-12.e1-2.

9. Natesan SA, Bladon AJ, Coskun S, Qubbaj W, Prates R, Munne S, et al. Genome-wide karyomapping accurately identifies the inheritance of single-gene defects in human preimplantation embryos in vitro. Genet Med. 2014;16(11): 838-45.
10. Treff NR, Tao X, Ferry KM, Su J, Taylor D, Scott RT Jr. Development and validation of an accurate quantitative real-time polymerase chain reaction-based assay for human blastocyst comprehensive chromosomal aneuploidy screening. Fertil Steril. 2012;97(4):819-24.
11. Martín J, Cervero A, Mir P, Martinez-Conejero JA, Pellicer A, Simón C. The impact of next-generation sequencing technology on preimplantation genetic diagnosis and screening. Fertil Steril. 2013;99(4):1054-61.e3.
12. Hou Y, Fan W, Yan L, Li R, Lian Y, Huang J, et al. Genome analyses of single human oocytes. Cell. 2013;155(7): 1492-506.
13. Scott RT Jr, Upham KM, Forman EJ, Hong KH, Scott KL, Taylor D, et al. Blastocyst biopsy with comprehensive chromosome screening and fresh embryo transfer significantly increases in vitro fertilization implantation and delivery rates: a randomized controlled trial. Fertil Steril. 2013;100(3):697-703.
14. Forman EJ, Hong KH, Ferry KM, Tao X, Taylor D, Levy B, et al. In vitro fertilization with single euploid blastocyst transfer: a randomized controlled trial. Fertil Steril. 2013; 100(1):100-7.e1.
15. Yang Z, Liu J, Collins GS, Salem SA, Liu X, Lyle SS, et al. Selection of single blastocysts for fresh transfer via standard morphology assessment alone and with array CGH for good prognosis IVF patients: results from a randomized pilot study. Mol Cytogenet. 2012;5(1):24.
16. Keltz MD, Vega M, Sirota I, Lederman M, Moshier EL, Gonzales E, et al. Preimplantation genetic screening (PGS) with Comparative genomic hybridization (CGH) following day 3 single cell blastomere biopsy markedly improves IVF outcomes while lowering multiple pregnancies and miscarriages. J Assist Reprod Genet. 2013;30(10):1333-9.
17. Assou S, Aït-Ahmed O, El Messaoudi S, Thierry AR, Hamamah S. Non-invasive preimplantation genetic diagnosis of X-linked disorders. Med Hypotheses. 2014; 83(4):506-8.
18. Galluzzi L, Palini S, Stefani S, Andreoni F, Primiterra M, Diotallevi A, et al. Extracellular embryo genomic DNA and its potential for genotyping applications. Future Sci OA. 2015;1(4):FSO62.
19. Palini S, Galluzzi L, De Stefani S, Bianchi M, Wells D, Magnani M, et al. Genomic DNA in human blastocoele fluid. Reprod Biomed Online. 2013;26(6):603-10.
20. Gianaroli L, Magli MC, Pomante A, Crivello AM, Cafueri G, Valerio M, et al. Blastocentesis: a source of DNA for preimplantation genetic testing. Results from a pilot study. Fertil Steril. 2014;102(6):1692-9.e6.
21. Stigliani S, Persico L, Lagazio C, Anserini P, Venturini PL, Scaruffi P. Mitochondrial DNA in Day 3 embryo culture medium is a novel, non-invasive biomarker of blastocyst potential and implantation outcome. Mol Hum Reprod. 2014;20(12):1238-46.
22. Wu H, Ding C, Shen X, Wang J, Li R, Cai B, et al. Medium-based noninvasive preimplantation genetic diagnosis for human α-thalassemias-SEA. Medicine. 2015;94(12): e669.
23. Hammond ER, McGillivray BC, Wicker SM, Peek JC, Shelling AN, Stone P, et al. Characterizing nuclear and mitochondrial DNA in spent embryo culture media: genetic contamination identified. Fertil Steril. 2017;107(1): 220-228.e5.
24. Vera-Rodriguez M, Diez-Juan A, Jimenez-Almazan J, Martinez S, Navarro R, Peinado V, et al. Origin and composition of cell-free DNA in spent medium from human embryo culture during preimplantation development. Hum Reprod. 2018;33(4):745-56.
25. Capalbo A, Romanelli V, Patassini C, Poli M, Girardi L, Giancani A, et al. Diagnostic efficacy of blastocoel fluid and spent media as sources of DNA for preimplantation genetic testing in standard clinical conditions. Fertil Steril. 2018;110(5):870-879.e5.
26. Xu J, Fang R, Chen L, Chen D, Xiao JP, Yang W, et al. Noninvasive chromosome screening of human embryos by genome sequencing of embryo culture medium for in vitro fertilization. Proc Natl Acad Sci U S A. 2016;113(42): 11907-12.
27. Poli M, Jaroudi S, Sarasa J, Spath K, Child T, Wells D. The blastocoel fluid as a source of DNA for preimplantation genetic diagnosis and screening. Fertil Steril 2013; 100(Suppl):S37.
28. Rubio C, Rienzi L, Navarro-Sanchez L, Cimadomo D, García-Pascual CM, Albricci L, et al. Embryonic cell-free DNA versus trophectoderm biopsy for aneuploidy testing: concordance rate and clinical implications. Fertil Steril. 2019;112:510-9.
29. Shamonki MI, Jin H, Haimowitz Z, Liu L. Proof of concept: preimplantation genetic screening without embryo biopsy through analysis of cell-free DNA in spent embryo culture media. Fertil Steril. 2016;106(6):1312-8.
30. Ho JR, Arrach N, Rhodes-Long K, Ahmady A, Ingles S, Chung K, et al. Pushing the limits of detection: investigation of cell-free DNA for aneuploidy screening in embryos. Fertil Steril. 2018;110(3):467-475.e2.
31. Kuznyetsov V, Madjunkova S, Abramov R, Antes R, Ibarrientos Z, Motamedi G, et al. Minimally invasive cell-free human embryo aneuploidy testing (miPGT-A) utilizing combined spent embryo culture medium and blastocoel fluid-towards development of a clinical assay. Sci Rep. 2020;10:7244.
32. Brouillet S, Martinez G, Coutton C, Hamamah S. Is cell-free DNA in spent embryo culture medium an alternative to embryo biopsy for preimplantation genetic testing? A systematic review. Reprod Biomed Online. 2020;40(6):779-96.

SECTION

Controversies and Challenges in Assisted Reproduction

Polycystic Ovarian Syndrome: Role of Insulin Sensitizers

Seema Pandey

INTRODUCTION

Polycystic ovarian syndrome (PCOS) is the most common disorder with both endocrine and metabolic dysfunction.[1] It impacts almost 20% of female patients of reproductive age. The symptoms of PCOS include androgen excess (hirsutism and/or hyperandrogenemia) and ovarian dysfunction (oligoovulation and/or polycystic ovarian morphology).[1] It also confirms the belief that PCOS is basically a metabolic disease with underlying ovarian defect. PCOS is diagnosed by ESHRE/ASRM (the European Society of Human Reproduction and Embryology/American Society for Reproductive Medicine) Rotterdam 2003 criteria.[2] Insulin resistance (IR) is an omnipresent finding of women with PCOS and differs between clinical phenotypes of PCOS. IR and compensatory hyperinsulinemia (HI) are present in 65–95% of women with PCOS including the vast majority of overweight and obese women and more than half of women of normal weight. IR is independent of but exacerbated by obesity.[3] Out of four phenotypes described in PCOS, IR is present in all phenotypes, and insulin sensitivity varies according to the PCOS phenotype. Classical phenotypes (types A and B) (80%) have the highest amount of IR, followed by ovulating PCOS (65%) and nonhyperandrogenic PCOS (38%).[4] Women with PCOS and IR have a significantly increased risk of adverse pregnancy outcomes[5] and chronic diseases, such as type 2 diabetes mellitus (T2DM), cardiovascular disease, and metabolic syndrome, which seriously affect the physical and mental health of women of childbearing age, increasing their social burden.[6-8] In spite of the knowledge of all this, the root cause of IR in PCOS is largely unknown and the underlying mechanism remains to be elucidated. IR and hyperandrogenism appear to be synergistic key factors in the pathogenesis of PCOS. Looking at the strong impact of IR on the occurrence and development of PCOS, accurate assessment of insulin sensitivity in the early stages of PCOS and effective treatment of IR are essential to reduce the risk of long-term complications.

UNDERSTANDING INSULIN RESISTANCE IN POLYCYSTIC OVARIAN SYNDROME

Insulin resistance in PCOS is caused by impaired insulin action in various target tissues, which is characterized by basal compensatory HI and a reduced insulin response to glucose overload. Insulin plays different roles in different tissues in balancing the supply and demand of nutrients. Insulin regulates glucose homeostasis by:

- Decreasing hepatic glucose synthesis
- Promoting glucose absorption by insulin-sensitive tissues, such as adipose tissue, skeletal muscle, the liver, and the heart.
- Inhibit lipolysis, which lowers levels of free fatty acids.

What is Insulin Resistance?

Insulin resistance is defined as the inability of insulin to exert a normal biological action at the level of its target tissues even when pancreatic function is normal **(Flowchart 1)**. It is *"a state (of a cell, tissue, or organism) in*

Flowchart 1: Insulin resistance (IR).

which a greater than normal amount of insulin is required to elicit a quantitatively normal response" and maintain glucose levels within the normal range. It is one of the principal pathogenetic defects of T2DM too.

KEY FEATURES OF INSULIN RESISTANCE IN POLYCYSTIC OVARIAN SYNDROME

- Insulin resistance in PCOS is endogenous and is worsened by the presence of obesity.
- Insulin resistance in PCOS is tissue selective and mutually affects metabolic or mitotic pathways in muscles, fat tissues, and the liver (classical insulin target tissues) and nonclassical insulin target tissues (e.g., ovary and pituitary gland).
- Androgen overload, lipid deposition, inflammatory cytokines, and other systemic factors are also involved in the IR of peripheral tissues.
- In most studies, its prevalence is between 44 and 75%, which is much higher than observed in young healthy individuals.
- The metabolic defect accounts for the 35–40% decrease in insulin-stimulated glucose utilization found in PCOS independent of obesity
- The degree of IR is modest in women with PCOS and may arise from either "natural" (genetic defects) or "acquired" (exogenous obesity) causes.

Hyperinsulinemia caused by tissue IR is central to PCOS pathology.[8-10]

How Does Insulin Resistance and Hyperinsulinemia Affect Polycystic Ovarian Syndrome?

Insulin functions both directly and indirectly by affecting the control of the hypothalamic-pituitary-ovarian axis. Insulin serves as a cogonadotropin, increasing luteinizing hormone (LH) activity by activating the expression of LH, insulin, and insulin-like growth factor (IGF) receptors on granulosa cells **(Flowchart 2)**. The levels of total and free androgen rise as a result of HIs increased adrenal steroid response to adrenocorticotropic hormone (ACTH) stimuli and decreased hepatic production of the sex hormone-binding globulin (SHBG).[3]

What Happens in PCOS Ovaries?

There is wide distribution of insulin receptors (InsRs) in stromal and follicular ovarian cells, and evidence shows the direct ovarian effect of insulin on steroid production. There is selective IR in PCOS ovaries. HI enhances intrathecal steroid production and leads to impaired follicular maturation. Under physiological conditions, insulin acts as a helper gonadotropin (cogonadotropin) through its homologous receptor to increase LH-induced androgen synthesis in membrane cells, and LH induces luteinization in granulosa cells. HI can lead to androgen-dependent anovulation via different mechanisms. By acting on the membrane cells of the ovary which are more sensitive to the hyperandrogenic effects of insulin than healthy women,

Flowchart 2: Disrupted insulin metabolism.

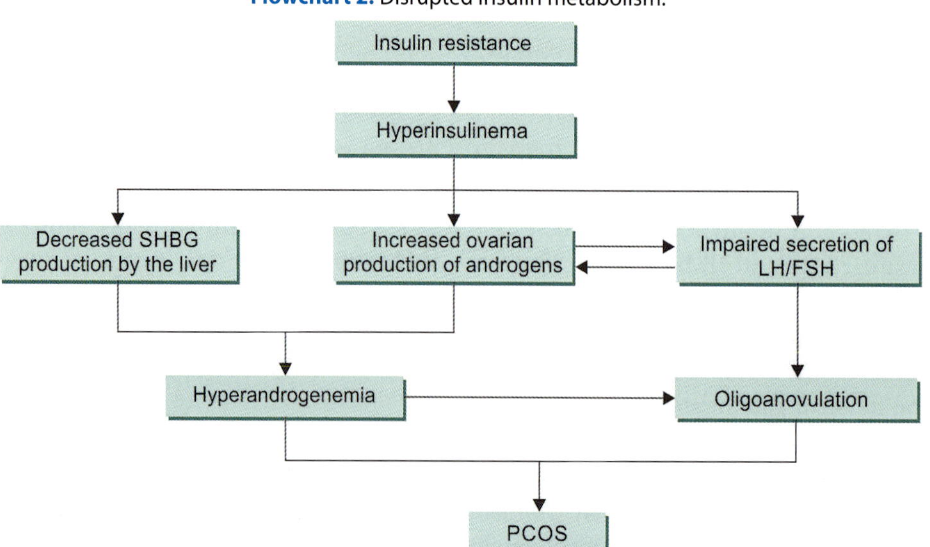

(FSH: follicle-stimulating hormone; LH: luteinizing hormone; PCOS: polycystic ovarian syndrome; SHBG: sex hormone-binding globulin)

insulin directly triggers androgen synthesis by increasing the activity of cytochrome P450c17α, a key enzyme that regulates androgen biosynthesis encoded by CYP17.[11] There is premature expression of LH receptors in small follicles, leading to premature differentiation of granulosa cells and follicular growth arrest in anovulatory PCOS. This is due to the synergistic effect of high insulin and LH levels.[12]

What Happens in the Uterus?

Studies have shown that IR and HI also negatively affect endometrial physiology. HI can impair decidualization of endometrial stromal cells in vitro through the transcriptional inhibition of FOXO1. The insulin-sensitizer metformin promotes glucose transporter type 4 (GLUT4) transcription by increasing adenosine monophosphate-activated protein kinase (AMPK), improves IR, and indirectly restores endometrial function in PCOS patients.[13,14]

The clinical manifestations of IR include:

- Hyperglycemia
- Hyperlipidemia
- Increased circulating inflammatory marker levels
- Diminished plasma adiponectin levels

The only clinical presentation of IR is overt diabetes.

How to Deal with Insulin Resistance and Hyperinsulinemia?

The present recommendations generally advise lifestyle changes (healthy eating and exercise) and weight loss to improve insulin sensitivity and thereby prevent or treat T2DM. Nonetheless, various antihyperglycemic medicines which are used to treat T2DM, can improve IR directly or indirectly.[15]

LIFESTYLE CHANGES

Lifestyle modification is the cornerstone of PCOS treatment and is the first line for obese PCOS as lifestyle plays a vital role in the development of PCOS. Looking at the vicious cycle of hyperandrogenism and HI and IR in PCOS, if we break this cycle we can achieve what is desired for these women. Lifestyle modification works by improving insulin sensitivity, by improving the SHBG level, and by restoration of ovulation and menstrual regularities by decreasing androgen production and its availability to the target tissues.

Lifestyle modification is based on three key components:

1. Dietary modifications
2. Physical exercises
3. Behavioral modifications.

Lifestyle modification is also important even for lean and normal weight PCOS as they also have an increased risk for metabolic disorders and chronic fatigue. Various studies have proven that these effects of lifestyle modification works for the patient whether it has been adopted alone or in combination of other medications like metformin and this benefit is extended toward those patients also whose concern is either hirsutism or only menstrual irregularities **(Box 1)**.[15]

Exercise Modification

Improvements in health outcomes are more likely to be linked to the exercise intensity rather than the exercise itself. Short-term goals of improving IR could be met by moderate aerobic exercise.

Vigorous aerobic exercise and resistance training bring better improvement in terms of insulin sensitivity and abnormal androgen level. Physical activity improves insulin sensitivity through:

- Increasing mitochondrial biogenesis
- GLUT4 protein content
- Glucose absorption in muscles
- Repartitioning intramyocellular lipid
- Decreasing fat mass.[16]

Diet Modifications

Very few studies have focused on the dietary preferences to combat IR and obesity exclusively in PCOS but there are certain recommendations as follows:

- Low-calorie diet is better than any other specific type of diet.
- Low-carbohydrate diet or carbohydrate intake <45% helps in losing weight [body mass index (BMI)] and restore cholesterol
- Adherence to low-carbohydrate diet is said to improve the levels of follicle-stimulating hormone (FSH) and SHBG.

It was reported that diet modifications could reduce IR and increase the serum levels of SHBGs when compared with metformin **(Table 1)**.[17]

Mood Modifications

Mood disorders are linked to excessive androgen secretion, IR as well as obesity. An appropriate and applicable mood modification for the two treatments is regarded as the potential modification which could help females with PCOS to lead a better life.

Box 1: Lifestyle modifications and their impact on women with PCOS.[16]

Exercise modifications	• Women with PCOS can improve insulin sensitivity and abnormal androgen level by involving exercises in their lifestyle • The minimum aerobic activity is advised (>150 min/week including intensive exercise for >90 minutes) • A 12-week exercise intervention increases branched chain amino acid catabolism in skeletal muscle and subcutaneous adipose tissue (SAT), which may explain why insulin sensitivity improves
Diet modifications	• Reduce insulin resistance and increase the serum levels of sex hormone-binding globulins when compared to metformin • The unsatisfactory long-term results of dietary modifications are regaining weight and fail to keep a normal body mass index (BMI)
Weight modifications	• Weight loss could improve the features of PCOS patients regardless of dietary composition • Even 5–10% of weight loss improves the IR, controls the HA and restores ovulation in obese PCOS, regulates menstruation and improves mood disorders • Obese PCOS have been recommended to improve their weight before going for infertility treatment as the obesity is linked to a higher risk of miscarriage and preeclampsia later in their pregnancies
Mood modifications	• PCOS women are prone to have mood disorders, such as depression, anxiety, and perceived stress • Screening and effective mood modification tools for these disorders should be used
Sleep modifications	• A positive association of sleep deprivation with an increased risk of insulin resistance and obesity as well as type 2 diabetes is observed • Studies reported that women are more likely to be disturbed by type 2 diabetes if the length of sleep is not >5 hours per night when compared with women whose length of sleep ranges from 7 to 8 hours per night

(HA: hyperandrogenemia; IR: insulin resistance; PCOS: polycystic ovarian syndrome)

TABLE 1: Advantages of low-carbohydrate diet.

Increased	***Decreased***
CPR	Miscarriage rates
Ovulation	AMH
Menstrual regularity	FAI
SHBG	Total testosterone
	Clinical hyperandrogenism

(AMH: anti-Müllerian hormone; CPR: clinical pregnancy rate; FAI: free androgen index; SHBG: sex hormone-binding globulin)

Sleep Modifications

Seven to eight hours sleep is mandatory for good melatonin secretion and its beneficial effect on overall well-being of PCOS.[16,18]

Bariatric Surgery

Bariatric surgery is the most effective antiobesity technique, resulting in significant and persistent body weight loss, increases in whole-body insulin sensitivity, and even T2DM remission.[17]

INSULIN SENSITIZERS IN POLYCYSTIC OVARIAN SYNDROME

Insulin sensitizers are drugs that improve the body's reaction to insulin, making it more effective at managing blood glucose levels. Based on the clinical evidence to date, the use of insulin sensitizers promises new treatment options for PCOS for both fertility and long-term disease prevention.

They operate by a variety of mechanisms including:
- *Improving insulin signaling:* Insulin sensitizers aid to restore cells' insulin sensitivity, allowing for improved glucose absorption and utilization.
- *Reducing androgen synthesis:* By increasing insulin sensitivity, these drugs help reduce the ovaries' excessive synthesis of androgens, addressing one of the fundamental reasons of PCOS.
- *Menstrual cycle regulation:* Insulin sensitizers can restore regular menstrual cycles and improve ovulation in PCOS women, boosting reproductive prospects.

There are several oral antihyperglycemic agents which are used as insulin sensitizers to treat women with PCOS:
- Metformin
- Inositols—myoinositol (MI) and D-chiroinositol (DCI)
- Thiazolidinedione
- Glucagon-like peptide-1 receptor agonists (GLP-1-RAs)
- Berberine (BBR)
- N-acetylcysteine
- Alpha-lipoic acid (ALA)
- Resveratrol
- Melatonin
- Other nutraceutical compounds
- Traditional Chinese herbal medicines.

Metformin

Metformin belongs to category of biguanides. It is an antihyperglycemic agent which enhances glucose tolerance by lowering both basal and postprandial plasma glucose in T2DM patients. It is known to act by inhibiting mitochondrial activity and improve insulin sensitivity by increasing peripheral glucose uptake and utilization which results in decreased hepatic glucose production and intestinal absorption.[19]

Metformin minimizes the proinflammatory response by inhibiting nuclear factor kappa B (NF-κB) through both liver-related AMPK-dependent and independent pathways, this suppresses the production of prostaglandin E2 (PGE2), nitric oxide (NO), and acute inflammatory markers (tumor necrosis factor-α, interleukin-1, and interleukin-6) **(Fig. 1)**.[20]

It has been shown to improve glucose-insulin metabolism by:
- Lowering intestinal glucose absorption, gluconeogenesis, and glycogenolysis
- Increasing glucose uptake in the liver, skeletal muscle, adipose tissue, and ovaries
- Increasing insulin receptor tyrosine kinase activity in liver
- An increase in the recruitment and activity of GLUT4 glucose transporters.

Role in PCOS: Metformin is the most extensively used insulin sensitizer in PCOS due to its efficiency and safety.

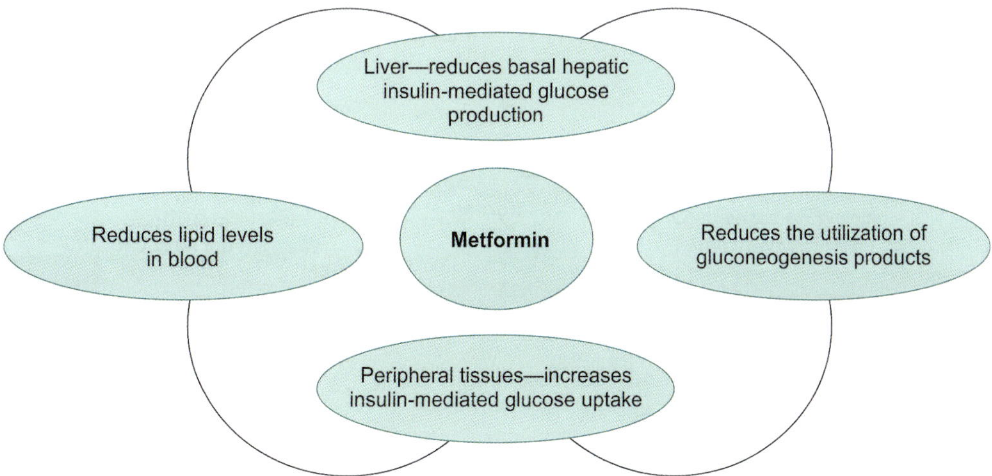

Fig. 1: Metformin: mechanism of action.

It is used in conjunction with oral contraceptives (COCs), especially in overweight or obese patients, or when COCs are contraindicated. This link is thought to be especially helpful in women from high metabolic danger categories, such as those who have diabetes risk factors, certain ethnic groups, and adolescents with BMI ≥25.[15]

Metformin on Bodyweight and Body Mass Index

Taking metformin can reduce BMI, waist circumference, FSH, LH, low-density lipoprotein (LDL) cholesterol, and testosterone levels in overweight women with PCOS. However, there is no improvement in fasting insulin levels, homeostatic model assessment for insulin resistance (HOMA-IR), LDL cholesterol levels, high-density lipoprotein (HDL) cholesterol levels, SHBG levels, fasting blood glucose (FBG) levels, androstenedione levels, total cholesterol (TC) levels, or triglyceride (TG) levels. Current results suggest that metformin may be the most effective intervention for PCOS in overweight women. The beneficial effects of metformin are becoming more apparent, especially when combined with lifestyle changes, improving the pathogenetic mechanisms underlying PCOS, restoring ovarian function, and improving metabolic profile, particularly insulin sensitivity and, unlike COCs and lipoprotein pattern.[20]

Metformin in Hyperandrogenemia

According to Cochrane review 2020, metformin is less effective in improving hirsutism compared to oral contraceptive pill (OCP) in women with BMI 25–30 kg/m^2 and uncertain in women with BMI <25 kg/m^2 and >30 kg/m^2. Either metformin or OCP alone may be less effective in improving hirsutism compared to its combination **(Fig. 2)**.

Metformin as Oral Ovulogen

- Metformin alone could be used as an oral ovulogen and is better than a placebo but it is least effective in terms of clinical pregnancy rates and live birth rates (LBRs) when compared with letrozole, clomiphene citrate (CC), and gonadotropins (grade A and B).
- There is good evidence though that metformin in combination with CC improves ovulation and CPR but does not improve LBR compared with CC alone in PCOS women (grade A). This also stands true for women with BMI >35 kg/m^2 those with CC resistance, although there is no evidence of a difference in LBR.
- Metformin alone does not increase the miscarriage rates when stopped at initiation of pregnancy.
- There is fair evidence that pretreatment with metformin for at least 3 months followed by addition of another ovulation inducing agent increases the LBR (grade B).
- Metformin can be administered with CC or gonadotropins in PCOS women who are anovulatory and are not sensitive to the ovulation induction agent to enhance ovulation, pregnancy, and LBRs. In a recent Cochrane review, authors have concluded that metformin may increase the LBR among women undergoing ovulation induction with gonadotropins and can be started before giving ovulation induction.[21]

Role in assisted reproductive technology (ART): In women with PCOS who are receiving in vitro fertilization/intracytoplasmic sperm injection (IVF/ICSI) therapy

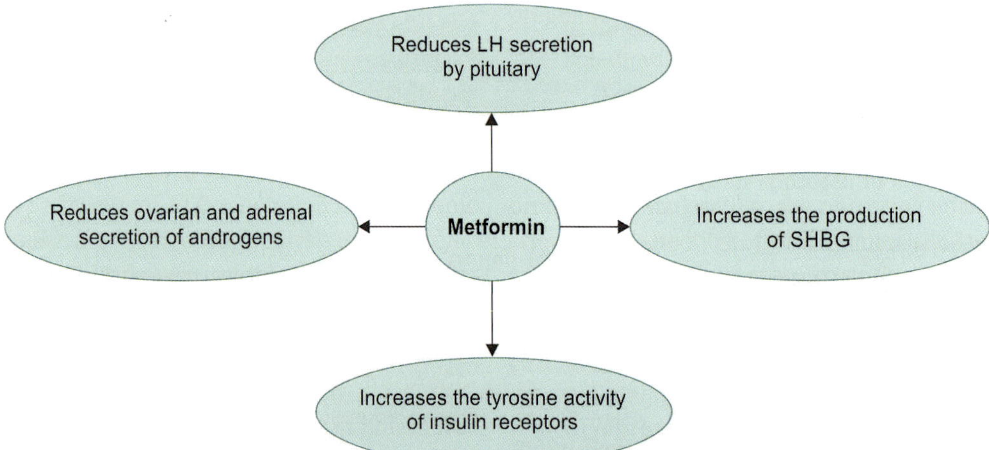

Fig. 2: Effect of metformin on hyperandrogenemia.
(LH: luteinizing hormone; SHBG: sex hormone-binding globulin)

for infertility, adjunct metformin medication is effective before and during ovarian stimulation to enhance clinical pregnancy rates and lower the risk of ovarian hyperstimulation syndrome (OHSS).[15]

The Cochrane study 2020 concluded that metformin treatment was associated with a decreased risk of OHSS but had no association with the overall clinical pregnancy rate or LBR among women with PCOS undergoing IVF/ICSI-ET and it should be preferred in obese or overweight PCOS.[22]

Metformin in Pregnancy

Metformin has a good safety profile during pregnancy. The continued use of metformin, during pregnancy in women with PCOS, had no effect on incidence of fetal abnormalities or fetal birth weight.[23] Greatest benefit of metformin during pregnancy is seen in obese women in terms of decreased miscarriage rates and LBR. Women with PCOS are at increased risk of pregnancy-related complications including gestational diabetes, pregnancy-induced hypertension, preeclampsia, and neonatal morbidity. The role of metformin in improving these complications or decreasing their rate is controversial. Metformin decreases the chances of late miscarriage and preterm deliveries if used from late first trimester until delivery.

Dosage: It is usually started in the dose of 500 mg once daily and increased gradually up to 1,500 mg and a maximum dose of 2,500 mg/day. The target dose is 500–850 mg thrice daily, with meals, in PCOS is sufficient and increases the frequency of spontaneous ovulation, menstrual cyclicity, and ovulatory response to clomiphene. Gradual increment in dose is advised. It should be given for 2–3 months minimum.

The various side effects include gastrointestinal (GI) intolerance, vitamin B deficiency, hypoglycemia, impaired kidney function, and lactic acidosis. Metformin should not be prescribed to patients with renal, hepatic, or major cardiovascular disease or hypoxia because these patients have a predisposition to elevated lactate levels.

Precautionary temporal withdrawal of metformin is advised in patients undergoing radiological procedures involving intravascular iodinated contrast materials and surgery.

Thiazolidinediones

According to a Cochrane study, pioglitazone may improve menstrual pattern in PCOS, but no change in anthropometric outcomes [BMI and waist-hip ratio (WHR)], endocrine outcomes (testosterone and SHBG), or metabolic results (fasting insulin) was reported between pioglitazone and placebo.[24]

Glitazones do not seem to possess significant metabolic or clinical advantages compared to metformin treatment; and therefore, the glitazones are not used routinely. The use is further complicated by the adverse effects on bone mineral density and probably cardiovascular compartment and the need for safe birth control.[25]

Inositols

Inositols are chemically identified as hexa-hydroxy-cyclohexanes ($C_6H_{12}O_6$) with a molecular weight of 180.16. They include a family of nine stereoisomers among, them MI is the most important and widely distributed in nature. In humans, inositols are primarily derived from dietary sources as MI. MI can be then converted to DCI by a nicotinamide adenine dinucleotide (NAD)–NADH-dependent epimerase, under the stimulus of insulin. Inositols help in the intracellular synthesis of insulin second messengers like phospho-myoinositol-3-phosphate (PIP3) and inositolphosphoglycan (IPG). Under physiological conditions, both MI and DCI (MI-IPG and DCI-IPG) are second messengers involved in insulin signaling and mediate different effects in humans.

The tissues with high glucose consumption, such as the brain and the heart have high concentration of MI. DCI concentration is elevated in tissues that store glycogen (i.e., liver, muscles, and fat) and low in tissues with high glucose utilization.[26]

The role of both these compounds is described in **Figure 3**.

Myoinositol

Myoinositol is ingested with food mostly from fruits, beans, grains, and nuts. Daily intake of MI from phytate-rich

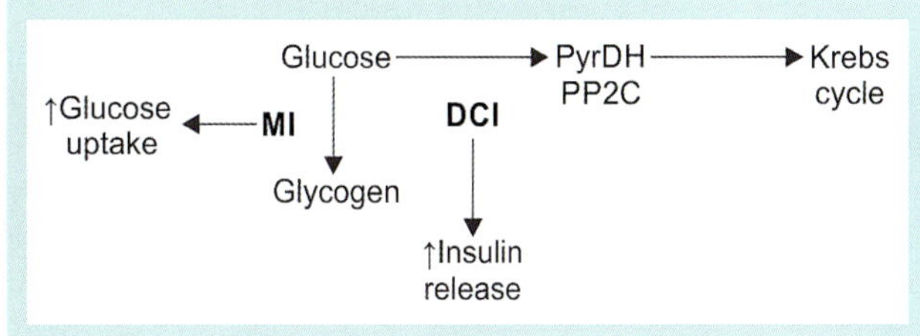

Fig. 3: Role of MI and DCI in body.
(DCI: D-chiroinositol; MI: myoinositol)

food does not exceed 500–700 mg/day for western diet. It is converted to DCI in cells and plays an important role in morphogenesis, cell growth, and lipid synthesis. MI improves ovarian function, decreases LH/FSH ratio, reduces serum androgens, increases SHBG, and decreases serum total and free testosterone. The ideal dose of MI has not yet been defined and the studies have used 1–4 g/day in different settings.

Both MI and DCI show insulin-mimetic properties and decrease postprandial blood glucose level **(Fig. 3)**. DCI increases glycogen synthesis and MI increases glucose catabolism.

Myoinositol and DCI both play important roles in glucose metabolism. MI participates in cellular glucose uptake, inducing GLUT4 translocation to the cell membrane and inhibiting the adenylate cyclase enzyme, reduces the release of free fatty acids from adipose tissues, whereas DCI engages in glycogen synthesis. MI and DCI are abundant in the ovaries and follicular fluid and have distinct roles in insulin signaling and follicular development. As a second messenger, MI enhances FSH signaling, whereas DCI is responsible for insulin-mediated androgen production and can function as an aromatase inhibitor **(Figs. 4 and 5)**. The equilibrium between these two isomers maintains proper hormone production and ovarian function in the normal ovary. The normal MI/DCI ratio is between 100:1 in the follicular fluid and 40:1 in plasma. HI increases the DCI-to-MI

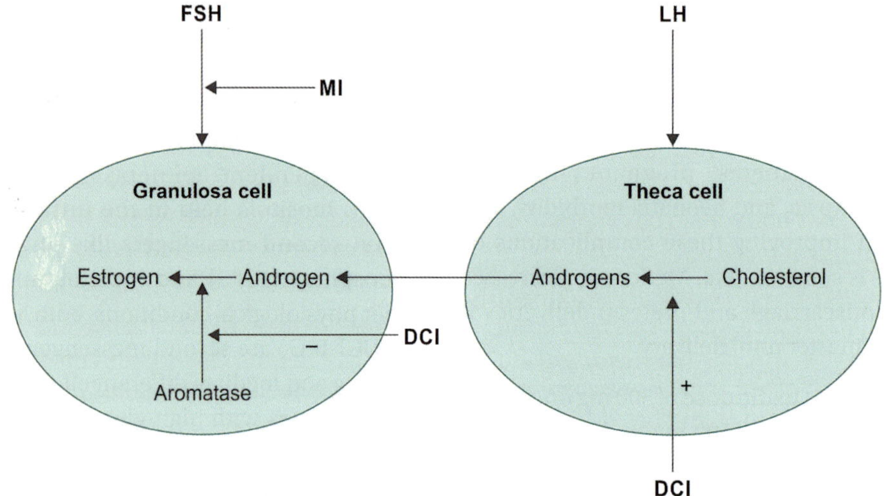

Fig. 4: MI and DCI role in androgen synthesis.
(DCI: D-chiroinositol; MI: myoinositol)

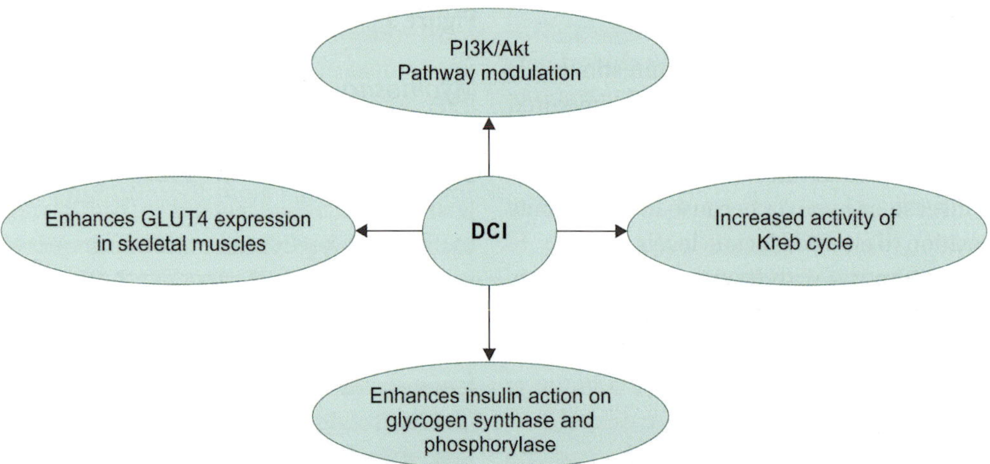

Fig. 5: Mechanism of action of DCI.
(DCI: D-chiroinositol; GLUT4: glucose transporter type 4)

ratio in individuals with PCOS and IR due to increased epimerase activity, which converts MI to DCI.[27,28]

Despite their molecular similarities and synergistic impact on insulin sensitivity, MI and DCI have separate roles in the ovary. MI can have the opposite effect on aromatase activity as DCI.

Higher MI/DCI ratios boost aromatase activity in the granulosa, raising estrogen levels, while lower MI/DCI ratios stimulate testosterone synthesis in theca cells. This results in hyperandrogenism and reduced FSH signaling. This process is implicated in what is known as the "ovarian paradox".

Studies have shown that MI treatment improved ovarian function and fertility, reduced the severity of hyperandrogenism, acne, and hirsutism, and positively affected metabolic parameters and modulated various hormonal parameters deeply involved in reproductive axis function and ovulation, making it a novel method to improve spontaneous ovulation or ovulation induction.[29]

They are given in several forms and combinations which are illustrated in **Table 1**.

With PCOS, 2 g of MI plus 200 µg of folic acid can be administered twice daily, or 1.2 g of DCI once daily for 6 months.

Alpha-lipoic Acid

Alpha-lipoic acid is a natural antioxidant lipophilic compound that acts as an essential cofactor for mitochondrial enzymes. ALA regulates glucose and lipid metabolism by boosting glucose absorption via an intracellular redistribution of GLUT1 and GLUT4 glucose transporters, comparable to insulin. Other than glucose metabolism, it has been proposed that ALA may enhance reproductive function and metabolic parameters in PCOS women.

Studies have also shown that combining ALA with inositols not only regulates insulin plasma levels, but also improves reproductive pathways via an influence on FSH signal transduction.[30]

Glucagon-like Peptide-1 Receptor Agonists

Mechanisms of action of Glucagon-like peptide-1 receptor agonists (GLP-1-RAs) include insulin secretion stimulation, glucagon secretion inhibition, and suppression of food intake and appetite, all of which work together to enhance glucose homoeostasis.

Based on their structure they are divided in two categories:

1. Human GLP-1 backbone:
    a. Dulaglutide
    b. Albiglutide
    c. Liraglutide
    d. Semaglutide
2. Exendin-4 backbone:
    a. Exenatide (two formulations)
    b. Lixisenatide

In several studies, the effect of liraglutide (which is a common GLP-RA) was evaluated and it was found that patients prescribed liraglutide showed considerable weight loss and testosterone decrease, with mixed results in terms of IR measures and menstrual patterns improvements. Looking at current evidence, it seems that body weight reduction is the primary mechanism of GLP-1RAs action in PCOS. Future studies are needed to evaluate other tissue-specific effects on GLP-1R, especially at the level of the hypothalamic-pituitary-gonadal (HPG) axis that goes beyond mere weight-lowering potential that would give further insight in identifying specific PCOS phenotypes that would be the most benefited candidates.[31]

Berberine

Berberine is an alkaloid and is a major active component of the Chinese herbal medicines Rhizoma coptidis, Cortex Phellodendri, and Cortex berberidis stems and roots of *Berberis vulgaris* (barberry).

Berberine is known to enhance InsRs and insulin receptor substrate-1 (IRS-1) expression that lowers fasting glucose level and decreases IR. In individuals who do not react to oral hypoglycemic medication, BBR improves the function of pancreatic islets even if it does not directly increase insulin secretion. BBR (300 mg, tid, 3 months) has been found like MET (500 mg, bid, 3 months) in enhancing pregnancy. The incidence of nausea, vomiting, diarrhea, abdominal pain, and other adverse reactions in BBR group are found lower than patients given metformin, but further studies are still needed to evaluate the adverse effects of BBR.[32]

Resveratrol

Resveratrol is a natural polyphenolic compound (trans-3,5,4′-trihydroxystilbene) which is found in a variety of plants, foods, and drinks, such as grapes, nuts, cranberries, and red wine. Resveratrol is known for its several benefits

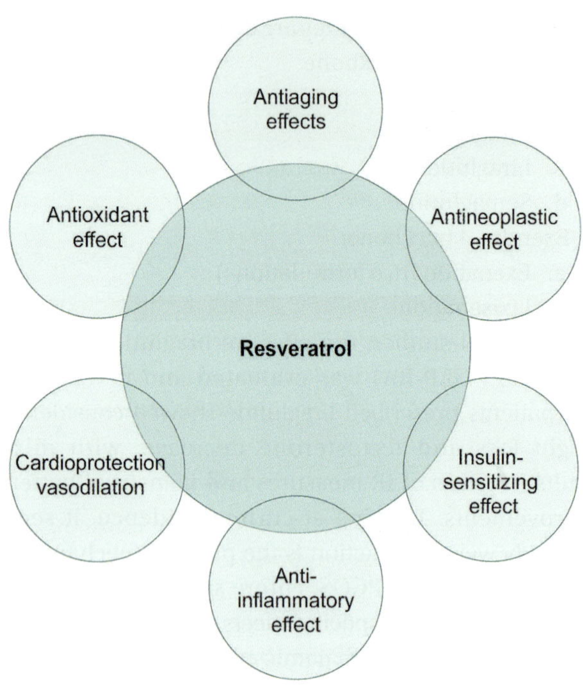

Fig. 6: Resveratrol and its functions.

(Fig. 6). Resveratrol is known to increase liver fatty acid oxidation and decrease oxidative stress which leads to improved insulin sensitivity.[33] Resveratrol can be given from 8 to 3,000 mg/day from 4 weeks to 12 months to show its effect.

Melatonin

Melatonin, or N-acetyl-5-methoxytryptamine, is always known for its role in sleep and circadian regulation including acute effects as well as circadian phase-shifting effects but in recent years its role in glucose control and in T2DM risk or treatment has increased. This is due to the recent discovery of T2DM risk variants in *MTNR1B (melatonin receptor 1b gene)*, and partly because of the compelling evidence for the adverse impact of circadian disruption on glucose metabolism.[34]

N-acetylcysteine

N-acetylcysteine increases the cellular levels of antioxidants, that is why it is considered to enhance insulin receptor activity in human erythrocytes and improve insulin secretion in response to glucose.[35] Recommended dose is 600–1,800 mg/day for a minimum of 6 weeks.

Nutraceuticals and Chinese Herbs

Chinese herbs, like Heyan Kuntai capsule (HYKT), Heqi San, Cangfudaotan decoction (CFD), etc. and nutraceutical have been used to increase insulin sensitivity. Other than these green tea, cinnamon, red onion and soy supplements, and nuts are also effective in IR.[36]

CONSIDERATIONS AND FUTURE DIRECTIONS

While insulin sensitizers have shown promising outcomes in the treatment of PCOS, numerous factors should be considered:

- *Individualized approach:* Treatment selections should be customized to each woman's unique needs, taking into account factors, such as BMI, metabolic profile, and reproductive objectives.
- *Combination therapy:* Insulin sensitizers are frequently used in conjunction with other therapy, such as lifestyle changes, oral contraceptives, and fertility medications, to achieve comprehensive PCOS management.
- *Long-term benefits and safety:* More studies are needed to investigate the long-term advantages and safety profiles of insulin sensitizers in PCOS women, especially in terms of cardiovascular health and pregnancy outcomes.

CONCLUSION

Insulin resistance is an inherent metabolic disorder which is linked to PCOS. Increased resistance toward insulin results into HI-induced hyperandrogenemia in PCOS. Lifestyle modifications and insulin sensitizers combined can improve the body's reaction to insulin, making it more effective at managing blood glucose levels and excessive synthesis of androgens, addressing one of the fundamental reasons of PCOS.

REFERENCES

1. De Leo V, Musacchio MC, Cappelli V, Massaro MG, Morgante G, Petraglia F. Genetic, hormonal and metabolic aspects of PCOS: an update. Reprod Biol Endocrinol. 2016; 14(1):38.
2. Rotterdam ESHRE/ASRM-Sponsored PCOS consensus workshop group. Revised 2003 consensus on diagnostic criteria and long-term health risks related to polycystic ovary syndrome (PCOS). Hum Reprod. 2004;19(1):41-7.
3. Flavia T, Enzo B, Paolo M. Insulin resistance in a large cohort of women with polycystic ovary syndrome: a comparison

between euglycaemic-hyperinsulinaemic clamp and surrogate indexes. Hum Reprod. 2017;32:2515-21.

4. Moghetti P, Tosi F, Bonin C, Di Sarra D, Fiers T, Kaufman JM, et al. Divergences in insulin resistance between the different phenotypes of the polycystic ovary syndrome. J Clin Endocrinol Metab. 2013;98:E628-E637.
5. Chen Y, Guo J, Zhang Q, Zhang C. Insulin Resistance is a Risk Factor for Early Miscarriage and Macrosomia in Patients With Polycystic Ovary Syndrome From the First Embryo Transfer Cycle: A Retrospective Cohort Study. Front Endocrinol. 2022;13:853473.
6. Rubin KH, Glintborg D, Nybo M, Abrahamsen B, Andersen M. Development and Risk Factors of Type 2 Diabetes in a Nationwide Population of Women With Polycystic Ovary Syndrome. J Clin Endocrinol Metab. 2017;102(10):3848-57.
7. Wekker V, van Dammen L, Koning A, Heida K, Painter R, Limpens J, et al. Long-term cardiometabolic disease risk in women with PCOS: a systematic review and meta-analysis. Hum Reprod Update. 2020;26:942-60.
8. Evanthia DK, Andrea D. Insulin resistance and the polycystic ovary syndrome revisited: an update on mechanisms and implications. Endocr Rev. 2012;6:981-1030.
9. Nestler JE, Jakubowicz DJ, Aida FDV, Brik C, Quintero N, Medina F. Insulin stimulates testosterone biosynthesis by human thecal cells from women with polycystic ovary syndrome by activating its own receptor and using inositolglycan mediators as the signal transduction system. J Clin Endocrinol Metab. 1998;83:2001-5.
10. Samuel Varman T, Shulman GI. Mechanisms for insulin resistance: common threads and missing links. Cell 2012; 148:852-71.
11. Rice S, Christoforidis N, Gadd C, Nikolaou D, Seyani L, Donaldson A, et al. Impaired insulin-dependent glucose metabolism in granulosa-lutein cells from anovulatory women with polycystic ovaries. Human Reprod. 2005;20:373-81.
12. Palomba S, Piltonen T, Giudice L. Endometrial function in women with polycystic ovary syndrome: a comprehensive review. Hum Reprod Update. 2021;27:584-618.
13. Zhang Y, Hu M, Yang F, Zhang Y, Ma S, Zhang D, et al. Increased uterine androgen receptor protein abundance results in implantation and mitochondrial defects in pregnant rats with hyperandrogenism and insulin resistance. J Mol Med. 2021;99:1427-46.
14. Xue J, Zhang H, Liu W, Liu M, Shi M, Wen Z, et al. Metformin inhibits growth of eutopic stromal cells from adenomyotic endometrium via AMPK activation and subsequent inhibition of AKT phosphorylation: a possible role in the treatment of adenomyosis. Reproduction. 2013; 146:397-406.
15. Teede HJ, Tay CT, Laven JJE, Dokras A, Moran LJ, Piltonen TT, et al. Recommendations from the 2023 international evidence-based guideline for the assessment and management of polycystic ovary syndrome. Eur J Endocrinol. 2023;189(2):G43-G64.
16. Gu Y, Zhou G, Zhou F, Wu Q, Ma C, Zhang Y, et al. Life Modifications and PCOS: Old Story But New Tales. Front Endocrinol (Lausanne). 2022;13:808898.
17. Rodriguez Paris V, Bertoldo MJ. The Mechanism of Androgen Actions in PCOS Etiology. Med Sci (Basel). 2019; 7(9):89.
18. 18. Shang Y, Zhou H, He R, Lu W. Dietary Modification for Reproductive Health in Women With Polycystic Ovary Syndrome: A Systematic Review and Meta-Analysis. Front Endocrinol (Lausanne). 2021;12:735954.
19. Amisi CA. Markers of insulin resistance in Polycystic ovary syndrome women: An update. World J Diabetes. 2022; 13(3):129-49.
20. Mastrototaro L, Roden M. Insulin resistance and insulin sensitizing agents. Metabolism. 2021;125:154892.
21. Morley LC, Tang T, Yasmin E, Norman RJ, Balen AH. Insulin-sensitising drugs (metformin, rosiglitazone, pioglitazone, D-chiro-inositol) for women with polycystic ovary syndrome, oligo amenorrhoea and subfertility. Cochrane Database Syst Rev. 2017;11(11):CD003053.
22. Tso LO, Costello MF, Albuquerque LET, Andriolo RB, Macedo CR. Metformin treatment before and during IVF or ICSI in women with polycystic ovary syndrome. Cochrane Database Syst Rev. 2020;12(12):CD006105.
23. Romualdi D, Versace V, Lanzone A. What is new in the landscape of insulin-sensitizing agents for polycystic ovary syndrome treatment. Ther Adv Reprod Health. 2020;14: 2633494120908709.
24. Eggleton JS, Jialal I. Thiazolidinediones. In: StatPearls. Treasure Island (FL): StatPearls Publishing; 2024.
25. van Genugten RE, Möller-Goede DL, van Raalte DH, Diamant M. Extra-pancreatic effects of incretin-based therapies: potential benefit for cardiovascular-risk management in type 2 diabetes. Diabetes Obes Metab. 2013;15(7):593-606.
26. Facchinetti F, Unfer V, Dewailly D, Kamenov ZA, Diamanti-Kandarakis E, Laganà AS, et al. Inositols in Polycystic Ovary Syndrome: An Overview on the Advances. Trends Endocrinol Metab. 2020;31(6):435-47.
27. Unfer V, Nestler JE, Kamenov ZA, Prapas N, Facchinetti F. Effects of Inositol(s) in Women with PCOS: A Systematic Review of Randomized Controlled Trials. Int J Endocrinol. 2016;2016:1849162.
28. Ijuin T, Takenawa T. Regulation of insulin signaling and glucose transporter 4 (GLUT4) exocytosis by phosphatidylinositol 3,4,5-trisphosphate (PIP3) phosphatase, skeletal muscle, and kidney enriched inositol polyphosphate phosphatase (SKIP). J Biol Chem. 2012;287(10):6991-9.
29. Taieb J, Grynberg M, Pierre A, Arouche N, Massart P, Belville C, et al. FSH and its second messenger cAMP stimulate the transcription of human anti-Müllerian hormone in cultured granulosa cells. Mol Endocrinol. 2011;25(4):645-55.

30. Guarano A, Capozzi A, Cristodoro M, Di Simone N, Lello S. Alpha Lipoic Acid Efficacy in PCOS Treatment: What Is the Truth? Nutrients. 2023;15(14):3209.
31. Jensterle M, Herman R, Janež A. Therapeutic Potential of Glucagon-like Peptide-1 Agonists in Polycystic Ovary Syndrome: From Current Clinical Evidence to Future Perspectives. Biomedicines. 2022;10(8):1989.
32. Li MF, Zhou XM, Li XL. The Effect of Berberine on Polycystic Ovary Syndrome Patients with Insulin Resistance (PCOS-IR): A Meta-Analysis and Systematic Review. Evid Based Complement Alternat Med. 2018;2018:2532935.
33. Karimi A, Tutunchi H, Naeini F, Vajdi M, Mobasseri M, Najafipour F. The therapeutic effects and mechanisms of action of resveratrol on polycystic ovary syndrome: a comprehensive systematic review of clinical, animal and in vitro studies. Clin Exp Pharmacol Physiol. 2022;49(9): 935-49.
34. Garaulet M, Qian J, Florez JC, Arendt J, Saxena R, Scheer FAJL. Melatonin Effects on Glucose Metabolism: Time To Unlock the Controversy. Trends Endocrinol Metab. 2020; 31:192-204.
35. Sandhu JK, Waqar A, Jain A, Joseph C, Srivastava K, Ochuba O, et al. Oxidative Stress in Polycystic Ovarian Syndrome and the Effect of Antioxidant N-Acetylcysteine on Ovulation and Pregnancy Rate. Cureus. 2021;13(9):e17887.
36. Sun J, Ren J, Hu X, Hou Y, Yang Y. Therapeutic effects of Chinese herbal medicines and their extracts on diabetes. Biomed Pharmacother. 2021;142:111977.

Chapter

Poor Responders: Is There an Ideal Protocol?

Pratik Tambe

INTRODUCTION

In vitro fertilization (IVF) has been used since the late 1970s to offer hope to childless couples struggling with infertility. Unfortunately, despite advances in IVF, laboratory technology, and improving success rates, a small subset of patients known as "poor responders" still presents a unique challenge even today. These poor responders have a compromised ovarian response, which is characterized by a suboptimal number of ovarian follicles and a lower number of retrieved oocytes during ovarian stimulation (OS).

Furthermore, the oocytes retrieved may be of poor quality and may not yield good-quality embryos, which further decreases the success rates in this population. Hence, this group of women requires special attention and personalized/individualized stimulation protocols to improve their chances of a successful outcome and higher clinical pregnancy rates. We evaluate whether there is an ideal stimulation protocol for poor responders in IVF based on the current evidence to date.

WHAT CONSTITUTES A "POOR RESPONDER"?

There are a multitude of definitions (41 in toto) in literature of poor responders including premature ovarian failure, poor ovarian response (POR), premature ovarian insufficiency, etc. Poor responders represent a complex and heterogeneous group, which can be classified and subdivided on the basis of various criteria including the patient's age, antral follicle count (AFC), oocytes retrieved at follicular aspiration, among others. Hence, identifying an ideal protocol that may suit all poor responders may be difficult. Individualized stimulation protocols probably are the way forward.

Various factors contribute to poor response, including advanced maternal age, diminished ovarian reserve, previous ovarian surgery, or exposure to radiotherapy or chemotherapy. These factors alter the ovarian response and necessitate an adaptable protocol that maximizes the chances of successfully retrieving a good number of high quality oocytes.

ESHRE CONSENSUS AND BOLOGNA CRITERIA[1]

Poor ovarian response to OS indicates a reduced ovarian follicular growth, resulting in a lesser number of retrieved oocytes than what would be expected with a standardized conventional stimulation.

According to the Bologna criteria proposed by Ferraretti et al. in 2011, to define a poor response in IVF, at least two of the following three criteria must be present:

1. Advanced maternal age or any other risk factor for POR
2. A previous POR
3. An abnormal ovarian reserve test (ORT).

By definition, the term POR refers to the ovarian response; therefore, at least one stimulated cycle is considered essential for the diagnosis of POR. Patients of advanced age with an abnormal ORT may be classified as poor responders since both advanced age and an abnormal ORT may indicate reduced ovarian reserve. These patients can be properly defined as an "expected poor responder".

This standardized definition proposed was of paramount importance as the minimal inclusion criterion needed to select patients for clinical trials was essential to allow comparisons and eliminate confusion resulting from the numerous conflicting definitions existing earlier. By reducing bias caused by spurious POR definitions, it would be possible to compare results and to draw reliable conclusions.[1]

POSEIDON CLASSIFICATION (TABLE 1)[2]

While the Bologna criteria were found to be useful in predicting the outcome of IVF and for counseling purposes, their use in clinical trials was questioned, because they grouped together women who differ significantly in their biological characteristics.

For example, according to the Bologna criteria, young women with a low ovarian reserve associated with a previous episode of POR, young women with a normal ovarian reserve and two POR episodes, and older women (≥40 years) with a normal ovarian reserve and a previous episode of POR would all be clumped together and included in the same category even though the clinical management of these patients requires different approaches and individualized therapy.

To tailor-make the treatment to the patient, various parameters that affect reproductive outcomes need to be considered while planning the treatment strategy including:

- Oocytes retrieved at previous stimulation
- Age-related embryo/blastocyst aneuploidy rate
- Ovarian "sensitivity" to exogenous gonadotropins, which has been demonstrated to vary depending on follicle-stimulating hormone (FSH) receptor (FSHR) profiles.

Hence, the POSEIDON (Patient-Oriented Strategies Encompassing IndividualizeD Oocyte Number) classification introduced clinically relevant criteria that can help to guide the fertility clinician in patient management.[2]

There are now two defined categories of impaired response:

1. A "suboptimal response" is defined as the retrieval of four to nine oocytes, which is associated, at any given age, with a significantly lower live birth rate (LBR) compared with normal responders who yield 10–15 oocytes.
2. A "hyporesponse," is when a higher dose of gonadotropins and more prolonged stimulation are required to obtain an adequate number of oocytes (more than three).

The other criteria which are relevant include the age of the patient and the expected aneuploidy rate and biomarkers and functional markers [i.e., anti-Müllerian hormone (AMH) and AFC].

A physiological classification which is clinically relevant has therefore been proposed:

Group 1 patients <35 years with sufficient prestimulation ovarian reserve parameters (AFC ≥5, AMH ≥1.2 ng/mL) and with an unexpected poor or suboptimal ovarian response; this group is further divided into:

- *1a:* Patients with <4 oocytes retrieved
- *1b:* 4–9 oocytes retrieved after standard OS

Group 2 patients ≥35 years with sufficient prestimulation ovarian reserve parameters (AFC ≥5, AMH ≥1.2 ng/mL) and with an unexpected poor or suboptimal ovarian response; This group is further divided into:

- *2a:* patients with <4 oocytes retrieved
- *2b:* 4–9 oocytes retrieved after standard OS

Group 3 patients <35 years with poor ovarian reserve prestimulation parameters (AFC <5, AMH <1.2 ng/mL)

Group 4 patients ≥35 years with poor ovarian reserve prestimulation parameters (AFC <5, AMH <1.2 ng/mL)

Personalization of treatment protocols can be at various points:

- Using different gonadotropin-releasing hormone (GnRH) analog regimens

TABLE 1: POSEIDON stratification.[2]

POSEIDON group 1	***POSEIDON group 2***
Young patients <35 years with adequate ovarian reserve parameters (AFC ≥5; AMH ≥1.2 ng/mL) and with an unexpected poor or suboptimal ovarian response *Subgroup 1a:* <4 oocytes* *Subgroup 1b:* 4–9 oocytes retrieved*	Older patients ≥35 years with adequate ovarian reserve parameters (AFC ≥ 5; AMH ≥ 1.2 ng/mL) and with an unexpected poor or suboptimal ovarian response *Subgroup 2a:* <4 oocytes* *Subgroup 2b:* 4–9 oocytes retrieved*
POSEIDON group 3	***POSEIDON group 4***
Young patients (<35 years) with poor ovarian reserve prestimulation parameters (AFC <5; AMH <1.2 ng/mL)	Older patients (≥35 years) with poor ovarian reserve prestimulation parameters (AFC <5; AMH <1.2 ng/mL)

*After standard ovarian stimulation

(AFC: antral follicle count; AMH: anti-Müllerian hormone; POSEIDON: Patient-Oriented Strategies Encompassing IndividualizeD Oocyte Number)

- Detecting polymorphisms of gonadotropins and their receptors
- Tailoring the FSH starting dose
- Personalizing gonadotropin doses [i.e., FSH monotherapy or addition of luteinizing hormone (LH)-containing drugs]
- Evaluating special regimens, including oocyte/embryo accumulation to maximize outcomes.

PROTOCOLS STUDIED IN POOR RESPONDERS

Conventional Stimulation

The conventional stimulation protocol involves initiating OS with injectable FSH on day 2/3 of the menstrual cycle, followed by serial ultrasound monitoring and hormone assays to guide dose adjustments until follicular maturation occurs. Unfortunately, this protocol with standardized dosages may not be the most suitable choice for poor responders, who have a limited ovarian reserve and/or reduced sensitivity to exogenous FSH stimulation.

High-dose Protocols

The high-dose stimulation protocols involve increasing the FSH dose in the follicular recruitment stage of OS in an attempt to recruit more follicles and improve oocyte yield. While conventional stimulation may not use dosages higher than 300 IU/day; in high-dose stimulation, up to 600 IU/day has been described. Increasing the dosage may not necessarily translate into a greater oocyte yield. Patients with diminished ovarian reserve and compromised egg quality may yield 1–2 extra oocytes with this approach, but they may not be of good quality, therefore not resulting in an improved clinical pregnancy rate.

Microdose Protocol

The microdose protocol utilizes lower doses of gonadotropins while concomitantly adding other medications such as GnRH agonists or antagonists. It aims to obtain a more controlled response, minimizes the possibility of OHSS, and maximizes oocyte quality. Although this protocol may be more favorable for poor responders, it requires careful monitoring and adjustments to achieve optimal results.

Natural Cycle or Mild Stimulation Protocol

The natural cycle does not use exogenous stimulation and mild stimulation protocol involves utilizing a mild OS approach, using oral ovulogens and without the use of exogenous gonadotropins. This protocol aims to work with the limited ovarian reserve and avoids additional risks or discomfort associated with high doses of gonadotropins. However, the success rates of this protocol are lower than those of conventional approaches.

Random-start Protocol

The random-start protocol involves initiating OS at any point of time in the menstrual cycle, as opposed to the conventional day 2/3 initiation. This variation allows for immediate treatment, even during the luteal phase of the previous cycle, without waiting for the next menstrual period. This protocol may benefit poor responders, who have more unpredictable and irregular menstrual cycles without waiting for their next cycle but further research is required to determine its efficacy.

Follicle to Oocyte Index[3,4]

The follicle to oocyte index (FOI) is a new model introduced to address the hyporesponsiveness or ovarian resistance to gonadotropins during OS and or insufficient ovulation trigger strategies. It assesses the ratio between the total number of oocytes retrieved at oocyte pickup to the number of antral follicles available at the beginning of stimulation. A low FOI is when <50% of the antral follicles yield oocytes at retrieval. A low FOI may also be seen in patients with "normal" ovarian reserve.

ART CALCULATOR[5]

The ART calculator developed by the POSEIDON group provides two predictions:

1. A pretreatment estimation of the number of mature oocytes needed to achieve at least one euploid blastocyst
2. Uses the actual number of collected mature oocytes to estimate the chances of having a euploid blastocyst using that oocyte cohort.

This can help clinicians counsel patients about their prognosis and individualize treatment regimens. The ART calculator takes into consideration a number of predictors including female partner age and type of sperm, which are the most important factors for blastocyst euploidy. The ART calculator is available online for free at http://www.members.groupposeidon.com/calculator.

MANAGEMENT STRATEGIES

POSEIDON Groups 1 and 2 (Table 2)[4]

The pathophysiology behind the POR in POSEIDON groups 1 and 2 is not fully understood. The decreased sensitivity of follicles to exogenous FSH may be the most plausible explanation. Specific genetic polymorphisms affecting gonadotropin receptors have been suggested. A common LH beta subunit variant has been noted to be associated with increased FSH consumption during stimulation. A systematic review and meta-analysis of 33 studies on FSHR polymorphisms showed that both serine carriers of FSHR (rs6166) and carriers of FSHR (rs1394205) are associated with ovarian resistance to stimulation.[6]

Environmental contaminants may be associated with POR, e.g., elevated intrafollicular levels of benzene and polychlorinated biphenyl congeners (PBC). It is believed that benzene leads to transduction deficiency in the FSHR. Oxidative stress might also affect both folliculogenesis and spermatogenesis. This leads to an increase in free radicals, e.g., reactive oxygen species (ROS), which influence the quality of oocytes, spermatozoa, and embryos with reduced assisted reproductive technology (ART) outcomes.

Best practice recommendations for these patients include:
- Use of recombinant FSH (rFSH) instead of urinary gonadotropins
- An increased FSH dosage
- The use of recombinant LH (rLH)
- Dehydroepiandrosterone (DHEA) supplementation before OS
- A double-stimulation (DuoStim) protocol.

POSEIDON Groups 3 and 4 (Flowchart 1)[4]

POSEIDON groups 3 and 4 are patients where there is an "expected" poor response to OS owing to their low ovarian reserve as defined by an AFC <5, and/or AMH <1.2 ng/mL. Group 4 women have a high risk of having poor oocyte quality in addition to a reduced quantity due to an age-related increase in oocyte aneuploidy. Group 3 constitutes 10% while group 4. 55% of all poor responders.

Group 4 patients have a significantly poorer prognosis owing to the increase in aneuploidy rates with consequent

TABLE 2: Recommendations for POSEIDON groups 1 and 2 patients.[7]

Best practice in POSEIDON groups 1 and 2		
Pretreatment protocol	• AFC ≥5 and/or AMH ≥1.2 ng/mL with a history of suboptimal or poor oocyte number after conventional stimulation • Consider ART calculator and genotype screening* • Consider androgens in selected patients (in particular, POSEIDON group 2 with ovarian reserve markers in the lower limits)	
Stimulation protocol	POSEIDON group 1 (age <35 years)	POSEIDON group 2 (age ≥35 years)
	Increase recombinant FSH dosage: • 50–75 IU if no variants • 75–100 IU if FSHR variants (maximum daily dose of 300 IU) *Consider adding rLH:* • 2:1 ratio of rFSH and rLH from the first stimulation day in women who consumed >3,000 IU or with a history of follicular stagnation	• Recombinant FSH dose of 300 IU daily • Consider Duo-Stim approach POSEIDON group 2 (age 35–39 years) rLH 150 IU daily from stimulation day 1 in both agonist and antagonist regimens
Trigger/retrieval	• Consider antagonist regimen, GnRHa trigger, and elective embryo freezing in cases of AFC >16 and/or AMH >3.36 ng/mL • Consider preimplantation genetic testing for aneuploidy (PGT-A) in POSEIDON group 2 (in particular, patients aged >38 years) • Consider single blastocyst embryo transfer	

*FSH receptor variants [FSHR (rs6165), FSHR (rs6166), FSHR (rs1394205)]; LH beta chain variants [LH beta (rs1800447, rs34349826)]; LHCG receptor (LHCGR) variants [(LHCGR (rs2293275) and LHCGR (rs12470652)].

(AFC: antral follicle count; AMH: anti-Müllerian hormone; FSH: follicle-stimulating hormone; FSHR: FSH receptor; GnRHa: gonadotropin-releasing hormone agonist; LH: luteinizing hormone; LHCG: luteinizing hormone choriogonadotropin; POSEIDON: Patient-Oriented Strategies Encompassing IndividualizeD Oocyte Number; rFSH: recombinant FSH; rLH: recombinant LH)

Flowchart 1: Recommendations for POSEIDON groups 3 and 4 patients.[5]

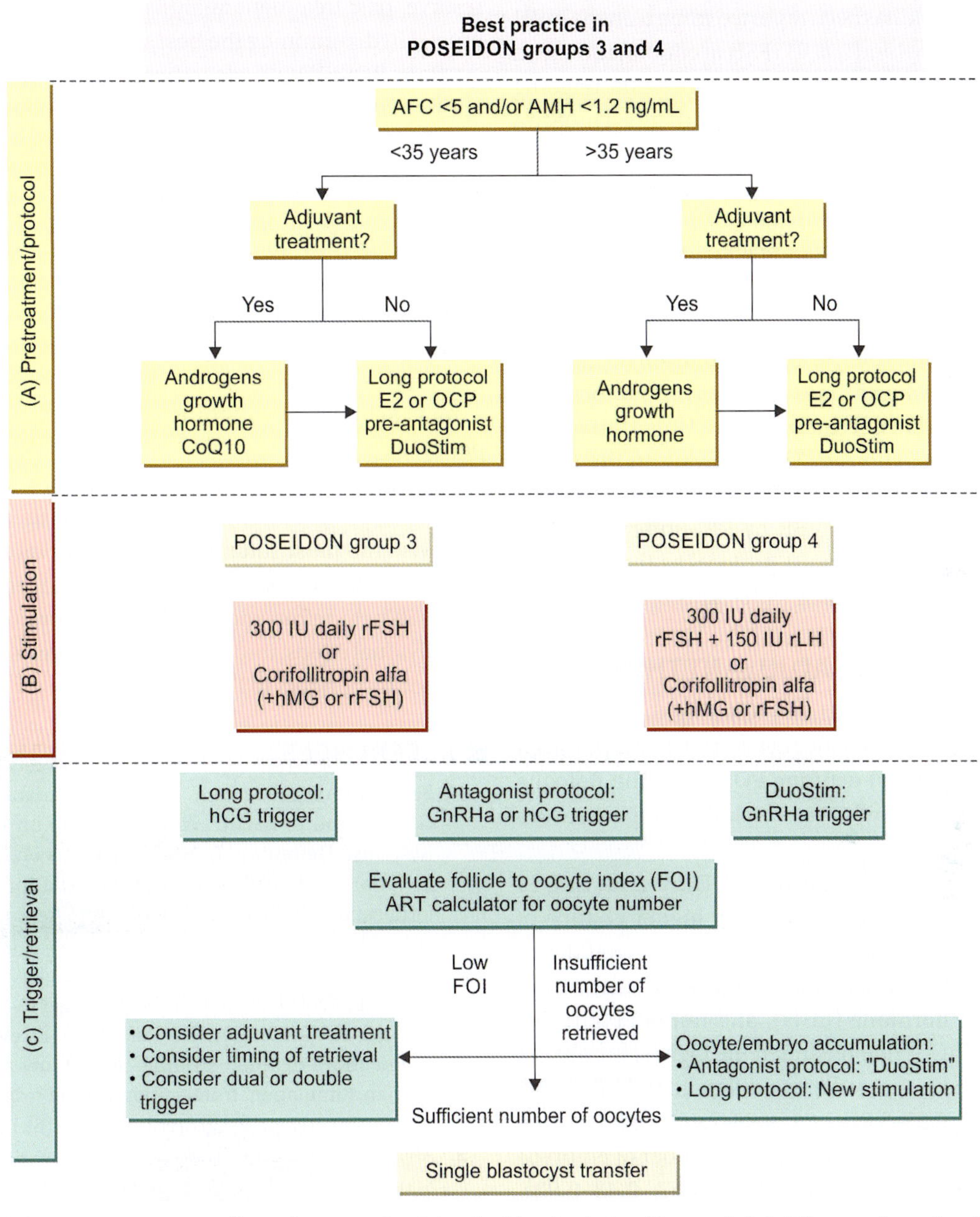

(AFC: antral follicle count; AMH: anti-Müllerian hormone; DuoStim: double-stimulation; E2: estradiol; GnRHa: gonadotropin-releasing hormone agonist; hCG: human chorionic gonadotropin; hMG: human menopausal gonadotropin; OCP: oral contraceptive pill; rFSH: recombinant follicle-stimulating hormone; rLH: recombinant luteinizing hormone)

aneuploid embryos, higher embryo transfer cancellation rates and the necessity of multiple IVF cycles. The management is difficult and the goal of treatment is to increase the probability of having at least one euploid blastocyst for embryo transfer.

The evidence-based strategies recommended include:

- Choosing an appropriate individualized stimulation protocol,
- Individualizing the ovulation trigger strategy
- Adding adjuvants prior to the initiation of OS.

CONTROVERSIES TO CONSENSUS

An 11% LBR per cycle has been reported when using a GnRH agonist long protocol and 300 IU rFSH in combination with 150 IU rLH daily from day 1 of stimulation. A 20% ongoing pregnancy rate has been reported with the DuoStim protocol. In comparison, the natural cycle IVF LBRs are only 2.6%. Hence, OS with exogenous gonadotropin stimulation at a maximum of 300 rFSH should be used rather than natural cycle IVF in POSEIDON groups 3 and 4 patients.[8,9]

A nonsignificant increase is seen in the number of mature oocytes by one oocyte, but a significant decrease in cancellation rates when a long GnRH agonist protocol was used in patients with POR compared to a GnRH antagonist protocol has been reported. This is owing to the better follicular synchronization after downregulation. The one extra oocyte increases the LBR by 5%, underlining the utility of the long GnRH agonist protocol as the preferred stimulation protocol in women with "expected" POR.[10,11]

META-ANALYSIS OF ADJUVANT THERAPIES[12]

Out of 1,124 studies, 46 trials including 6,312 women were included in a systematic review and 19 randomized controlled trials (RCTs) defining POR using the Bologna criteria with 2,677 women were included in the network meta-analysis.

When compared to controls, DHEA and CoQ10 treatments resulted in a significantly higher chance of clinical pregnancy [odds ratio (OR): 2.46, 95% confidence interval (CI): 1.16–5.23; 2.22, 1.08–4.58]. Estradiol, human growth hormone (hGH), and human chorionic gonadotropin (hCG) demonstrated the highest number of oocytes retrieved [weighted mean difference (WMD) 2.08, 0.72–3.44; 2.02, 0.23–3.81; 1.72, 0.98–2.46]. Testosterone and hGH treatment led to the highest number of embryos transferred (WMD: 0.72, 0.11–1.33; 0.67, 0.43–0.92). Significantly, hGH resulted in the highest estradiol level on the hCG day (WMD: 797.63, 466.45–1,128.81). CoQ10 led to the lowest global cancellation rate (OR: 0.33, 0.15–0.74).

CONCLUSION

Optimizing the stimulation protocol for poor responders in IVF remains a challenge owing to the multifactorial nature of POR. Different protocols exist to address variations in individual patients' ovarian reserve and response. Personalization, individualization, and a thorough evaluation of each patient, including their age, ovarian reserve, past treatment analysis, and medical history, are crucial in determining the best stimulation protocol.

Post-POSEIDON classification, an individualized approach at all steps of treatment, including a targeted pretreatment evaluation, the choice of GnRH analogs, gonadotropin type and dose, ovulation trigger, and adjuvant therapies are of paramount importance. Tools such as FOI and the ART calculator can help develop individualized treatment regimens and most importantly help counsel patients about their reproductive prognosis. With such individualized treatment approaches, even the very poor prognosis patients in POSEIDON group 4 may achieve an ongoing pregnancy rate of >20% per cycle.[13]

Collaborative efforts between physicians, embryologists, and reproductive endocrinologists are essential to devise the most suitable stimulation protocol for each patient. Continuous research and advancements in the field will help refine and develop novel protocols tailored to individual needs, improving success rates and outcomes for poor responders in IVF.

REFERENCES

1. Ferraretti AP, La Marca A, Fauser BC, Tarlatzis B, Nargund G, Gianaroli L; ESHRE Working Group on Poor Ovarian Response Definition. ESHRE consensus on the definition of 'poor response' to ovarian stimulation for in vitro fertilization: the Bologna criteria. Hum Reprod. 2011;26(7): 1616-24.
2. Poseidon Group (Patient-Oriented Strategies Encompassing IndividualizeD Oocyte Number); Alviggi C, Andersen CY, Buehler K, Conforti A, De Placido G, Esteves SC, et al. A new more detailed stratification of low responders to ovarian stimulation: from a poor ovarian response to a low prognosis concept. Fertil Steril. 2016;105(6):1452-3.
3. Alviggi C, Conforti A, Esteves SC, Vallone R, Venturella R, Staiano S, et al. Understanding Ovarian Hypo-Response to Exogenous Gonadotropin in Ovarian Stimulation and Its New Proposed Marker—The Follicle-To-Oocyte (FOI) Index. Front Endocrinol. (Lausanne). 2018;9:589.
4. Abu-Musa A, Haahr T, Humaidan P. Novel physiology and definition of poor ovarian response; clinical recommendations. Int J Mol Sci. 2020;21(6):2110.
5. Esteves SC, Carvalho JF, Bento FC, Santos J. A novel predictive model to estimate the number of mature oocytes required for obtaining at least one euploid blastocyst for transfer in couples undergoing in vitro fertilization/ intracytoplasmic sperm injection: The ART Calculator. Front Endocrinol (Lausanne). 2019;10:99.

6. Alviggi C, Conforti A, Santi D, Esteves SC, Andersen CY, Humaidan P, et al. Clinical relevance of genetic variants of gonadotrophins and their receptors in controlled ovarian stimulation: a systematic review and meta-analysis. Hum Reprod Update. 2018;24:599-614.
7. Conforti A, Esteves SC, Cimadomo D, Vaiarelli A, Di Rella F, Ubaldi FM, et al. Management of women with an unexpected low ovarian response to gonadotropin. Front Endocrinol (Lausanne). 2019;10:387.
8. Humaidan P, Chin W, Rogoff D, D'Hooghe T, Longobardi S, Hubbard J, et al. Efficacy and safety of follitropin alfa/lutropin alfa in ART: a randomized controlled trial in poor ovarian responders. Hum Reprod. 2017;32: 544-55.
9. Alsbjerg B, Haahr T, Elbaek HO, Laursen R, Povlsen BB, Humaidan P. Dual stimulation using corifollitropin alfa in 54 Bologna criteria poor ovarian responders—a case series. Reprod Biomed Online. 2019;38:677-82.
10. Sunkara SK, Coomarasamy A, Faris R, Braude P, Khalaf Y. Long gonadotropin-releasing hormone agonist versus short agonist versus antagonist regimens in poor responders undergoing in vitro fertilization: A randomized controlled trial. Fertil Steril. 2014;101:147-53.
11. De Geyter C, Fehr P, Moffat R, Gruber IM, von Wolff M. Twenty years' experience with the Swiss data registry for assisted reproductive medicine: outcomes, key trends and recommendations for improved practice. Swiss Med Wkly. 2015;145:w14087.
12. Zhang Y, Zhang C, Shu J, Guo J, Chang HM, Leung PCK, et al. Adjuvant treatment strategies in ovarian stimulation for poor responders undergoing IVF: a systematic review and network meta-analysis. Hum Reprod Update. 2020;26(2): 247-63.
13. Haahr T, Esteves SC, Humaidan P. Individualized controlled ovarian stimulation in expected poor-responders: an update. Reprod Biol Endocrinol. 2018;16(1):20.

Total Fertilization Failure: What Next?

Keshav Malhotra

INTRODUCTION

In the realm of assisted reproductive technologies (ART), in vitro fertilization (IVF) and intracytoplasmic sperm injection (ICSI) stand as groundbreaking methods designed to overcome various infertility challenges. These techniques, which involve the fusion of sperm and egg outside the body, have offered hope to countless individuals and couples aspiring to build families. However, even in the face of technological advancements, not every IVF or ICSI attempt results in the anticipated fertilization. Total fertilization failure (TFF) represents a perplexing and disheartening outcome that warrants comprehensive exploration.

Despite the high success rates reported in ART procedures, TFF emerges as a rare but formidable challenge. TFF is characterized by the absence of fertilized eggs, commonly known as zygotes, following the attempted union of sperm and egg. This unforeseen outcome can be emotionally distressing for individuals and couples who have invested not only their hope but also their substantial resources into the process.

While TFF is considered rare, the precise incidence varies across different studies.[1] The understanding of contributing factors is crucial in managing expectations and tailoring treatment plans for those facing this unique challenge.

MECHANISMS OF FERTILIZATION FAILURE

Fertilization, the intricate dance between sperm and egg, is a finely orchestrated process governed by numerous factors. When this intricate ballet falters, TFF may ensue, leaving individuals and couples grappling with the complexities of infertility. Understanding the mechanisms behind fertilization failure is pivotal in unraveling the mysteries surrounding TFF.

Before delving into the aberrations leading to TFF, it is imperative to grasp the delicacy of the normal fertilization cascade which includes:

- *Sperm maturation and capacitation:* Sperms undergo a series of changes, known as capacitation, during their journey through the female reproductive tract. This process primes them for penetration of the egg's protective layers.
- *Egg activation:* Upon encountering a mature sperm, the egg undergoes activation, initiating a series of events that culminate in the formation of a zygote. Key among these events is the fusion of the sperm and egg pronuclei, uniting the genetic material.
- *Zygote formation:* The fusion of genetic material results in the formation of a zygote, the first step in embryonic development.

Understanding the intricacies of normal fertilization allows us to identify the deviations that lead to TFF.[2] Fertilization failure can be attributed to factors related to sperm, egg, laboratory conditions, and the complex interplay between these elements. **Box 1** summarizes the various factors that can be associated with TFF.[3,4]

Sperm-related factors:

- *Abnormalities in sperm count:* In cases of oligospermia (low sperm count) or severe asthenospermia (poor sperm motility), the chances of successful fertilization diminish.
- *Sperm morphology issues:* Abnormal sperm morphology, characterized by structural defects, can impede the sperm's ability to penetrate the egg.
- *Sperm dysfunction:* Impaired sperm function, including deficient acrosomal reaction or compromised DNA integrity, may hinder successful fertilization.

BOX 1: Factors contributing to total fertilization failure (TFF).

Mechanisms and factors contributing to TFF:
- *Sperm-related factors:* Abnormalities in sperm count, motility, or morphology
- *Egg-related factors:* Oocyte quality, maturation issues, or abnormalities in the zona pellucida
- *Laboratory and technical factors:* Inadequate culture conditions, errors in gamete handling, or issues during the insemination process
- *Interaction factors:* Complex interactions between sperm and egg that may not align optimally

Egg-related factors:
- *Oocyte quality:* The quality of the egg is paramount. Age-related decline in egg quality, as well as abnormalities in oocyte maturation, can lead to fertilization failure.
- *Zona pellucida abnormalities:* The zona pellucida, the protective layer surrounding the egg, plays a crucial role. Abnormalities in its structure or composition may prevent sperm penetration.

Laboratory and technical factors:
- *Culture conditions:* Inadequate culture conditions in the laboratory can compromise the viability of both sperm and eggs, leading to TFF.
- *Gamete handling errors:* Mishandling of gametes during the various stages of IVF or ICSI, from retrieval to insemination, can result in fertilization failure.

Interaction factors:
- *Failure of sperm–egg recognition:* Complex interactions between sperm and egg involve intricate signaling.[5] Failure in the recognition and binding process can impede fertilization.
- *Deficient sperm–egg fusion:* Even if recognition occurs, abnormalities in the fusion process may hinder the formation of a zygote.

CLINICAL IMPLICATIONS OF TOTAL FERTILIZATION FAILURE

The occurrence of TFF introduces a spectrum of clinical considerations, spanning from diagnostic challenges to emotional repercussions on individuals and couples navigating the intricate landscape of infertility.
- *Diagnostic dilemmas in identifying TFF:*
    - *Assessment of fertilization rates:* The initial challenge lies in accurately assessing fertilization rates, distinguishing TFF from cases of low fertilization.
    - *Confirmation of TFF:* The use of advanced imaging techniques, like time-lapse imaging, provides valuable insights into the dynamics of fertilization and aids in confirming TFF.
- *Psychological impact on patients:* The emotional toll of TFF extends beyond the clinical realm, impacting the mental well-being of those hoping for success in their fertility journey. Understanding and addressing the psychological aspects of TFF is integral to holistic patient care.
- *Ethical considerations in communicating TFF:* Open and transparent communication about TFF is essential, raising ethical considerations related to informed consent, patient autonomy, and the delicate balance between hope and realism.

INCIDENCE AND RISK FACTORS OF TOTAL FERTILIZATION FAILURE

Understanding the incidence and risk factors associated with TFF is essential for both clinicians and individuals undergoing ART. A nuanced comprehension of these aspects allows for better-informed decision-making, personalized treatment plans, and improved counseling for those navigating the challenges of infertility.

Prevalence of Total Fertilization Failure

Varied incidence rates:
- The incidence of TFF varies across different studies and clinical settings.
- Reported rates range from <1% to around 5%,[1] highlighting the rarity of this outcome but emphasizing the need for awareness.

Impact of treatment centers:
- Differences in laboratory techniques, equipment, and expertise among ART centers contribute to variations in TFF rates.
- Centers with advanced technologies and experienced staff may exhibit lower incidences.

Demographic and Clinical Risk Factors

Female age as a predominant factor:
- Advanced maternal age is a well-established risk factor for TFF.
- Declining egg quality and increased chromosomal abnormalities in eggs contribute to higher failure rates.

Male factor infertility:
- Male-related factors, like poor sperm quality, may contribute to fertilization failure.

- Techniques like ICSI may be employed to address specific male infertility issues.

Ovulatory dysfunction: Irregularities in ovulation, hormonal imbalances, or disorders affecting egg release may increase the risk of TFF.

Previous ART cycles:
- Individuals with a history of TFF in previous ART cycles may be at a higher risk of recurrence.
- Tailored interventions and adjustments may be considered for subsequent cycles.

Impact of Female Age on Fertilization Success

Age-related decline in fertility:
- Female fertility declines with advancing age, with a notable drop after the age of 35 years.
- Increased chromosomal abnormalities in eggs contribute to a higher likelihood of TFF in older women.

Optimal reproductive age: The age range of 20–35 years is generally associated with the highest fertility rates and lower risks of TFF.

Individualized counseling: The impact of female age on fertility underscores the importance of individualized counseling for couples, considering both partners' age and reproductive health.

STRATEGIES FOR PREVENTION OF TOTAL FERTILIZATION FAILURE

Preventing TFF in ART is a multifaceted challenge that requires a comprehensive approach. Strategies encompass pre-IVF screening, optimization of laboratory conditions, and the integration of innovative techniques.[6] Understanding and addressing potential risk factors are central to designing preventive measures and enhancing the overall success rates of ART cycles.

Pre-IVF Screening and Counseling

Comprehensive health assessment:
- Conduct a thorough health assessment of both partners, including medical history, lifestyle factors, and any preexisting conditions.
- Identify and address potential risk factors that may contribute to TFF.

Genetic screening: Perform genetic screening to assess chromosomal abnormalities and potential genetic factors that may impact fertilization.

- Provide counseling on the implications of identified genetic factors and potential alternative reproductive options.

Hormonal evaluation:
- Assess hormonal levels to identify any imbalances or irregularities in ovulation.
- Optimize hormonal balance through medication or lifestyle modifications as needed.

Individualized counseling:
- Offer individualized counseling sessions to discuss the risks associated with age, lifestyle factors, and potential challenges in the ART process.
- Set realistic expectations and explore alternative reproductive options when necessary.

Optimization of Laboratory Conditions

Quality control measures:
- Implement stringent quality control measures in the laboratory, including regular equipment maintenance and calibration.
- Monitor and maintain optimal temperature, humidity, and gas levels to create an ideal environment for gametes.

Staff training and certification:
- Ensure that laboratory staff receives ongoing training and certification in the latest ART techniques and best practices.
- Foster a culture of continuous improvement and adherence to standardized protocols.

Innovative techniques to improve fertilization rates:
- Integrate advanced technologies such as time-lapse imaging to monitor and optimize embryo development in real-time.
- Consider intracytoplasmic morphologically selected sperm injection (IMSI) for cases of male factor infertility to enhance sperm selection.

Addressing Male Factor Infertility

Sperm quality improvement:
- Implement lifestyle changes such as a balanced diet, regular exercise, and avoidance of tobacco and excessive alcohol to enhance sperm quality.
- Consider antioxidant supplementation to mitigate oxidative stress on sperm.

Intracytoplasmic sperm injection for male factor infertility:

- In cases of known male factor infertility, opt for ICSI to directly inject a morphologically selected sperm into the egg.
- This targeted approach increases the chances of successful fertilization.

Continuous Monitoring and Adjustment

Feedback mechanisms:

- Establish regular feedback mechanisms between clinical and laboratory teams to identify and address any challenges or anomalies during the ART process.
- Conduct regular reviews of clinical outcomes to inform adjustments in protocols.

Adaptive protocols:

- Develop adaptive protocols that can be tailored to individual patient profiles and specific challenges identified during the ART process.
- Modify stimulation protocols, culture conditions, or insemination techniques based on ongoing assessments.

MANAGEMENT APPROACHES AFTER TOTAL FERTILIZATION FAILURE

Total fertilization failure in ART can be emotionally challenging for individuals and couples aspiring to build a family. Effective management strategies following TFF involve a thorough understanding of the causes, personalized assessment, and the development of a tailored plan for future ART cycles. The outlines various approaches to guide clinicians and individuals through the post-TFF phase are outlined below.

Review of Treatment Options

Root cause analysis:

- Conduct a comprehensive review of the factors contributing to TFF, including sperm and egg quality, laboratory conditions, and any identified issues during the ART cycle.
- Collaborate with both clinical and laboratory teams to identify specific points of failure.

Consultation with fertility specialists:

- Schedule a consultation with fertility specialists to discuss the implications of TFF and explore potential modifications to treatment plans.
- Consider additional diagnostic tests, such as genetic or hormonal assessments, to gather more information.

Considerations for Future In Vitro Fertilization/Intracytoplasmic Sperm Injection Cycles

Tailored treatment plans:

- Develop personalized treatment plans based on the insights gained from the analysis of the previous TFF cycle.
- Modify stimulation protocols, culture conditions, or insemination techniques to address identified challenges.

Advanced techniques and technologies:

- Integrate advanced technologies, such as time-lapse imaging or IMSI, to enhance fertilization success in subsequent cycles.
- Consider additional interventions, like preimplantation genetic testing (PGT), to identify embryos with the highest developmental potential.

Oocyte Activation

Oocyte activation refers to the process by which an oocyte is stimulated to undergo the events leading to the formation of a zygote after fertilization. In the context of TFF, where fertilization does not occur despite the introduction of sperm and oocytes in ART procedures like IVF or ICSI, oocyte activation mechanisms become particularly relevant.

When TFF occurs, it is crucial to explore and address potential issues related to the activation of the oocyte. In conventional IVF, fertilization involves the natural penetration of the sperm through the zona pellucida and the fusion with the oocyte. In the cases of TFF, ICSI is often employed as an alternative. During ICSI, a single sperm is directly injected into the oocyte to facilitate fertilization. However, even with ICSI, the subsequent steps of oocyte activation must occur for successful fertilization.

Oocyte activation agents: Some cases of TFF may be associated with abnormalities in the oocyte activation process. Oocyte activation agents are substances or techniques used to stimulate the activation of an oocyte, leading to the initiation of events that result in the formation of a zygote. These agents are particularly relevant in cases of ART, such as IVF or ICSI, where fertilization failure has occurred, and additional measures are needed to promote successful oocyte activation. One commonly used oocyte activation agent is a calcium ionophore. This agent can trigger the rise of intracellular calcium levels in the oocyte, mimicking the natural activation process that occurs after sperm penetration.

Calcium ionophores: Calcium ionophores facilitate the influx of calcium ions into the oocyte, triggering the intracellular signaling cascades that are essential for oocyte activation. In natural fertilization, the sperm-induced rise in intracellular calcium is a crucial step for the oocyte to resume meiosis and progress to the formation of a diploid zygote. When fertilization fails to occur after standard insemination or ICSI, calcium ionophores can be used to artificially induce the rise in intracellular calcium levels, mimicking the physiological process triggered by sperm entry.

Calcium ionophores are typically administered shortly after the ICSI procedure or after insemination to coincide with the expected time of natural oocyte activation. Studies have suggested that the use of calcium ionophores can improve fertilization rates in cases where previous fertilization failures have occurred.[7] However, the success may vary, and careful patient selection is crucial. The safety of using calcium ionophores is an area of ongoing research. While they have been shown to be effective in certain cases, concerns have been raised about potential adverse effects on embryo development, and further studies are needed to assess their safety profile.

Alternative Reproductive Options

Donor gametes:
- Discuss the possibility of using donor sperm or eggs in cases where TFF is attributed to severe male or female factor infertility.
- Provide comprehensive counseling regarding the implications of using donor gametes and address any emotional or ethical concerns.

Surrogacy:
- Explore the option of surrogacy, especially in cases where both partners face challenges in carrying a pregnancy to term.
- Ensure legal and ethical considerations are thoroughly discussed with all parties involved.

Emotional Support and Counseling

Psychological counseling:
- Offer psychological counseling to individuals and couples experiencing the emotional impact of TFF.
- Address feelings of grief, disappointment, and anxiety while providing support in navigating future decisions.

Support groups:
- Facilitate participation in support groups where individuals can share experiences, coping strategies, and insights.
- Create a supportive community to alleviate the sense of isolation often associated with fertility challenges.

Ethical Considerations and Informed Decision-making

Informed consent:
- Prioritize open and transparent communication during the informed consent process for future ART cycles.
- Ensure individuals and couples have a comprehensive understanding of the risks, alternatives, and potential outcomes.

Patient autonomy:
- Empower individuals and couples to make informed decisions about their reproductive journey.
- Respect patient autonomy in choosing alternative reproductive options or pursuing further ART cycles.

Research Participation and Future Options

Clinical trials and research participation:
- Discuss the option of participating in clinical trials or ongoing research studies focused on addressing fertilization challenges.
- Contribute to the advancement of ART by exploring innovative interventions and techniques.

Exploration of new options:
- Stay informed about emerging technologies and interventions in the field of reproductive medicine.
- Consider exploring novel options as they become available and undergo rigorous evaluation.

CONCLUSION

The management of individuals and couples after TFF involves a thorough review of previous cycles, personalized treatment planning, emotional support, and exploration of alternative reproductive options. By addressing the physical, emotional, and ethical dimensions of the post-TFF phase, clinicians and individuals can collaboratively navigate the complexities of infertility and make informed decisions about their reproductive journey.

REFERENCES

1. Goksan Pabuccu E, Sinem Caglar G, Dogus Demirkiran O, Pabuccu R. Uncommon but devastating event: total fertilisation failure following intracytoplasmic sperm injection. Andrologia. 2016;48:164-70.
2. Kahyaoglu I, Demir B, Turkkanı A, Cınar O, Dilbaz S, Dilbaz B, et al. Total fertilization failure: is it the end of the story? J Assist Reprod Genet. 2014;31:1155-60.
3. Swain JE, Pool TB. ART failure: oocyte contributions to unsuccessful fertilization. Hum Reprod Update. 2008;14: 431-46.
4. Flaherty SP, Payne D, Matthews CD. Fertilization failures and abnormal fertilization after intracytoplasmic sperm injection. Hum Reprod. 1998;13 Suppl 1:155-64.
5. Combelles CM, Morozumi K, Yanagimachi R, Zhu L, Fox JH, Racowsky C. Diagnosing cellular defects in an unexplained case of total fertilization failure. Hum Reprod. 2010;25:1666-71.
6. Centers for Disease Control and Prevention; American Society for Reproductive Medicine; Society for Assisted Reproductive Technology. 2010 Assisted Reproductive Technology National Summary Report. Atlanta: US Department of Health and Human Services; 2012.
7. Campos G, Sciorio R, Esteves SC. Total fertilization failure after ICSI: insights into pathophysiology, diagnosis, and management through artificial oocyte activation. Hum Reprod Update. 2023;29:369-94.

16 Chapter

Empty Follicle Syndrome: Causes and Further Line of Treatment

Sonia Malik, Aneesha M Grover

INTRODUCTION

The term empty follicle syndrome (EFS) was first coined by Coulam et al. in 1986. They defined EFS as failure to retrieve oocytes from normally growing follicles after ovarian stimulation.[1]

Empty follicle syndrome is an extremely rare condition occurring in women undergoing in vitro fertilization (IVF) treatment. Its incidence as reported in literature is 0.045–3.5% of IVF cycles.[2] It is associated with a recurrence rate of 15% in subsequent cycles.[3] The risk for recurrence increases with increasing age and is as high as 57% in women over 40 years of age.[4]

ETIOPATHOGENESIS OF EMPTY FOLLICLE SYNDROME

Many theories have been put forward to explain the occurrence of EFS.

Age is one of the major associated factors for the occurrence of EFS. The incidence of EFS increases with increasing age due to ovarian aging and altered folliculogenesis. In fact, Revelli et al. found that the prevalence of EFS is five times higher in women >40 years of age compared to younger women.[5]

Inan et al. suggested that alteration in folliculogenesis due to ovarian aging leads to EFS. In altered folliculogenesis, there is early atresia of the oocyte but with continued growth of the follicle.[6] They also found alteration in 160 genes in a patient who had developed EFS.[6]

There is a mixed opinion regarding association of EFS with *ovarian reserve*. While some studies found a higher prevalence of EFS in patients with low ovarian reserve, there were others who found a higher occurrence of EFS in polycystic ovary syndrome (PCOS) patients with antral follicle count (AFC) >15 and anti-Müllerian hormone (AMH) >5 ng/mL.[2] Madani et al. found higher occurrence of EFS in patients with poor ovarian reserve with AMH <1 ng/mL and AFC <4.[7]

Studies have also been conducted to evaluate the role of the *stimulation protocol* in the occurrence of EFS. While Singh et al. and Baum et al. found the incidence highest in antagonist protocols, Madani et al. found its occurrence maximum in microdose flare protocols.[2,7,8]

The physiopathology of EFS varies with the *type of trigger injection* used. Human chorionic gonadotropin (hCG) has a direct action on the ovary and thus EFS with hCG trigger may be due to altered folliculogenesis or abnormal response of the ovary to the hCG.[9] Inadequate exposure to hCG to cause oocyte detachment from the follicular wall and variation in the efficacy of the hCG due to batch-to-batch variations are some other theories for the occurrence of EFS.[2] It is believed that when there is insufficient amounts of bioactive hCG, oocyte meiotic maturation is not triggered, cumulus expansion does not ensue, and the immature oocyte-cumulus complexes are resistant to follicular aspiration, thereby resulting in EFS.[10]

On the other hand, EFS with gonadotropin-releasing hormone (GnRH) agonist trigger may be due to the inability of the pituitary to release luteinizing hormone (LH) which is sufficient to trigger ovulation, or there is failure in one of the mediators/receptors of the ovary.[9]

Genetic basis for EFS is one more theory which has been postulated. It has been found that EFS is associated with paternally transmitted heterozygous missense mutation of c.400 G>A (p.Ala134Thr) in zona pellucida glycoprotein 3 (ZP3).[11] It was found that the oocytes in females carrying this mutation lacked zona pellucida. When mutant and wild ZP3 are coexpressed, there is decreased interaction between the ZP2 and ZP3, leading to absent communication between cumulus cells and the oocyte, which ultimately resulted in oocyte degeneration and empty follicles.[11]

Another genetic cause of EFS can be due to the loss-of-function mutations of LHCGR (luteinizing hormone/choriogonadotropin receptor), which is a glycoprotein hormone receptor belonging to the G-protein coupled receptor family. It is inherited as a recessive genetic trait. There is defective beta-hCG binding to its receptor and is associated with defective folliculogenesis and ovulation.[12]

Patients with GnRH receptor polymorphism or hypogonadotropic/hypogonadal patient with endogenous levels of LH and follicle-stimulating hormone (FSH) below 1.2 IU/L are also at risk of EFS if they are given GnRH agonist as trigger. This occurs due to inadequate surge of gonadotropins after receiving GnRH agonist trigger.[12]

TYPES OF EMPTY FOLLICLE SYNDROMES

Grossly, EFS has been subclassified into two subtypes: Genuine EFS (G-EFS) and false EFS (F-EFS).

Genuine Empty Follicle Syndrome

Failure to retrieve oocytes in spite of good hCG levels on day of ovum pickup (OPU) is considered to be G-EFS. The cause of G-EFS may be due to some genetic mutation. While Yuan et al.[13] found a homozygous mutation in LHCGR gene, Chen et al. found a heterozygous missense mutation of c.400 G>A (p.Ala134Thr) in ZP3 as possible reason for EFS.[2] G-EFS accounts for 33% of all cases of EFS.[14] Diagnosis is made when serum hCG at time of oocyte retrieval (OCR) is >40 IU/L at time of occurrence of EFS.[15] Since in G-EFS there is failure to retrieve oocytes from mature ovarian follicles after ovulation induction for IVF, in spite of apparently normal follicular development and steroidogenesis and in the presence of optimal hCG levels on the day of OCR, these patients are unlikely to respond to a rescue protocol.[14] Also, the chances of recurrence of EFS is high in subsequent cycle.

False Empty Follicle Syndrome

Failure to retrieve oocytes in patients who are diagnosed to have a low hCG (hCG <40 IU/L) on the day of OPU is considered as false type of EFS.[15] The low levels may be due to either low bioavailability of the hCG or improper method of administration of the hCG in the form of wrong timing, wrong method of administration, or problems in manufacturing, packaging, and storage of the drug.[9] F-EFS accounts for 67% of all EFS cases.[14] Diagnosis is made when serum hCG at time of OCR is <40 IU/L at time of occurrence of EFS.[15] Since, in F-EFS, there is failure to retrieve oocytes in the presence of low hCG due to an error in the administration or the bioavailability of hCG on the day of OCR, these patients are more likely to respond to a rescue protocol.[12] Also, the chances of recurrence of EFS in subsequent cycle are very low.

Table 1 summarizes the basic differences between G-EFS and F-EFS.

PREDICTION OF EMPTY FOLLICLE SYNDROME

Some of the factors which may be used as red flags to warn us about the possibility of encountering EFS at the time of OCR are:

- Ovarian aging/advanced maternal age
- Poor ovarian reserve

TABLE 1: A comparison between genuine and false empty follicle syndrome (EFS).

	False EFS	*Genuine EFS*
Definition	Failure to retrieve oocytes in spite of good serum human chorionic gonadotropin (hCG) levels at the time of ovum pickup	Failure to retrieve oocytes due to insufficient levels of serum hCG at the time of ovum pickup
Incidence	33% of all EFS	67% of all EFS
Causes	• Genetic mutation • Advanced maternal age with oocyte aging • Decreased ovarian reserve	Low bioavailability of hCG due to: • Fault in drug manufacturing, packaging, transport, storage • Fault in time of administration
Diagnosis	Circulating hCG at time of oocyte retrieval is >40 IU/L	Circulating hCG at time of oocyte retrieval is <40 IU/L
Prognosis	Unlikely to respond to rescue protocol	Likely to retrieve oocytes with rescue protocol
Risk of recurrence	High	Low

- Long duration of stimulation
- High doses of gonadotropins
- Slower response to stimulation
- Premature luteinization of follicles due to a premature LH surge
- High progesterone (P) levels on the day of hCG injection
- Too short an interval between the onset of preovulatory follicular changes and follicular aspiration
- History of EFS in previous IVF cycle.

MANAGEMENT (FLOWCHART 1)

After GnRH agonist trigger, LH levels peak at 4 hours and then onward decreases. If LH is <15 IU/L and progesterone (P4) <3.5 ng/mL at 8–12 hours after trigger, then the chances of encountering EFS are high.[9]

Preventive measures for occurrence of F-EFS is taking a blood sample at 12–24 hours after triggering, or measurement of urine LH 4-6 hours after triggering and taking appropriate action in case of abnormal results.[12]

At time of OCR, if there is occurrence of empty follicles, measures which can be taken for further management include the following:[12]

- Check the functioning and pressures of the suction pump.
- Do a urinary LH or urinary hCG test on the operation table. If negative, blood sample to be drawn for further testing.
- Measure the serum LH level in case of a GnRH agonist trigger. If LH at 36 hours after trigger is <8 IU/L, it indicates that the trigger was not taken 36 hours before. In case of hCG trigger, serum hCG of <6 IU/L indicates negative result.[12,15]
- Rescue of the cycle may be attempted with a second trigger with hCG and a retrieval done 24–36 hours after the repeat trigger.
- Determine hCG levels after 24 hours after the trigger and if negative, repeat hCG trigger followed by OPU after 24–36 hours.

The concept of rescue cycle in case of EFS was introduced in 1997 by Ndukwe et al.[16] Many studies have been conducted to evaluate the usefulness of this novel technique of rescue trigger. Stevenson et al. conducted a literature review on this and found that 42.8% of cycles undergoing rescue trigger followed by repeat OCR procedure resulted in a healthy newborn baby.[14] However, Reichman et al. in 2010 conducted a large, single case series study and their results were not so promising.[10] They found this protocol was associated with lower egg yield, postmaturity of oocytes, higher incidence of triploidy, and lower implantation rates.[10] However, in 2012, Reichman et al. conducted another study to evaluate the effectiveness of rescue cycle. In patients with negative serum hCG in the morning after trigger injection, a second intramuscular (IM) hCG trigger was administered, and retrieval was

Flowchart 1: Management options in empty follicle syndrome (EFS).[11]

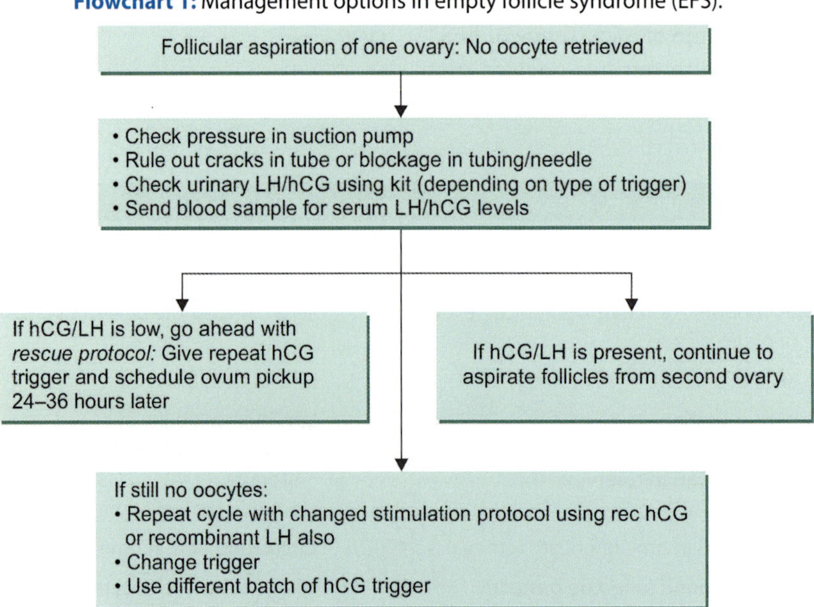

(hCG: human chorionic gonadotropin; LH: luteinizing hormone)

postponed by 24 hours. The live birth rate was 39.0% in this cohort of patients. They concluded that early detection and repeat trigger injection successfully prevented EFS and salvaged the IVF cycle.[17]

ROLE OF DUAL TRIGGER

It is known that oocyte maturation and follicular rupture are time-bound processes and may vary in different women. Some women may exhibit a delayed expansion of cumulus and detachment of oocyte, which may ultimately result in empty follicles at the time of OCR. It was theorized that addition of an agonist trigger to conventional hCG trigger may induce FSH surge along with LH surge, which is more physiological and mimics a natural cycle, unlike hCG trigger which causes only LH surge. This FSH surge not only helps in nuclear maturation, resumption of meiosis, and cumulus expansion but also induces LH receptor formation on the granulosa cells.

Noushin et al. conducted a study to evaluate whether sequential administration of GnRH agonist and hCG as a trigger at 40 hours and 36 hours, respectively, before OCR could correct G-EFS.[18] All women who had G-EFS in their first cycle were given dual trigger in their next cycle. They were administered GnRH agonist (Decapeptyl 0.4 mg; Ferring) and recombinant hCG (Ovitrelle 250 μg; Merck Serono) subcutaneously at 40 hours and 36 hours, respectively, as the trigger before OCR. Post trigger, their LH and beta-hCG values were evaluated at 8 hours and 12 hours, respectively, to confirm the action of the trigger. They were able to successfully retrieve oocytes in 92.31% of their cases and none of the patients had premature rupture of follicles or ovarian hyperstimulation syndrome (OHSS). Their study found a positive role of dual trigger in the management of G-EFS.

Similar findings were found by Lok et al., and they postulated that GnRH agonist provides a more physiological stimulus with an endogenous LH surge, which is more effective than the pharmacological stimulus provided by the LH surge subsequent to the hCG administration.[19,20]

CONCLUSION

Empty follicle syndrome is a rare condition encountered at the time of OCR in an IVF cycle.

It is important to recognize the high-risk factors for occurrence of EFS such as advanced maternal age, prolonged duration of stimulation, and requirement of high doses of gonadotropins for stimulation. In such cases, adequacy of LH surge should be checked in the morning after the trigger injection and repeat trigger to be given if found to be inadequate.

Timely on-table diagnosis is also important with urinary kit for LH/hCG in order to decide regarding *rescue protocol*. As per literature, a pregnancy rate of 39% is seen after rescue protocol and thus it may be a useful modality to salvage the cycle.

In patients undergoing a repeat IVF cycle and who had EFS in previous cycle, it may be useful to change the protocol and the trigger injection. Careful monitoring post trigger also needs to be done to check for adequacy of LH surge.

Also, counseling of the patients regarding the possibility of recurrence and future poor prognosis is imperative.

The optimal treatment and the prognosis in case of EFS are still not understood completely and large, multicenter studies are required to increase our understanding of this condition.

REFERENCES

1. Coulam CB, Bustillo M, Schulman JD. Empty follicle syndrome. Fertil Steril. 1986;46:1153-5.
2. Singh N, Dalal V, Kriplani A, Malhotra N, Mahey R, Perumal V. Empty follicle syndrome: a challenge to physician. J Hum Reprod Sci. 2018;11:274-8.
3. Baum M, Machtinger R, Yerushalmi GM, Maman E, Seidman DS, Dor J, et al. Recurrence of empty follicle syndrome with stimulated IVF cycles. Gynecol Endocrinol. 2012;28:293-5.
4. Zreik TG, Garcia-Velasco JA, Vergara TM, Arici A, Olive D, Jones EE. Empty follicle syndrome: evidence for recurrence. Hum Reprod. 2000;15:999-1002.
5. Revelli A, Carosso A, Grassi G, Gennarelli G, Canosa S, Benedetto C, et al. Empty follicle syndrome revisited: definition, incidence, aetiology, early diagnosis and treatment. Reprod Biomed Online. 2017;35:132-8.
6. Inan MS, Al-Hassan S, Ozand P, Coskun S. Transcriptional profiling of granulosa cells from a patient with recurrent empty follicle syndrome. Reprod Biomed Online. 2006; 13:481-91.
7. Madani T, Jahangiri N. Empty follicle syndrome: The possible cause of occurrence. Oman Med J. 2015;30:417-20.
8. Baum M, Machtinger R, Yerushalmi GM, Maman E, Seidman DS, Dor J, et al. Recurrence of empty follicle syndrome with stimulated IVF cycles. Gynecol Endocrinol. 2012;28:293-5.
9. Blazquez A, Guillén JJ, Colomé C, Coll O, Vassena R, Vernaeve V. Empty follicle syndrome prevalence and management in oocyte donors. Hum Reprod. 2014;29(10):2221-7.

10. Reichman DE, Hornstein MD, Jackson KV, Racowsky C. Empty follicle syndrome—does repeat administration of hCG really work? Fertil Steril. 2010;94(1):375-7.
11. Chen T, Bian Y, Liu X, Zhao S, Wu K, Yan L, et al. A Recurrent Missense Mutation in ZP3 Causes Empty Follicle Syndrome and Female Infertility. Am J Hum Genet. 2017;101(3):459-65.
12. Choudhary SD, Mishra V. Empty Follicular Syndrome: Understanding Controversial Entity. J South Asian Feder Obst Gynae. 2017;9(2):113-7.
13. Yuan P, He Z, Zheng L, Wang W, Li Y, Zhao H, et al. Genetic evidence of "genuine" empty follicle syndrome: a novel effective mutation in the LHCGR gene and review of the literature. Hum Reprod. 2017;32:944–53.
14. Stevenson TL, Lashen H. Empty follicle syndrome: the reality of a controversial syndrome, a systematic review. Fertil Steril. 2008;90:691-8.
15. Doyle JO, Attaman JA, Styer AK, Sabatini ME, Petrozza JC, Toth TL. Rescue human chorionic gonadotropin for false empty follicle syndrome: optimism for successful pregnancy outcome. Fertil Steril. 2012;98(2):450-2.
16. Ndukwe G, Thornton S, Fishel S, Dowell K, Aloum M, Green S. 'Curing' empty follicle syndrome. Hum Reprod. 1997;12: 21-3.
17. Reichman DE, Greenwood E, Meyer L, Kligman I, Rosenwaks Z. Can in vitro fertilization cycles be salvaged by repeat administration of intramuscular human chorionic gonadotropin the day after failed injection? Fertil Steril. 2012;98(3):671-4.
18. Noushin AM, Singh S, Sonia A, Singh S, Basheer R, Ashraf R, et al. Genuine empty follicle syndrome: role of double trigger and delayed oocyte retrieval (DTDO). J Hum Reprod Sci. 2021;14:36-41.
19. Lok F, Pritchard J, Lashen H. Successful treatment of empty follicle syndrome by triggering endogenous LH surge using GnRH agonist in an antagonist down-regulated IVF cycle. Hum Reprod. 2003;18:2079-81.
20. Revelli A, Carosso A, Grassi G, Gennarelli G, Canosa S, Benedetto C. Empty follicle syndrome revisited: definition, incidence, aetiology, early diagnosis and treatment. Reprod Biomed Online. 2017;35(2):132-8.

Chapter

Supplements to Enhance Male Infertility: Are They Actually Needed?

Kedar N Ganla, Rana Choudhary

INTRODUCTION

Male infertility is still a Pandora's box.[1] Exposure to radiation, smoking, varicocele, infection, urinary tract infection, environmental factors, nutritional deficiencies, and oxidative stress contribute to male infertility.[2,3] Oxidative stress to the sperms occurs if there is increase in reactive oxygen species (ROS) as compared to the natural antioxidant defenses of body.[4] This could be due to various reasons, such as exposure to raised temperature, electromagnetic waves, air pollution, insecticides, consumption of excessive tobacco and alcohol, obesity as well as malnutrition.[5]

Sperms are adversely affected by ROS and oxidative stress.[6-9] The plasma membrane of sperms consists of high levels of polyunsaturated fatty acids (PUFAs). This is required for flexibility. However, this also increases their vulnerability to ROS.[10,11] The sperm motility is adversely affected by lipid peroxidation and leads to reduced functional integrity of membrane cells. Further, increased ROS causes increase in sperm deoxyribonucleic acid (DNA) damage and mitochondrial membrane changes.[12]

The human semen contains various antioxidants naturally, like vitamins E and C, superoxide dismutase, glutathione, etc. These help in neutralization of free radical and have a protective effect on sperms.[4] Recent literature shows that oxidative injury leads to increase in male infertility (low sperm count and motility). This suggests that oral antioxidants may benefit in improving semen parameters of infertile men. However, some studies revealed paradoxical results.

Of the 90+ ingredients and combinations available in market, only 20 (22%) had any published evidence regarding sperm parameters and live birth rates as seen in **Table 1**. And only 15 (17%) showed a positive effect in one or more randomized controlled trial.[13]

TABLE 1: Common ingredients in supplements for improving sperm parameters.

Zinc	*Vitamin D*
Folate	Omega-3 fatty acids
Coenzyme Q10 (CoQ10)	Lycopene
Vitamin E	Selenium
Vitamin C	B-carotene
L-carnitine	Vitamin B_{12}
Arginine	

Other substances like N-acetyl cysteine (NAC), cryptoxanthin, inositol, α-lipoic acid, D-aspartic acid, PQQ, ashwagandha, and shilajit are also commonly seen.

COMPOSITION OF SUPPLEMENTS

These are a mixture of many vitamins, minerals, herbs, amino acids, and antioxidants. As these do not fall in the category of medicines, they are not subject to Food and Drug Administration (FDA) scrutiny.[14] Hence, the marketing and manufacturers can make all sorts of claims and sell these which may or may not work.[14] It has been seen that the content and dosage vary widely. While most supplements often contain naturally occurring compounds that may not harm the health but sometimes overdosage can do harm as seen in **Box 1**. Many do not even work in increasing the sperm count or pregnancy rates.[14] Unfortunately, there are not many randomized control trials (RCTs) in this area. These RCTs are expensive and complex to conduct.[14] **Box 2** enumerates the ingredients that have the most studies and seem to work best.

BOX 1: Side effects of excess supplements.

- High levels of iron, zinc, and calcium—gastrointestinal problems
- Excess of vitamin D—increased risk of kidney stones
- High vitamin B_6—neuropathy
- Excessively high levels of antioxidants can itself lead to infertility. When antioxidants in the body outnumber reactive oxygen species (ROS), unbalancing of body's natural homeostasis occurs leading to reductive stress. This is detrimental to sperms and adversely affects embryogenesis

BOX 2: Ingredients with the best-proven effectiveness.

- Vitamin E
- Vitamin C
- L-carnitine
- Coenzyme Q10 (CoQ10)
- Zinc

Vitamin C and Vitamin E

Vitamin C is a water-soluble vitamin and a good antioxidant and is important in hydroxylation and amidation processes. Ascorbic acid is needed in the synthesis of collagen, proteoglycan, and formation of the intercellular matrix. The seminal plasma contains high levels of vitamin C.[15] High levels of vitamin C in seminal fluid prevent damage to sperm DNA. Unlike vitamin C, vitamin E is a fat-soluble antioxidant. It neutralizes free radicals and also protects cellular membrane against O_2 free radical injury. Vitamin E has additive antioxidant action with other agents and prevents peroxidation of lipids.[16]

In a recent study, 1 g of vitamin E and vitamin C was given to infertile men for 2 months. At the end of 2 months, the sperm DNA fragmentation improved significantly in these men (p <0.001). Unfortunately, the other semen parameters remained unchanged.[17] It is a well-known fact that lesser DNA fragmented sperms gave better results in intracytoplasmic sperm injection (ICSI) and in vitro fertilization (IVF). Greco et al. concluded that 2 months therapy with these vitamins improved ICSI success rate.[18]

Carnitine

Carnitine, also known as 3-aminobutyric acid, is a semi-essential vitamin like substance. It is involved in intermediary metabolism for bioenergetic processes. It helps information of long-chain fatty acids. The epididymis contains 2,000 times higher concentration of carnitine through an active secretory process. A double-blind controlled clinical trial (2004) included 60 infertile men with oligoasthenoteratozoospermia (OATS). The intervention group received 2 g/day L-carnitine (LC) and 1 g/day L-acetyl carnitine (LAC) for 6 months. At the end of 6 months, the sperm motility was significantly increased particularly in men with baseline severe asthenozoospermia.[19] Another RCT by Balercia et al. including 60 men with idiopathic asthenoteratospermia also showed improvement in sperm motility. Nine women became pregnant in carnitine-treated men and five after LC plus LAC.[20] However, a study by Sigman et al. (2006) did not find any difference with carnitine supplementation.[21]

Coenzyme Q10/Ubiquinone

Coenzyme Q (CoQ) is a part of electron transport chain and helps in energy generation. It is an oil-soluble substance present in lipoproteins and membranes of cells. In a double-blind controlled trial by Balercia, it was observed that coQ10 supplementation increases sperm motility.[22] This was supplemented by a similar study by Safarinejad et al. (2012). However, trial by Nadjarzadeh et al. (2014) showed nonsignificant changes in semen parameters, such as density, motility, or morphology while total antioxidant capacity was increased significantly (p <0.05).[23] Other studies also proved that the concentration of CoQ10 was correlated with major semen parameters, such as count, motility, and morphology. A recent meta-analysis showed that CoQ10 does not increase pregnancy rates or live births, but there is an improvement in sperm parameters such as concentration and motility.[24]

Zinc

It is important in development of testis and maturation of sperms. Its deficiency can cause hypogonadism and problems with secondary sexual characteristics. It also causes a reduction in sperm fertilization. Zinc in seminal plasma binds with three types of protein (low molecular weight ligands, average molecular weight ligands, and high molecular weight ligands). Ebisch et al. found that 66 mg of zinc improved sperm count without any increase in motility.[25] Hadwan et al. gave 440 mg/day of zinc to OATS men for 3 months. This increased the volume, motility as well as sperm count. However, some studies found no improvement. Infertile men had higher peroxynitrite levels and nitric oxide (NO) synthase activity, which can be normalized after zinc supplementation.

Selenium and N-acetyl Cysteine

Selenium is important in sperm and testosterone biosynthesis. These selenoproteins are required for sperm structure integrity. NAC is a naturally occurring compound of amino acid L-cysteine. It is a precursor of glutathione peroxidase. It increases sperm counts, concentration, motility, and morphology in subfertile men.[26] A study of 468 men with idiopathic OATS supplemented with 30 weeks of selenium and NAC found reduction in serum follicle-stimulating hormone (FSH) and increase in testosterone and inhibin B along with improvement in all semen parameters. Administering selenium plus NAC resulted in further beneficial effects in semen parameters.[26]

MULTIPLE ANTIOXIDANT SUPPLEMENTATIONS

The role of multiple antioxidant supplementations for synergistic action is being studied in male infertility. Many studies have shown benefit of this combination therapy using 1,500 mg of LC, 60 mg vitamin C, 20 mg CoQ10, 10 mg vitamin E, 10 mg zinc, 200 µg folic acid, 50 µg selenium, and 1 µg vitamin B_{12} for 3 months. Antioxidant treatment improves sperm quality and maintains sperm DNA integrity.[27,28]

Many authors have studied the effect of LC on sperms and proved a positive relationship. A meta-analysis by Lafuente et al. demonstarted that CoQ10 supplementation results in significant improvement in motility and sperm count. However, there was no change in pregnancy rates.[6,28] Vitamin E and C did not increase the sperm count or motility, but improved sperm DNA damage. Use of multiple antioxidants leads to an increase in semen parameters.

CONCLUSION

Use of LC, vitamin C, vitamin E, and selenium may increase sperm count, motility, and morphology and can improve sperm DNA fragmentation too.[28] However, future research is needed to know the appropriate antioxidant composition, combinations, and dosage. Also, these should be taken with caution to prevent overdosage and its side effects.

REFERENCES

1. Irvine DS. Epidemiology and aetiology of male infertility. Hum Reprod. 1998;13 (Suppl 1):33-44.
2. Olayemi FO. A review on some causes of male infertility. Afr J Biotech. 2010;9(20):2834-42.
3. Wong WY, Thomas CM, Merkus JM, Zielhuis GA, Steegers-Theunissen RP. Male factor subfertility: possible causes and the impact of nutritional factors. Fertil Steril. 2000;73:435-42.
4. Tremellen K. Oxidative stress and male infertility-a clinical perspective. Hum Reprod Update. 2008;14:243-58.
5. Aitken RJ, De Iuliis GN. Origins and consequences of DNA damage in male germ cells. Reprod Biomed Online. 2007; 14:727-33.
6. Lafuente R, González-Comadrán M, Solà I, López G, Brassesco M, Carreras R, et al. Coenzyme Q10 and male infertility: a meta-analysis. J Assis Reprod Gen. 2013;30: 1147-56.
7. Makker K, Agarwal A, Sharma R. Oxidative stress and male infertility. Ind J Med Res. 2009;129:357-367.
8. Agarwal A, Said TM. Oxidative stress, DNA damage and apoptosis in male infertility: a clinical approach. BJU Int. 2005;95:503-7.
9. Saleh RA, HCLD AA. Oxidative stress and male infertility: from research bench to clinical practice. J Androl. 2002;23: 737-52.
10. Eskenazi B, Kidd S, Marks A, Sloter E, Block G, Wyrobek A. Antioxidant intake is associated with semen quality in healthy men. Hum Reprod. 2005;20:1006-12.
11. Sheweita SA, Tilmisany AM, Al-Sawaf H. Mechanisms of male infertility: role of antioxidants. Curr Drug Metab. 2005;6:495-501.
12. Hosen MB, Islam MR, Begum F, Kabir Y, Howlader MZH. Oxidative stress induced sperm DNA damage, a possible reason for male infertility. Iran J Reprod Med. 2015;13: 525-32.
13. Agarwal A, Baskaran S, Parekh N, Cho CL, Henkel R, Vij S, et al. Male infertility. Lancet. 2021;397(10271):319-33.
14. Ahmadi S, Bashiri R, Ghadiri-Anari A, Nadjarzadeh A. Antioxidant supplements and semen parameters: An evidence based review. Int J Reprod Biomed. 2016; 14(12):729-36.
15. Ko EY, Sabanegh ES. The Role of Over-the-Counter Supplements for the Treatment of Male Infertility-Fact or Fiction? J Androl. 2012;33:292-308.
16. Ross C, Morriss A, Khairy M, Khalaf Y, Braude P, Coomarasamy A, et al. A systematic review of the effect of oral antioxidants on male infertility. Reprod Biomed Online. 2010;20:711-23.
17. Greco E, Iacobelli M, Rienzi L, Ubaldi F, Ferrero S, Tesarik J. Reduction of the incidence of sperm DNA fragmentation by oral antioxidant treatment. J Androl. 2005;26:349-53.
18. Greco E, Romano S, Iacobelli M, Ferrero S, Baroni E ,Minasi MG, et al. ICSI in cases of sperm DNA damage: beneficial effect of oral antioxidant treatment. Hum Reprod. 2005;20: 2590-4.
19. Lenzi A, Sgro P, Salacone P, Paoli D, Gilio B, Lombardo F, et al. A placebo-controlled double-blind randomized trial of the use of combined l-carnitine and l-acetyl-carnitine treatment in men with asthenozoospermia. Fertil Steril. 2004;81:1578-84.

20. Balercia G, Regoli F, Armeni T, Koverech A, Mantero F, Boscaro M. Placebo-controlled double-blind randomized trial on the use of L-carnitine, Lacetylcarnitine, or combined L-carnitine and Lacetylcarnitine in men with idiopathic asthenozoospermia. Fertil Steril. 2005;84: 662-71.
21. Sigman M, Glass S, Campagnone J, Pryor JL. Carnitine for the treatment of idiopathic asthenospermia: a randomized, double-blind, placebo-controlled trial. Fertil Steril. 2006; 85:1409-14.
22. Balercia G, Buldreghini E, Vignini A, Tiano L, Paggi F, Amoroso S, et al. Coenzyme Q 10 treatment in infertile men with idiopathic asthenozoospermia: a placebo-controlled, double-blind randomized trial. Fertil Steril. 2009;91: 1785-92.
23. Nadjarzadeh A, Shidfar F, Amirjannati N, Vafa M, Motevalian S, Gohari M, et al. Effect of Coenzyme Q10 supplementation on antioxidant enzymes activity and oxidative stress of seminal plasma: a double-blind randomised clinical trial. Andrologia. 2014;46:177-83.
24. Lafuente R, González-Comadrán M, Solà I, López G, Brassesco M, Carreras R, et al. Coenzyme Q10 and male infertility: a meta-analysis. J Assis Reprod Gen. 2013;30: 1147-56.
25. Ebisch I, Pierik F, De Jong F, Thomas C, Steegers-Theunissen R. Does folic acid and zinc sulphate intervention affect endocrine parameters and sperm characteristics in men? Int J Androl. 2006;29:339-45.
26. Safarinejad MR, Safarinejad S. Efficacy of selenium and/ or N-acetyl-cysteine for improving semen parameters in infertile men: a double-blind, placebo controlled, randomized study. J Urol. 2009;181:741-51.
27. Abad C, Amengual M, Gosálvez J, Coward K, Hannaoui N, Benet J, et al. Effects of oral antioxidant treatment upon the dynamics of human sperm DNA fragmentation and subpopulations of sperm with highly degraded DNA. Andrologia. 2013;45:211-6.
28. Ahmadi S, Bashiri R, Ghadiri-Anari A, Nadjarzadeh A. Antioxidant supplements and semen parameters: an evidence based review. Int J Reprod Biomed. 2016;14(12): 729-36.

18

Chapter

Advanced Sperm Selection Techniques

Rahul Ramesh Salve

INTRODUCTION

The evolution of intracytoplasmic sperm injection (ICSI) has revolutionized the field of infertility treatment and has proven to be a boon for couples with male-factor infertility. The process of ICSI, however, bypasses the natural sperm selection, during its journey from the vagina to the ampulla of the fallopian tubes, and thus it is of utmost importance to select the most morphologically and functionally normal sperm, which would result in an euploid embryo with a good implantation potential. The sperm selection in ICSI is however subjective. A miniscule proportion of sperms out of the millions present are assessed, and this may be the reason for conflicting studies on the sperm morphology. Most studies have shown that during ICSI, normal forms are not predictive of either fertilization rates or pregnancy rates. It has also been observed that men with a complete absence of normal sperm morphology exhibited high rates of spontaneous pregnancy without assisted reproduction. Cases of globozoospermia, macrocephaly, decapitated sperm syndrome, and fibrous sheath dysplasia can be easily diagnosed with the conventional sperm parameters on fresh sample, but sperm morphology assessment has a very poor clinical impact not only in diagnostic investigation but also in the choice of ART (assisted reproductive technology) techniques.[1]

There is mounting evidence that suggests that an impairment of sperm DNA integrity causes a reduction of ART outcomes. For this reason, the selection of the most competent sperm cells, i.e., those with the highest fertilizing ability—is crucial to improve both laboratory and clinical outcomes following ART. In this regard, it is worth noticing that sperm selection based on physiological or molecular features has gained much interest from researchers. While traditional sperm selection techniques, mainly based on sedimentation or migration [swim-up and density-gradient centrifugation (DGC)], are useful to select motile, morphologically normal sperm, there is still room for improvement regarding their efficiency. For this reason, novel selection methods based on other sperm features, such as ultrastructure, surface cell proteins, or DNA integrity, have been developed in the last years. These approaches increase the likelihood of selecting structurally intact, viable, and mature sperm with an intact DNA prior to ART, thus enhancing fertilization, embryo development, and pregnancy rates. This provides the background for advanced sperm selection techniques, which may filter sperms as in the natural course and provide a better pool of sperms representative of the entire semen volume. These advanced techniques include IMSI (intracytoplasmic morphologically selected sperm injection), PICSI (physiological intracytoplasmic sperm injection), microfluidics, and MACS (magnetic-activated cell sorting).

THE NORMAL SPERM

According to the World Health Organization (WHO) Laboratory Manual for the Examination and Processing of Human Semen, sixth edition 2021, the normal sperm should have following characteristics[2] **(Fig. 1)**.

Head: Normal (ideal/typical) appearance of the head should be smooth, regularly contoured and generally oval in shape. There should be a well-defined acrosomal region comprising 40–70% of the head area. The acrosomal region should contain no large vacuoles, and not more than two small vacuoles, which should not occupy more than one-fifth of the sperm head. The postacrosomal region should not contain any vacuoles.

Midpiece: The midpiece should be slender, regular, and about the same length as the sperm head. The major axis

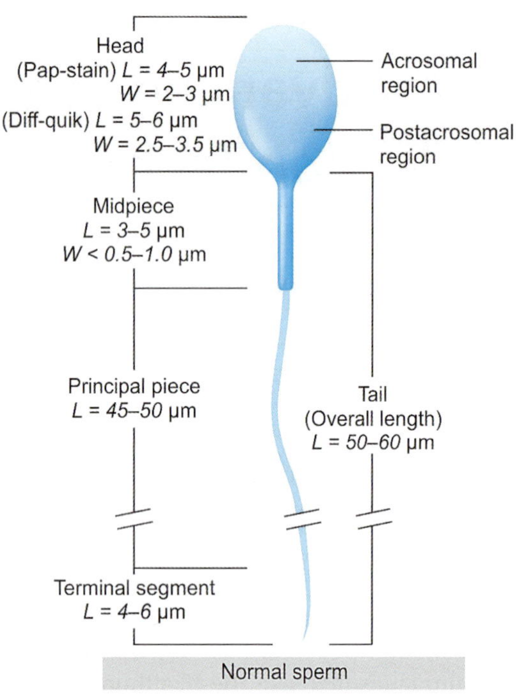

Fig. 1: Normal sperm. (L: length; W: width)

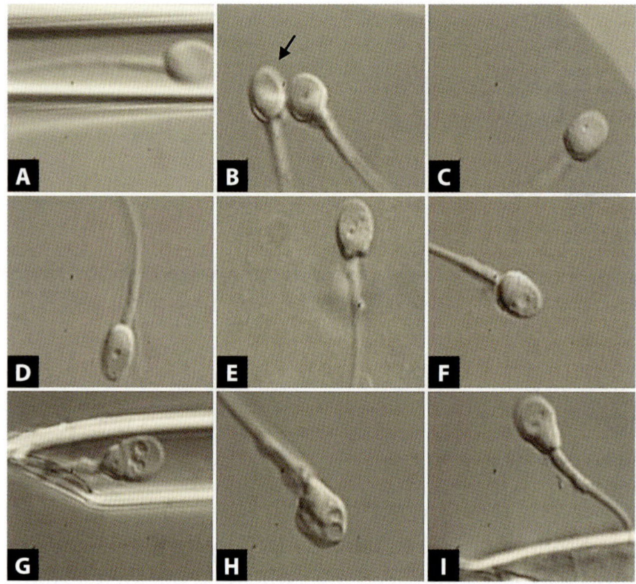

Figs. 2A to I: Classification of spermatozoa selected at 6,000 × magnification into three different categories. Class I (A, B, C)—spermatozoa of good quality; class II (D, E, F)—spermatozoa of poor quality; and class III (G, H, I)—spermatozoa of worse quality.[4]

of the midpiece should be aligned with the major axis of the sperm head.

Tail: The principal piece should have a uniform caliber along its length, be thinner than the midpiece, and be approximately 45 μm long (about 10 times the head length). It may be looped back on itself, provided there is no sharp angulation indicative of a broken flagellum.

Cytoplasmic residue: Cytoplasmic droplets (less than one-third of a normal sperm head size) are normal.

INTRACYTOPLASMIC MORPHOLOGICALLY SELECTED SPERM INJECTION/MOTILE SPERM ORGANELLE MORPHOLOGY EXAMINATION

The conventional ICSI uses 200–400 × magnification, which gives little details about the sperm morphology, especially about the sperm nucleus. IMSI or MSOME (motile sperm organelle morphology examination) was introduced by Bartoov et al. in 2001, by which the fine nuclear morphology of motile spermatozoa is examined in real time with an inverted light microscope equipped with high-power differential interference contrast (DIC) (Nomarski/DIC) optics (150 × magnification) enhanced by digital imaging (44 × magnification) to achieve a total magnification of over 6,000. This method can identify a motile spermatozoon with a normal nucleus, defined by an oval shape with a smooth configuration (length, 4.75 ± 0.28 μm; width, 3.28 ± 0.20 μm) and a normal nuclear content (with <4% of the nucleus occupied by vacuoles.[3]

The point of interest in this region is the number and size of vacuoles, especially the small ones. MSOME initially assessed six sperm organelles—namely, acrosome, postacrosomal lamina, nucleus, neck, tail, and mitochondria.[3] However, the sperm nucleus seems to be the important influencing factor. In addition to the normal shape and size, the presence of the nuclear vacuoles in the sperm head plays an important role in the outcomes **(Figs. 2A to I)**.

A sperm with a normal nuclear content is defined as having <4% of the nucleus occupied by vacuoles.[5] The prevalence of vacuoles is observed in both the normal as well as the abnormal-shaped spermatozoa, though some controversy exists about their distribution. Vacuoles were mainly located in the tip or middle area of the sperm.[6]

It has been suggested that sperm vacuoles should be regarded as normal features of the sperm head that occur naturally during the process of condensation of sperm nuclei, and should not be regarded as degeneration but as physiological changes that do not compromise the sperm quality.[7,8] Meanwhile, studies suggest that the presence of sperm vacuoles is related to male subfertility,[9]

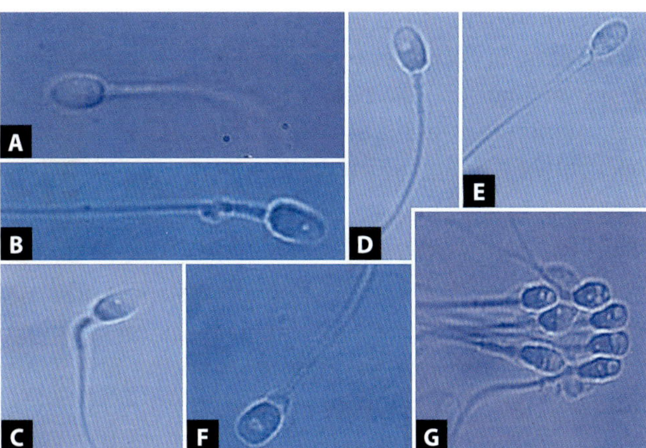

Figs. 3A to G: Grading of spermatozoa into four groups according to the presence or size of vacuoles. Grade I: Normal form and no vacuoles (A); Grade II: Normal form with less than or equal to two small vacuoles (B, C); Grade III: Normal form with more than two small vacuoles or at least one large vacuole (D, E); Grade IV: Large vacuole and abnormal head shapes or other abnormalities (F, G).[14]

lower mitochondrial membrane potential,[10] higher incidence of chromosomal abnormalities,[10,11] and sperm chromatin packaging/DNA abnormalities. Large vacuole was identified as an abnormal, "thumbprint"-like nuclear concavity covered by acrosomal and plasmic membranes.[12]

Although sperm count and motility were found to have no effect on the outcome of ICSI, scanning, and transmission electron microscopy indicated that the achievement of pregnancy may depend on normal morphology of the sperm nucleus.[13]

Based on the presence of vacuoles, sperm samples can be classified as (Vanderzwalmen's criteria) **(Figs. 3A to G)**:[5]

Grade I: Normal sperm without vacuoles

Grade II: Normal sperm with ≤2 small vacuoles covering <4% of the head

Grade III: Normal sperm with >2 small vacuoles and at least one large vacuole covering >4% of the head area

Grade IV: Large vacuole with other abnormalities.

INTRACYTOPLASMIC MORPHOLOGICALLY SELECTED SPERM INJECTION VERSUS CONVENTIONAL INTRACYTOPLASMIC SPERM INJECTION

IMSI in Male Factor Patients

Few randomized trials have evaluated the efficacy of IMSI over ICSI in couples with male-factor infertility. Souza Setti et al. and El Khattabi et al. observed a significantly higher clinical pregnancy rates with IMSI in patients with teratozoospermia.[15,16] Balaban et al. saw a significant progress in implantation rate (IR) after IMSI in male factor patients.[17] Contrary to these, Oliveira et al. did not observe a significant difference between IMSI and ICSI in terms of fertilization, embryo quality, and IRs and pregnancy rates, although a trend toward better outcomes in ongoing pregnancy rates, miscarriage rates (MRs), and live birth rates (LBRs) was reported.[18]

Few other studies observed that in patients with oligoasthenoteratozoospermia (OATS), IMSI was better to ICSI in terms of higher pregnancy rates and lower MRs.[11,19] Additionally, it was observed that in patients with sperm count <0.1 million, IMSI had a better influence on fertilization, IRs, and pregnancy rates. Mangoli et al. observed that sperm selection with MSOME criteria and IMSI can improve the embryo morphokinetics and clinical outcomes in couples with male-factor infertility.[20]

Intracytoplasmic morphologically selected sperm injection was observed to be beneficial over conventional ICSI in patients with abnormal sperms like globozoospermia[21] and macrocephalic sperm head[22] syndrome.

IMSI in Repeated Implantation Failure

Bartoov et al. was the first to compare IMSI versus conventional ICSI in patients with prior ICSI failures.[23] Though there was no difference in fertilization rate and number of embryos in both groups, higher pregnancy rates and lower MRs were observed in the IMSI group (66.0% vs. 30.0%; p <0.01; 33.0% vs. 9.0%; p <0.01, respectively). Following this, several other studies showed patients with two or more previous ICSI failure benefit more from IMSI in terms of not only increased pregnancy, but also lower MRs.[4,24,25]

In contrast to the above, Gatimel et al. did not find IMSI superior to ICSI in patients with previous two ICSI failures.[26] Unsuitable magnification at which ICSI was done and characteristics of male population are the plausible reasons for these contradictory conclusions. More prospective studies are needed to confirm these findings.

IMSI in Unselected Patients

Intracytoplasmic morphologically selected sperm injection has not been found to be superior to ICSI in improving ART outcomes in patients with unexplained infertility. No differences in fertilization rates, IRs, or pregnancy rates were observed between the two groups.[27] Additionally, patients with poor ovarian response to controlled ovarian stimulation (COS) did not benefit from sperm selection under high magnification prior to ICSI.[28] Thus, IMSI is not recommended for normozoospermic patients or couples undergoing in vitro fertilization (IVF) for the first time.

IMSI in Increased Sperm DNA Fragmentation Index

Hazout et al. measured sperm DNA integrity in 72 patients under IMSI and ICSI treatment. They observed improvement of IRs and birth rates, not only in patients with sperm DNA damage, but also in those with normal sperm DNA status.[25] Also, others recorded similar results in fertilization and good-quality embryos in patients with sperm DNA damage between sibling oocytes split into ICSI and IMSI groups.[29]

IMSI in Advanced Maternal Age

Advancing age has an effect on the quality of oocytes, which can affect the ICSI results. So, women with advanced age tend to have poor-quality oocytes and thus embryos after conventional fertilization. Cassuto et al. observed that the percentage of good-quality embryos was similar in young and old women (below and above 30 years) after IMSI, as the top-quality sperms selected by IMSI needed no repair.[30] Figueira Rde et al. studied the chromosomal status of embryos from couples with advanced maternal age in preimplantation genetic screening (PGS) cycles and observed that the incidence of sex chromosomal aneuploidy and chaotic embryos was significantly higher in ICSI embryos than in IMSI (23.5% vs. 15.0%, 27.5% vs. 18.8%, respectively).[31] Similarly, Luna et al. showed that IMSI procedure significantly improved the embryo quality and the IRs without affecting the chromosomal status of the embryos.[32]

IMSI in Advanced Paternal Age

It has been observed that the sperm parameters deteriorate with increasing age. A decrease in semen volume (3–22%), sperm motility (3–37%), and normal morphology (4–18%) have been observed between sperm samples of 30- and 50-year-old men.[33,34] Silva et al. observed that percentage of sperms with large nuclear vacuoles increase, and there is reduction in normal sperms with age.[35] Thus, a decrease in semen quality is observed with increasing age, and this may support the routine usage of IMSI/MSOME for sperm selection in ICSI for older men.

IMSI for Surgically Retrieved Sperms

Ai et al. evaluated the efficacy of IMSI for surgically retrieved sperms in patients with azoospermia. Though they did not observe any difference in the pregnancy rates, the MR was significantly less in the IMSI group (4.5% compared from 11.8%, respectively).[36] Gong et al. demonstrated that in patients with obstructive azoospermia and teratozoospermia, IMSI improves the fertilization rates and blastocyst formation rates.[37]

PHYSIOLOGICAL INTRACYTOPLASMIC SPERM INJECTION

Hyaluronan, a high-molecular-weight glycosaminoglycan, is a major component of the cumulus oophorus matrix surrounding the human oocyte. Similar to the binding observed between sperm and the zona pellucida, developmentally mature sperm bind to cross-linked hyaluronan gels and to hyaluronan chemically attached to a base structure.[38] The in vitro binding of sperm to hyaluronan is a selective process. Research has demonstrated that not all motile sperm bind to hyaluronan.[39] The understanding of the physiology underlying the binding of sperm to hyaluronan has been enhanced by the study of biochemical markers of human sperm development and function. Markers of human sperm development and function are enhanced in hyaluronan-bound (HB) sperm when compared with those parameters found in unbound sperm.[14,39-45]

Hyaluronan-bound sperm are devoid of DNA fragmentation (fDNA) and the apoptotic marker, caspase-3.[44] Most significantly, sperm bound to hyaluronan display a reduced frequency of chromosomal aneuploidies in comparison to their nonbinding counterparts.[43] Each of these biochemical and molecular parameters of developmental maturity play a critical role in the paternal contribution to successful preimplantation embryogenesis. The combined impact of fDNA and compromised levels of nuclear and cytoplasmic sperm maturation will adversely influence the developing embryo.

Hyaluronan Binding Assay®

The hyaluronan binding assay (HBA) is a diagnostic tool with dual hyaluronan-coated chambers for sperm sample evaluation. The sperm-HBA is designed to provide a qualitative assessment of sperm quality, maturity, and fertilizing potential. It allows to distinguish between mature sperm that express hyaluronan receptors and those that do not. Assessing the proportion of sperm with hyaluronan receptors can then be used to decide which treatment is best for a patient.

Each HBA slide **(Fig. 4)** has two identical chambers with a molecular layer of hyaluronan covalently attached to the chamber surface. These slides help to determine the hyaluronan-binding fraction of motile sperm in a semen sample. Mature, motile sperm bind with hyaluronan through specific receptors. 10 µL of semen sample is put in the chamber and covered by a cover slip. The chamber is incubated for 10 minutes, at room temperature (18°–28°C) to allow for complete binding. The number of bound and unbound motile sperms are then counted under the microscope. Bound motile sperm appear as ones with rapidly beating tails, but their heads showed no forward progressive movement, while unbound motile sperm swim around freely. The HBA score (%) is calculated as # bound motile sperm/# total motile sperm. The value of the HBA is based on the proposition that a low level of sperm binding to hyaluronan is suggestive that there is a low proportion of mature sperm in the sample.[46]

Interpretation of the HBA® Score Results

- *≥80% binding:* Normal maturity and physiological function
- *<80% binding:* Diminished maturity and physiological function.

The HBA® assay is shown to have good specificity and positive predictive values, although sensitivity was only 40%. Therefore, at a cutoff of <80% binding, it detects less than half of semen samples with truly low morphology, but among those detected as low HBA® score there is a strong prediction (>80%) of poor morphology. In a subsequent clinical trial with human outcomes, an HBA® score of 65% was used as the key cutoff.[47]

Hyaluronic acid (HA) has been shown to be capable of selecting spermatozoa with greater DNA integrity and normal morphology. Nasr-Esfahani et al. used HA-coated dishes **(Figs. 5A and B)** and found that the percentage of HA-bound (HB) spermatozoa were inversely correlated with abnormal sperm morphology, fDNA, and protamine deficiency in the semen sample.[48]

While Razavi et al. found hardly any difference in the fDNA in the sperms bound to hyaluronan with

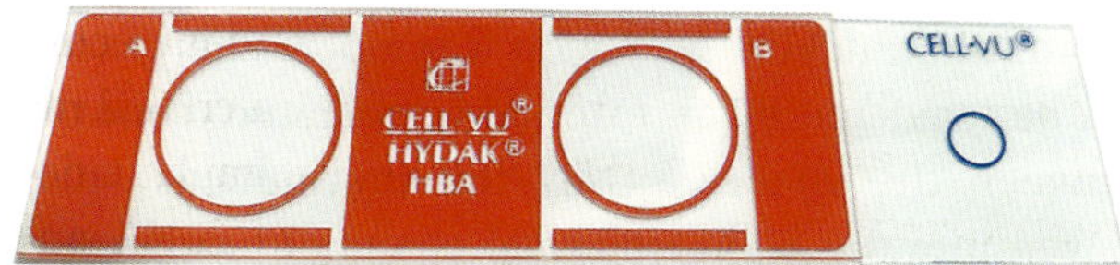

Fig. 4: Hyaluronan binding assay (HBA) chamber and the Cell-Vu grid cover slip.
Courtesy: NOVA IVF Fertility

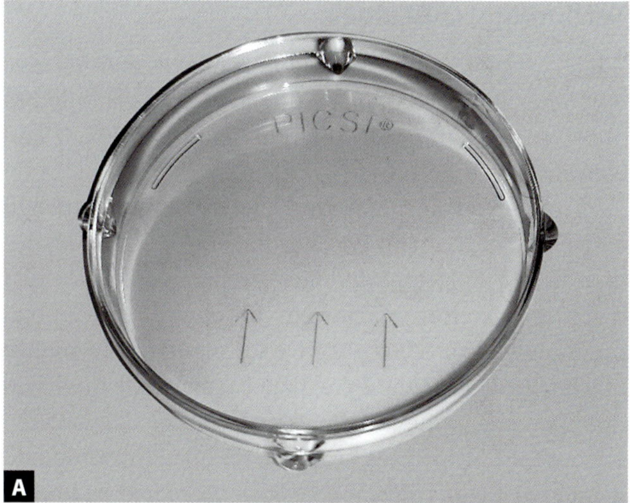

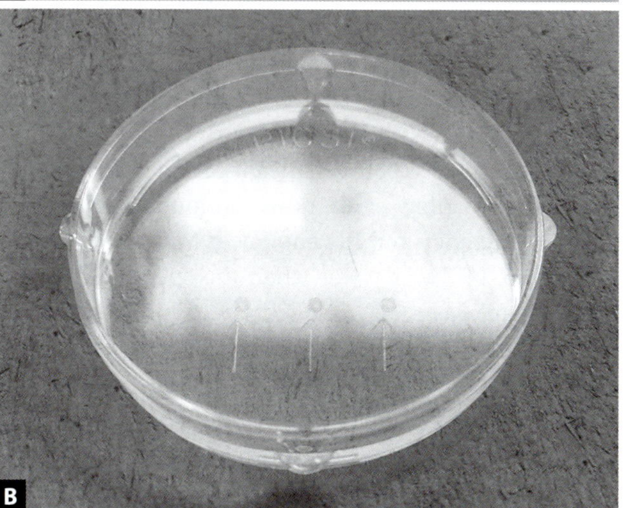

Figs. 5A and B: (A) Physiological intracytoplasmic sperm injection (PICSI) dish and (B) Hyaluronan dots in PICSI dish.
Courtesy (A): NOVA IVF Fertility

the unselected sperms,[49] others found lower fDNA in spermatozoa selected by HA-binding methods.[50-52]

Parmegiani et al.[50] and Huang et al.[53] compared the fDNA between the HB sperms and sperms obtained after swim-up and density-gradient (DG) processing techniques and reported lower fDNA in spermatozoa selected in HA solution compared to swim-up and DG continuous column. Mongkolchaipak[52] did DG on all the samples and then compared the fDNA between HB sperms and IMSI-selected sperms, no any difference was found. This may show that any added selection method is effective to some extent than no intervention.

Physiological Intracytoplasmic Sperm Injection and Assisted Reproductive Technology Outcomes

While few studies observed improvement in reproductive outcomes with PICSI, many other researchers failed to observe any significant difference between PICSI and conventional ICSI.

Erberelli et al. compared the outcomes between conventional ICSI and PICSI in patients with moderate-to-severe male-factor infertility. The parameters assessed were fertilization, cleavage, biochemical, clinical pregnancy, and MRs. PICSI had significantly higher biochemical and clinical pregnancy rates, while there was no difference in the abortion rate.[54] Kim et al. evaluated effect of PICSI in cases of severe teratozoospermia and compared it with conventional ICSI. PICSI had an impact in improvement of fertilization and embryo quality in cases with severe teratozoospermia.[55]

Contrary to these, Choe et al. did not observe any difference in blastulation rate, fertilization rate, and number of embryos between the PICSI and ICSI on sibling oocytes.[56] Worrilow et al., however, found significantly higher pregnancy and IRs and lower MRs in PICSI over ICSI. Also, LBR was lower when the sperm binding to hyaluronan was ≤65% in hyaluronan binding assay.[47] Similar findings were observed by Mokánszki et al.[57]

Liu et al. performed a sibling oocyte study by comparing polyvinylpyrrolidone (PVP)-ICSI and PICSI and observed that PVP-ICSI and PICSI had similar good-quality embryos while abnormal fertilization was higher in the PVP-ICSI group.[58] In a meta-analysis, Beck-Fruchter et al. did not find improved fertilization or clinical pregnancy rates with HA-ICSI, but did find improved embryo quality.[59] The meta-analysis included both randomized controlled trials and three sibling oocyte studies with varying inclusion criteria.

A recent Cochrane Review evaluating the effect of various advanced sperm selection techniques on IVF results did not find any difference between HA-ICSI and standard ICSI in LBR per woman randomized; however, a decrease in MR was observed with HA-ICSI.[60] The largest contributor to this meta-analysis was Miller et al. in which 2,772 couples undergoing ICSI were randomly assigned to receive either HA-ICSI or ICSI. The authors did not find any difference in LBR (the primary outcome), but a lower MR (secondary outcome) was observed.[61]

MICROFLUIDICS IN SPERM SELECTION

Microfluidics is the science which studies the behavior of fluids through microchannels and the technology of manufacturing microminiaturized devices containing chambers and tunnels through which fluids flow or/are confined. Fluids behave very differently on the micrometric scale than they do in everyday life: These unique features are the key for new scientific experiments and innovations. The key concept related to microfluidics is to integrate in a simple microsized system operations that commonly solicit a whole laboratory.

Mechanism of Action

A few million sperms reach the oocyte in the ampulla of the fallopian tube to fertilize it, after >200 million released after ejaculation in vagina during a normal intercourse. The sperms' journey is guided by mainly three mechanisms, i.e., chemotaxis, thermotaxis, and rheotaxis.[62-64] In an experiment by Xie et al., they used a microfluidic system where the chemoattractant (cumulus cells) in a double-way channel retrieved only about 10% of motile sperm cells.[65]

Thermotaxis mechanism refers to the movement of good quality sperm cells to a higher temperature gradient. Li et al. incorporated an interfacial valve in a microfluidic device by which a temperature gradient can be regulated by an external temperature controller between the spaces.[66] Only the thermotaxis sperm moved into the higher thermal chamber, while others move in other directions. In rheotaxis sperm move up long distance against a flow unlike chemotaxis and thermotaxis, which are short distance. Zaferani et al. used

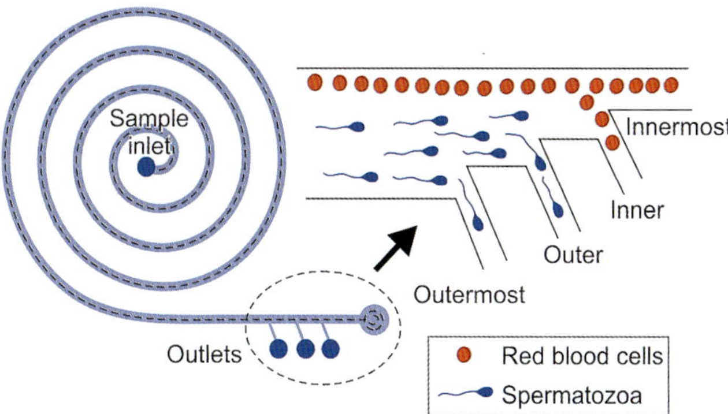

Fig. 6: Diagrammatic representation of the principle of passive microfluidics.
Source: Adaptation from Nsamela A. (2021). Microfluidics for sperm sorting: a review.

a rheotaxis microfluidic system to differentiate active from inactive sperms.[67]

Passive Selection in Microfluidic Sperm Sorting

Passive selection **(Fig. 6)** means cell separation based on density and size. Cells of different sizes and densities that will combat varying intensity of inertial forces in a circular microchannel. Larger cells move outward, while smaller cells remain inward toward the center.

Microfluidic Chips

A microfluidic chip is a pattern of microchannels, molded or engraved and linked to the macroenvironment by several holes of different dimensions hollowed out through the chip. It is through these pathways that fluids are injected into and evacuated from the microfluidic chip. Microfluidics allow the analysis and use of less volume of samples, chemicals, and reagents reducing the global fees of applications.[68]

An early insightful opinion on miniaturization and mini machines for biological applications was presented by Professor Richard P. Feynman (Nobel Laureate in Physics, 1965).[69] Droplet-based microfluidics manipulates and controls individual sections of fluid, rather than the bulk fluid flow. The main attractions of droplet-based microfluidics include a reduction in sample/reagents, faster reaction times, and increased control over dispersion, mixing, and separation.[70] Based on the fabrication and handling technique, the field itself can be further divided into two groups: Emulsion-based droplet microfluidics and digital microfluidics (DMF).

Emulsion-based Droplet Microfluidics

In emulsion-based droplet microfluidics, microdroplets are formed from the interaction of two immiscible fluids (such as oil and water- in continuous and dispersed phases, respectively). For ART application, this branch of microfluidics is very similar to what embryologists perform in clinical IVF, i.e., encapsulating the gamete in microdroplets covered with an oil overlay. Moreover, the technology can overcome many handling difficulties involving microdroplets in such clinical settings.[70]

Digital Microfluidics

Digital microfluidics is an emerging and very promising field in droplet-based microfluidics. Here, individual droplets (either in open or confined channels) can be precisely manipulated by noncontact forces such as electrical, magnetic, or thermal ones. The noncontact forces are of great benefit, especially for ART and IVF applications. DMF has a range of discrete fluidic operations for the manipulation of nanoliter to microliter droplets containing samples and reagents. Here, electric potential has been applied in series to array of patterned electrodes, which are coated with a hydrophobic insulator. DMF can address each reagent individually with no need for complicated networks of tubing or microvalves; it has the ability to control liquids relative to solids with no risk of clogging, and it is compatible with a large range of volumes, making it useful for preparative-scale sample handling.[71]

Fluids at the microscale are likely to suffer from forces that are typically insignificant at scales present in our everyday lives. Fluid at the scale of our typical environment is turbulent (undergoing irregular fluctuations), which leads to a particle within a stream of fluid moving in an unpredictable pattern. Turbulent flow depends on specific fluid characteristics (viscosity, density, and velocity) and the geometry of the channel, leading to the calculation of a value known as Reynold's number. As the scale of the channel reaches micrometer levels, the Reynold's number decreases. A decrease in Reynold's number below a threshold value brings the fluid flow in a laminar fashion, so that the flow within a channel becomes streamlined and predictable. Some of the advantages of utilizing a microfluidics platform include scalability, increased automation, and reduced turnaround times for male infertility diagnosis and treatment.[72,73]

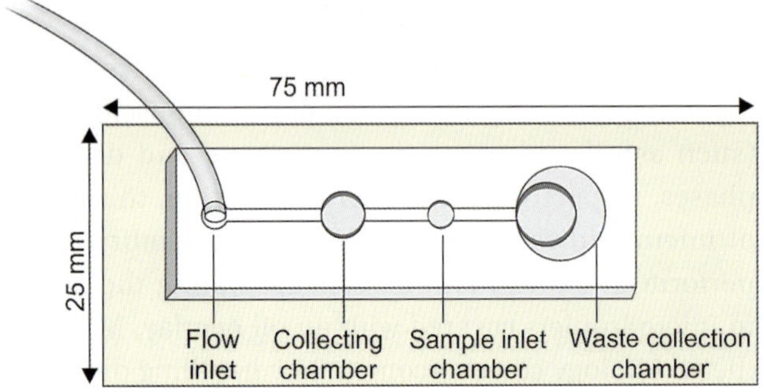

Fig. 7: Microfluidic chip for sperm selection.

A polydimethylsiloxane (PDMS) microfluidic biochip for sperm sorting is shown in **Figure 7**. This method collects highly active sperm from semen sample with the characteristic of laminar flow. A syringe pump with a small flow rate is combined with a microfluidic chip. Laminar flow is generated on a microscale and applied to sperm samples of varied concentration and mobility. A "flow cytometry analysis" of a PDMS microfluidic biochip was performed to verify the viability of sorted sperm from semen with the characteristic of laminar flow.[74] The result was more significant by at least 10% for both regular and oligozoospermia samples. Huang et al. explains a microfluidic system with three inlets and outlets for sorting motile sperm **(Figs. 8A and B)**.[75] The laminar flow characteristics have three parallel flows within a microfluidic chip. Only motile sperm can break through the boundary layer from their original laminar flow through the main channel because of their free-swimming property. This mechanism can, thus, separate motile sperm from nonmotile sperm and other particles. The velocity of the sperm is typically 70 µm/s. The motile sperm from the upper and lower inlets in the explained device can break through the stream boundary to the collection reservoir. The microfluidic system was designed to separate motile sperm, whereas nonmotile spermatozoa and debris flow along their initial streamlines and exit through outlet. In contrast, motile spermatozoa have an opportunity to swim into a parallel stream and exits through a separate outlet.

The Microfluidic Sperm Sorter Qualis (MSSQ) contains four chambers A, B, C, and D. These four chambers are connected by two parallel channels A–D and B–C. Media is added in chambers B, C, and D and laminar flow channels are allowed to form between the chambers. Sperm sample is added to chamber A. The laminar flow will help separate motile sperms form immotile sperms. The immotile sperms would passively flow in the direction

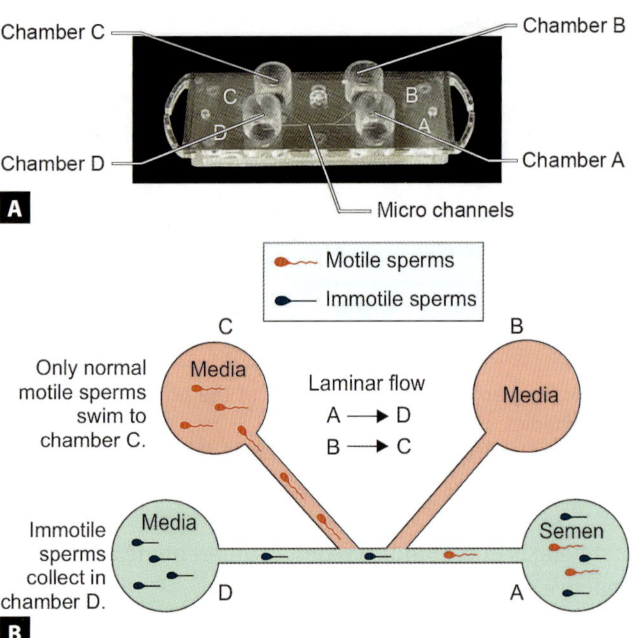

Figs. 8A and B: (A) Microfluidic device for isolation of motile sperm qualis and (B) Diagrammatic representation of the principle of the microfluidic sperm selection (MFSS) qualis.

of laminar flow A to D and thus collect in chamber D. While the motile sperms that can swim will swim up into the chamber C. After some time, only motile sperms would collect in chamber C, while immotile sperms would collect in chamber D.

Wu et al. explains, in the context of a microfluidic system, a "flowing upstream sperm sorter" (FUSS) device that is designed to replicate the selection mechanism found in the female body when sperm swims into the uterus **(Figs. 9A and B)**.[76] They proposed a microfluidic device capable of generating a retarding flow field for the sorting and separation of human motile sperm in a high-throughput manner. The proposed sorting/separation process begins with a rapid flow field in a straight-flow zone to carry sperm into a sorting zone to maintain the sperm's mobility. The sorting zone consists of a diffuser-type sperm sorter to differentiate sperm with different motilities based on the flowing upstream nature of human sperm in a retarding flow field. The dead sperm will then be separated from the live ones by passing through a dumbbell flow field to the outlet for disposal. The proposed FUSS is designed to imitate the selection mechanism found in the female body when sperm swim into the uterus. The experimental results demonstrate the utility of this device with regard to throughput (approximately

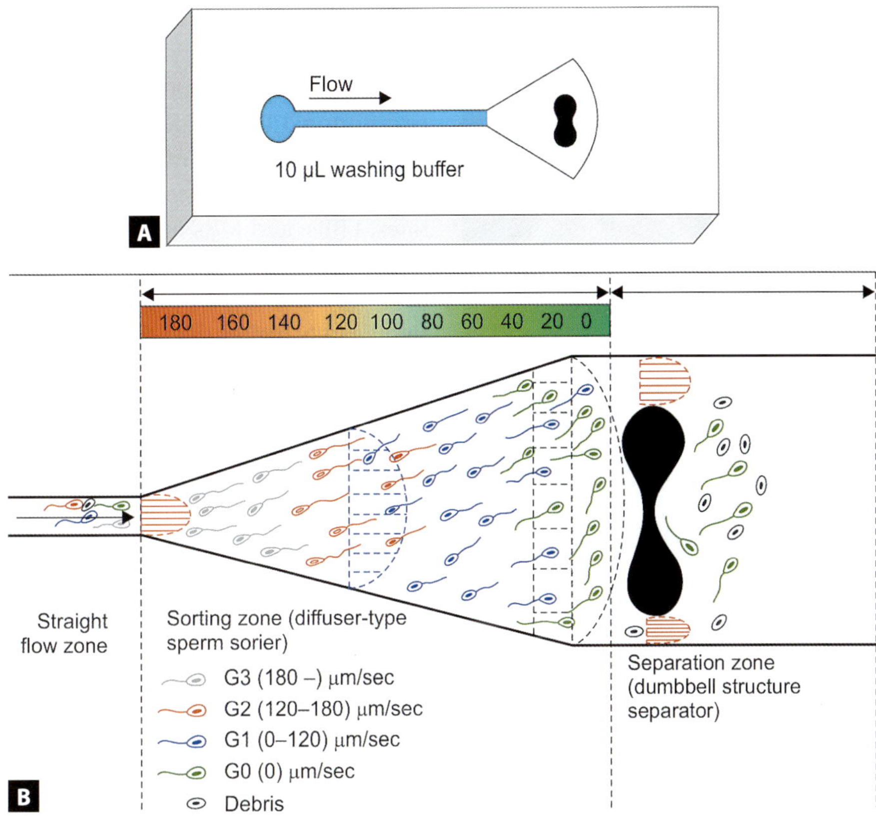

Figs. 9A and B: (A) Flowing upstream sperm sorter device and (B) Principle of flowing upstream sperm sorter.[77]

200,000 sperm/min and a maximum of 200 million cells/mL), efficiency (90% of selected sperm are mobile), and the ability to select sperm with high motility (~20% of sperm with a velocity exceeding 120 µm/s). The proposed device is suitable for intrauterine insemination as well as in vitro fertilization thanks to the highly efficient sorting process not interfering with the natural function and energy resource of human sperm. This system can rapidly (in 15 minutes) and gently sort sperm according to their motilities by a flow upstream sorting method that involves the retarding of the flow field.

ZyMōt MULTI (850 µL) SPERM SEPARATION DEVICE

ZyMōt devices separate sperm based on motility. Robles et al. did a study to determine if the use of the ZyMōt microfluidics sperm sorting device improves embryo development and euploidy rates compared to conventional DGC in patients undergoing ICSI with preimplantation genetic testing for aneuploidies (PGT-A).[78] Sample size of 86 patients were identified who had a prior ICSI/PGT-A cycle using DG for sperm preparation followed by an ICSI/PGT-A cycle using the ZyMōt microfluidics device for sperm preparation. A 1:1 comparison was performed that demonstrated a statistically significant difference in the average number of blastocysts as well as blastocyst rates obtained in the ZyMōt cycles versus the DG cycles. There was also a statistically significant difference in the euploidy rate in the ZyMōt cycles compared to the DG cycles **(Fig. 10)**.

Pujol et al. assessed whether the microfluidic-based device FertileChip® (now ZyMot®ICSI) can diminish the proportion of sperm with dsSDF.[79] This was a blinded split pilot study in which semen of nine patients diagnosed with ≥60% dsSDF (double-stranded sperm DNA fragmentation), was divided into three aliquots: Not processed, processed with FertileChip®, and processed with swim-up. The three aliquots were all analyzed using neutral COMET for the detection of dsSDF, resulting in a reduction of 46% (p <0.001) with FertileChip® (dsSDF: 34.9%) compared with the ejaculate and the swim up (dsSDF: 65%).

Kocur et al., studied if a sperm selection by ZYMOT can improve embryo ploidy. The basis of their study was that spermatozoa with the highest motility retain

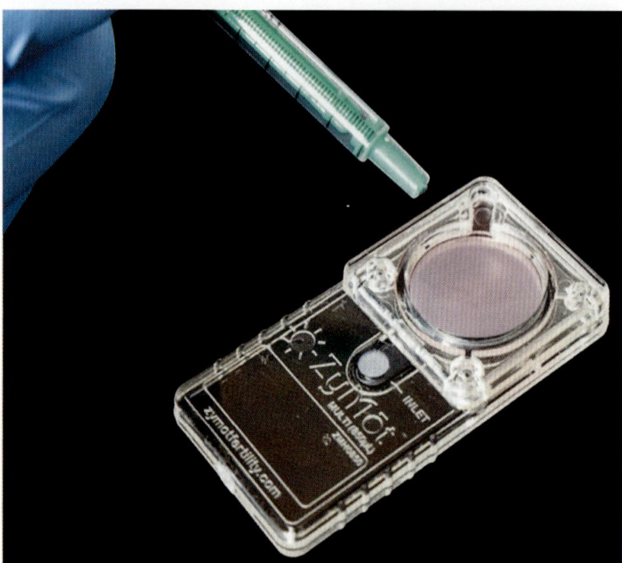

Fig. 10: ZyMōt device.

a superior genomic integrity and sperms with elevated sperm chromatin fragmentation (SCF) have been linked to poor reproductive outcomes.[80] Therefore, the utilization of a sperm selection method, such as microfluidic sperm selection (MFSS) (ZYMOT), is capable of reducing the SCF by yielding the most motile fraction of spermatozoa with the highest embryo developmental competence. Couples with a high incidence of embryo aneuploidy in a previous ICSI cycle with PGT-A were identified. These couples underwent subsequent ICSI/PGT-A cycles with MFSS. It was observed that MFSS prepared samples had significantly low SCF, and dsDNA compared to DG. The embryo euploidy rates remarkable improved from 25.3% in the DG cycles to 42.9% in the MFSS cycles ($p < 0.001$). Similarly, the IRs and clinical pregnancy rates were significantly higher in MFSS. They came to a conclusion, given the inverse relationship between SCF and motility, a selection of the most motile gamete by MFSS enhanced the proportion of spermatozoa with an intact genome, contributing to the generation of more euploid embryos that are capable of implanting and yielding increased term pregnancies.

Though MFSS helps in getting better-quality sperms with less fDNA, the overall impact on reproductive outcomes has not been conclusive. A study conducted by Yildiz et al. concluded that use of microfluidics in patients with previous failures results in better fertilization rates, but there is no significant improvement in pregnancy rates.[81]

Similarly, Ozcan et al. did not observe any difference in clinical pregnancy and ongoing pregnancy rates when microfluidic sperm selection was compared to conventional DG.[82] Yalcinkaya Kalyan et al. investigated the putative impact of microfluidics on sibling oocytes and did not find any significant difference in clinical pregnancy rates, LBRs, and MRs between the two groups.[77] Yetkinel et al. analyzed the microfluidics impact in unexplained infertility and observed that good-quality embryos are significantly higher than the control ICSI group, but there was no effect on fertilization rate, cleavage rate, or number of transferred embryos.[83]

A systematic review and meta-analysis by Ferreira Aderaldo et al. concluded that MFSS demonstrated marginal positive outcomes compared to standard sperm selection techniques in term of increasing pregnancy rates and decreasing MRs, but the difference is not statistically significant.[84]

MAGNETIC-ACTIVATED CELL SORTING

Magnetic-activated cell sorting is a method of sperm selection, which helps in identifying and removing apoptotic cells from the ejaculate. Apoptosis in testis removes abnormal spermatozoa and helps in maintaining testicular homeostasis of germ-cell population and testicular-nutrient availability.[85] Apoptotic mechanisms activate nuclear endonucleases, which lead to double-strand breaks on sperm DNA. Sperms with apoptotic DNA are implicated in implantation failure and miscarriages.[86] Sertoli cells help in eliminating sperms with apoptotic changes. Impairment in the clearing of apoptotic sperms by Sertoli cells or overactivity of testicular apoptosis can increase the population of apoptotic sperms in the ejaculate **(Figs. 11A to F)**.[87]

Phagocytes in the female genital tract can clear the apoptotic sperms by recognizing the externalized phosphatidylserine (PS) residues, and thus prevent the oocyte fertilization by these sperms.[88] However, this process is bypassed in ART. DGC or sperm swim-up cannot clear the apoptotic sperms because of their design to select motile sperm. Thus, the selection of nonapoptotic sperm relies solely at the subjective preference of the embryologist based on morphology which cannot differentiate between nonfunctional and viable sperm.

This issue is addressed by MACS technique, which identifies and eliminates apoptotic sperm cells[89] with externalized PS residues by annexin V-conjugated

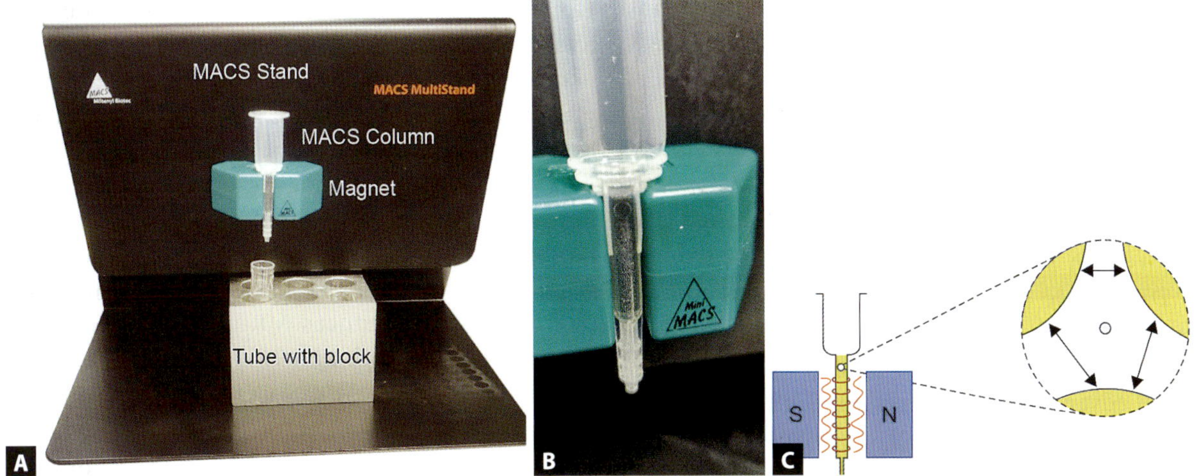

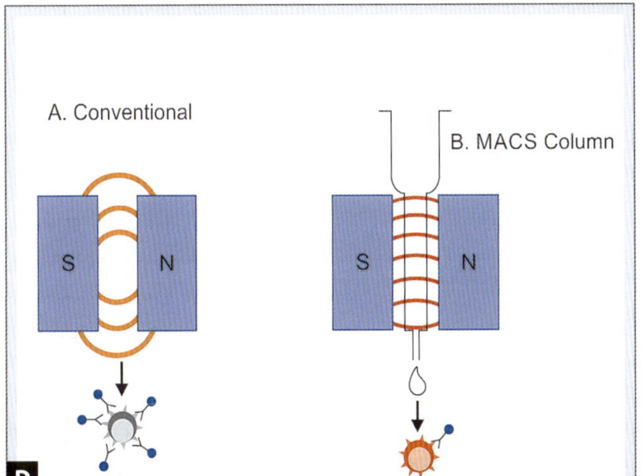

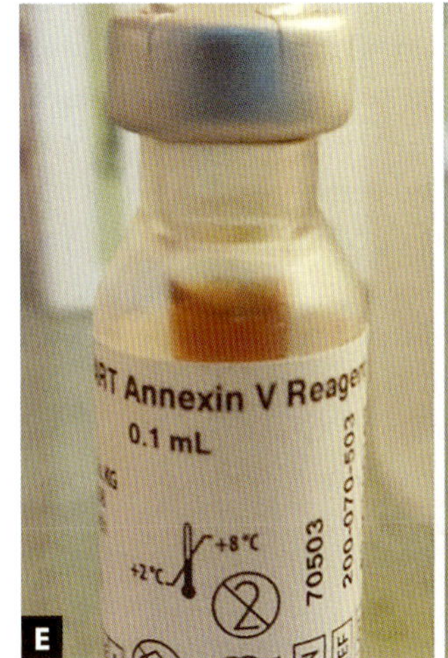

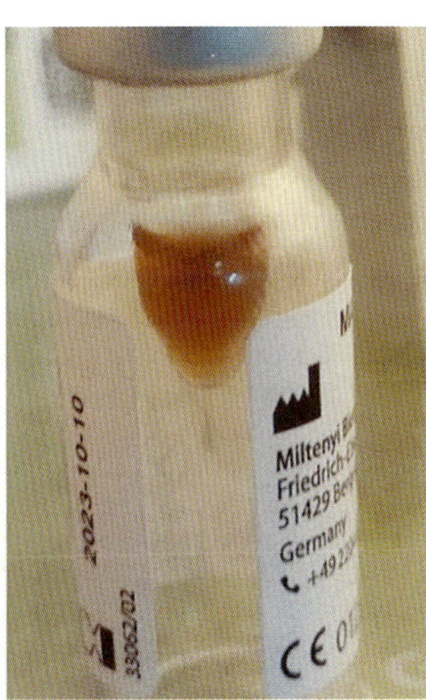

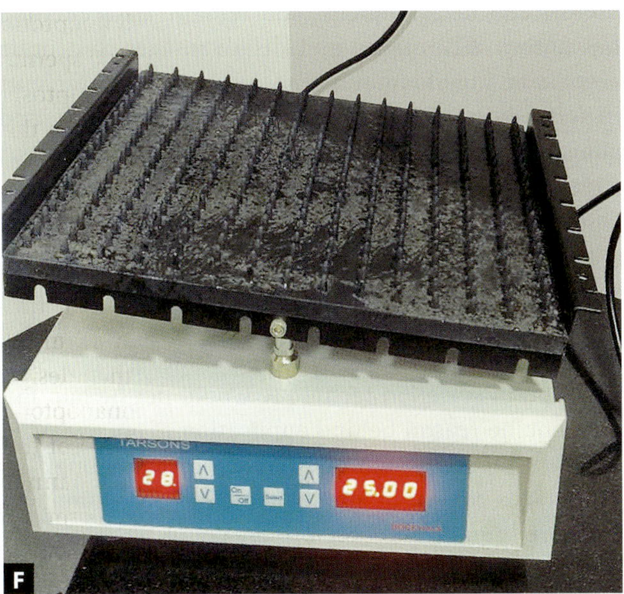

Figs. 11A to F: (A) Magnetic-activated cell sorting (MACS) assembly: MACS multistand, magnetic supporter, MACS column and test tube in a block; (B) MACS column with ferromagnetic spheres (close view); (C) Movement of sperms bound to beads between the ferromagnetic spheres in the column; (D) Comparison of magnetic field without column and in the presence of MACS column (magnetic field is 10,000 times stronger); (E) Annexin MicroBeads vial; (F) Shaker for thorough mixing of annexin beads with sperms.
Note: MACS MicroBeads are 50 nm in size and thus smaller than any other commercially available immunomagnetic beads for cell isolation. MACS MicroBeads are superparamagnetic, and therefore colloidal, i.e., they become magnetic when placed in a magnetic field. When removed from the magnetic field, they do not retain any residual magnetism. This feature of MACS MicroBeads is crucial, as particles with residual magnetism would aggregate quickly. MACS MicroBeads are biodegradable and nontoxic. Moreover, they have been designed to be compatible with any downstream application. MACS MicroBeads are conjugated to highly specific antibodies against a certain cell surface antigen. They bind specifically to cells expressing this antigen, thus preventing nonspecific labeling.[93]

superparamagnetic microbeads.[90-92] Population of sperms with fragmented DNA is reduced by MACS before ART procedures.

Magnetic-activated Cell Sorting and Assisted Reproductive Technology Outcomes

Magnetic-activated cell sorting is frequently suggested to patients with a high spermatic DNA fragmentation index (DFI), more than two unexplained ICSI failures and in certain cases, more than two miscarriages with an unknown female cause. The benefits of MACS as a method of advanced sperm selection technique on ART outcomes, however, is conflicting. Though some authors confirmed that MACS is useful in reducing the number of apoptotic sperms and thus improves overall embryo quality and pregnancy outcomes, many others did not observe any difference in the reproductive outcomes. Such discrepancies may be due to the great variability and low number of patients included in these studies.

Magnetic-activated cell sorting combined with DGC has been associated with a higher recovery of motile sperms, lower DFI, and an increase in the percentage of sperm with normal morphology.[94] Sperm selection via MACS have showed a reduction in spermatic fDNA when compared to the neat ejaculate from asthenoteratozoospermic, teratozoospermic, and normozoospermic men.[95,96] However, another study reported no significant improvement of sperm morphology, motility, fDNA, or markers of fertilization capability comparing MACS combined with swim-up or DGC against controls.[91]

A retrospective study by Pacheco et al. observed that the use of MACS group resulted in significantly lower MRs in autologous ICSI cycles, higher pregnancy rates in oocyte donation cycles, and a significant increase in LBRs in both autologous and oocyte donation cycles.[97] A systematic review and meta-analysis of only prospective randomized trials by Gil et al., to determine whether the use of MACS improves success rates in couples undergoing ART, found a statistically significant difference in pregnancy rate when compared with sperm preparation by DGC or swim-up, while IR and MR were statistically comparable.[98]

Gil Juliá et al. did a retrospective multicenter cohort study to determine the safety of MACS procedure in terms of obstetric and perinatal outcomes compared to conventional ICSI. There were no significant differences between the main obstetric and perinatal morbidities affecting the mothers and newborns' well-being between groups using either donated or autologous oocytes.[99] Similarly, Romany and colleagues compared obstetric and perinatal outcomes of MACS-ICSI cycles with swim-up-ICSI and concluded that MACS had no clinically relevant adverse effects for either mother or child.[85]

The Cochrane Database of Systematic Reviews for advanced sperm selection techniques for assisted reproduction, however, concluded that it is uncertain whether MACS improves either LBR or clinical pregnant rate, or if MACS reduces MR per woman or clinical pregnancy.[60] More high-quality and well-designed studies are required before MACS can be recommended for routine clinical use.

European Society of Human Reproduction and Embryology (ESHRE) good practice recommendations on add-ons in reproductive medicine recommend that there is insufficient evidence of an impact of MACS on pregnancy and LBRs compared to traditional sperm preparation methods.[100] Additionally, there are no data available regarding the safety of using MACS. So, MACS is currently not recommended for routine clinical use.

CONCLUSION

Selection of competent sperm with the highest fertilization potential is of utmost importance in ART. A number of methods have now been developed some of which mimic the natural selection processes that exist in the female reproductive tract. Although many studies have been conducted to identify the best technique, many doubts and disagreements still remain. Each method has shown advantages and disadvantages, but none seem to be superior at this time. Although improvements in fertilization, blastocyst formation, pregnancy, and clinical pregnancy is seen in some studies with all four sperm processing techniques, very few studies have shown significant improvement in LBRs. Also, very few studies have large sample size studies showing a positive outcome.

As seen in majority of the studies that female age is a major determinant of the outcome, drawing conclusion on a sperm selection technique would not be fair. But the genuine reason behind application of an advanced sperm selection technique could be that though its advantages cannot be predicted, there is definitely no negative impact. Another reason could be that these selection strategies provide a small number of potentially better sperms to choose from to inject into the oocyte.

Another very important scenario, in cases with very few or one mature oocyte for injection, it becomes even more wise to choose a selection strategy to justify the physical, psychological, and economical stress of the couple for a positive outcome.

Scientifically to say that one processing/selection technique is superior to other or to conventional ICSI, a large randomized control study has to be done, which is scarce at present. It is wise to choose a technique based on availability, affordability, and the expertise of the embryologist.

REFERENCES

1. Kovac JR, Smith RP, Cajipe M, Lamb DJ, Lipshultz LI. Men with a complete absence of normal sperm morphology exhibit high rates of success without assisted reproduction. Asian J Androl. 2017;19:39-42.
2. World Health Organization. WHO laboratory manual for the examination and processing of human semen, 5th edition.
3. Bartoov B, Berkovitz A, Eltes F, Kogosowski A, Menezo Y, Barak Y. Real-time fine morphology of motile human sperm cells is associated with IVF-ICSI outcome. J Androl. 2002;23:1-8.
4. Setti AS, Braga DP, Figueira RC, Iaconelli A Jr, Borges E. Intracytoplasmic morphologically selected sperm injection results in improved clinical outcomes in couples with previous ICSI failures or male factor infertility: a meta-analysis. Eur J Obstet Gynecol Reprod Biol. 2014;183:96-103.
5. Vanderzwalmen P, Hiemer A, Rubner P, Bach M, Neyer A, Stecher A, et al. Blastocyst development after sperm selection at high magnification is associated with size and number of nuclear vacuoles. Reprod Biomed Online. 2008;17:617-27.
6. Perdrix A, Travers A, Chelli MH, Escalier D, Do Rego JL, Milazzo JP, et al. Assessment of acrosome and nuclear abnormalities in human spermatozoa with large vacuoles. Hum Reprod. 2011;26:47-58.
7. Tanaka A, Nagayoshi M, Tanaka I, Kusunoki H. Human sperm head vacuoles are physiological structures formed during the sperm development and maturation process. Fertil Steril. 2012;98:315-20.
8. Watanabe S, Tanaka A, Fujii S, Mizunuma H, Fukui A, Fukuhara R, et al. An investigation of the potential effect of vacuoles in human sperm on DNA damage using a chromosome assay and the TUNEL assay. Hum Reprod. 2011;26:978-86.
9. Zhang S, Wang N, He B, Cheng J, Xi S, Wang SM, et al. Sperm head vacuoles–light microscopic and ultrastructural observations: a case report. Ultrastruct Pathol. 2012;36: 185-8.
10. Garolla A, Fortini D, Menegazzo M, De Toni L, Nicoletti V, Moretti A, et al. High-power microscopy for selecting spermatozoa for ICSI by physiological status. Reprod Biomed Online. 2008;17:610-6.
11. Antinori M, Licata E, Dani G, Cerusico F, Versaci C, d'Angelo D, et al. Intracytoplasmic Morphologically Selected Sperm Injection: A Prospective Randomized Trial. Reprod Biomed Online. 2008;16:835-41.
12. Boitrelle F, Ferfouri F, Petit JM, Segretain D, Tourain C, Bergere M, et al. Large human sperm vacuoles observed in motile spermatozoa under high magnification: nuclear thumbprints linked to failure of chromatin condensation. Hum Reprod. 2011;26:1650-8.
13. Berkovitz A, Eltes F, Ellenbogen A, Peer S, Feldberg D, Bartoov B. Does the Presence of Nuclear Vacuoles in Human Sperm Selected for ICSI Affect Pregnancy Outcome? Hum Reprod. 2006;21:1787-90.
14. Huszar G, Sbracia M, Vigue L, Miller DJ, Shur BD. Sperm plasma membrane remodeling during spermiogenetic maturation in men: relationship among plasma membrane beta 1,4-galactosyltransferase, cytoplasmic creatine phosphokinase, and creatine phosphokinase isoform ratios. Biol Reprod. 1997;56:1020-24.
15. Souza Setti A, Ferreira RC, Paes de Almeida Ferreira Braga D, de Cássia Sávio Figueira R, Iaconelli A Jr, Borges E Jr. Intracytoplasmic sperm injection outcome versus intracytoplasmic morphologically selected sperm injection outcome: a meta-analysis. Reprod Biomed Online. 2010;21(4):450-5.
16. El Khattabi L, Dupont C, Sermondade N, Hugues JN, Poncelet C, Porcher R, et al. Is intracytoplasmic morphologically selected sperm injection effective in patients with infertility related to teratozoospermia or repeated implantation failure? Fertil Steril. 2013;100(1):62-8.
17. Balaban B, Yakin K, Alatas C, Oktem O, Isiklar A, Urman B. Clinical outcome of intracytoplasmic injection of spermatozoa morphologically selected under high magnification: a prospective randomized study. Reprod Biomed Online. 2011;22(5):472-6.
18. Oliveira JB, Cavagna M, Petersen CG, Mauri AL, Massaro FC, Silva LF, et al. Pregnancy outcomes in women with repeated implantation failures after intracytoplasmic morphologically selected sperm injection (IMSI). Reprod Biol Endocrinol. 2011;9:99.
19. Goswami G, Sharma M, Jugga D, Gouri DM. Can intracytoplasmic morphologically selected spermatozoa injection be used as first choice of treatment for severe male factor infertility patients? J Hum Reprod Sci. 2018; 11(1):40-4.
20. Mangoli E, Khalili MA, Talebi AR, Agha-Rahimi A, Soleimani M, Faramarzi A, et al. IMSI procedure improves clinical outcomes and embryo morphokinetics in patients

with different aetiologies of male infertility. Andrologia. 2019;51:e13340.

21. Sermondade N, Hafhouf E, Dupont C, Bechoua S, Palacios C, Eustache F, et al. Successful childbirth after intracytoplasmic morphologically selected sperm injection without assisted oocyte activation in a patient with globozoospermia. Hum Reprod. 2011;26:2944-9.
22. Chelli MH, Albert M, Ray PF, Guthauser B, Izard V, Hammoud I, et al. Can intracytoplasmic morphologically selected sperm injection be used to select normal-sized sperm heads in infertile patients with macrocephalic sperm head syndrome? Fertil Steril. 2010;93:1347.e1-5.
23. Bartoov B, Berkovitz A, Eltes F, Kogosovsky A, Yagoda A, Lederman H, et al. Pregnancy rates are higher with intracytoplasmic morphologically selected sperm injection than with conventional intracytoplasmic injection. Fertil Steril. 2003;80(6):1413-9.
24. Delaroche L, Yazbeck C, Gout C, Kahn V, Oger P, Rougier N. Intracytoplasmic morphologically selected sperm injection (IMSI) after repeated IVF or ICSI failures: a prospective comparative study. Eur J Obstet Gynecol Reprod Biol. 2013;167(1):76-80.
25. Hazout A, Dumont-Hassan M, Junca AM, Cohen Bacrie P, Tesarik J. High-magnification ICSI overcomes paternal effect resistant to conventional ICSI. Reprod Biomed Online. 2006;12(1):19-25.
26. Gatimel N, Parinaud J, Leandri RD. Intracytoplasmic morphologically selected sperm injection (IMSI) does not improve outcome in patients with two successive IVF-ICSI failures. J Assist Reprod Genet. 2016;33(3):349-55.
27. Marci R, Murisier F, Lo Monte G, Soave I, Chanson A, Urner F, et al. Clinical outcome after IMSI procedure in an unselected infertile population: a pilot study. Reprod Health. 2013;10:16.
28. Setti AS, Braga DP, Figueira RC, Iaconelli A Jr, Borges E Jr. Poor-responder patients do not benefit from intracytoplasmic morphologically selected sperm injection. J Assist Reprod Genet. 2015;32(3):445-50.
29. de Almeida Ferreira Braga DP, Setti AS, Figueira RC, Nichi M, Martinhago CD, Iaconelli A Jr, et al. Sperm organelle morphologic abnormalities: contributing factors and effects on intracytoplasmic sperm injection cycles outcomes. Urology. 2011;78(4):786-91.
30. Cassuto NG, Bouret D, Plouchart JM, Jellad S, Vanderzwalmen P, Balet R, et al. A new real-time morphology classification for human spermatozoa: a link for fertilization and improved embryo quality. Fertil Steril. 2009;92(5):1616-25.
31. Figueira Rde C, Braga DP, Setti AS, Iaconelli A Jr, Borges E Jr. Morphological nuclear integrity of sperm cells is associated with preimplantation genetic aneuploidy screening cycle outcomes. Fertil Steril. 2011;95(3):990-3.
32. Luna D, Hilario R, Dueñas-Chacón J, Romero R, Zavala P, Villegas L, et al. The IMSI procedure improves laboratory and clinical outcomes without compromising the aneuploidy rate when compared to the classical ICSI procedure. Clin Med Insights Reprod Health. 2015;9: 29-37.
33. Kidd SA, Eskenazi B, Wyrobek AJ. Effects of male age on semen quality and fertility: a review of the literature. Fertil Steril. 2001;75:237-48.
34. Petersen CG, Mauri AL, Vagnini LD, Renzi A, Petersen B, Mattila M, et al. The effects of male age on sperm DNA damage: an evaluation of 2,178 semen samples. JBRA Assist Reprod. 2018;22:323-30.
35. Silva LF, Oliveira JB, Petersen CG, Mauri AL, Massaro FC, Cavagna M, et al. The effects of male age on sperm analysis by motile sperm organelle morphology examination (MSOME). Reprod Biol Endocrinol. 2012;10:19.
36. Ai L, Liu SY, Huang J, Chen SW, Liu J, Zhong Y. Intracytoplasmic morphologically selected sperm injection of testicular sperm: clinical outcome in azoospermia patients. Zhonghua Nan Ke Xue. 2010;16:826-9.
37. Gong Y, Meng XQ, Liu M, Wang J, Xiong F, Zhong Y, et al. Intracytoplasmic injection of morphologically selected spermatozoa from patients with male factor infertility: clinical and embryo development outcomes. Nan Fang Yi Ke Da Xue Xue Bao. 2015;35:1428-33.
38. Huszar G. Process and system for selection of mature sperm by surface membrane determinants for assisted reproduction. U.S. Patent 5,897,988, 1999.
39. Huszar G, Ozenci C, Cayli S, Zavaczki Z, Hansch E, Vique L. Hyaluronic acid binding by human sperm indicates cellular maturity, viability, and unreacted acrosomal status. Fertil Steril. 2003;79:1616-24.
40. Huszar G, Vique L, Oehninger S. Creatine kinase immunocytochemistry of human sperm-hemizona complexes: selective binding of sperm with mature creatine kinase-staining pattern. Fertil Steril. 1994;61: 136-42.
41. Huszar G, Vigue L. Incomplete development of human spermatozoa is associated with increased creatine phosphokinase concentration and abnormal head morphology. Mol Reprod Dev. 1993;34:292-8.
42. Sakkas D, Mariethoz E, St John JC. Abnormal sperm parameters in humans are indicative of an abortive apoptotic mechanism linked to the Fas-mediated pathway. Exp Cell Res. 1999;251:350-5.
43. Kovanci E, Kovacs T, Moretti E, Vigue L, Bray-Ward P, Ward DC, et al. FISH assessment of aneuploidy frequencies in mature and immature human spermatozoa classified by the absence or presence of cytoplasmic retention. Hum Reprod. 2001;16:1209-17.
44. Cayli S, Sakkas D, Vigue L, Demir R, Huszar G. Cellular maturity and apoptosis in human sperm: creatine kinase, caspase-3 and Bcl-XL levels in mature and diminished maturity sperm. Mol Hum Reprod. 2004;10: 365-72.

45. Huszar G. Sperm testing and ICSI selection by hyaluronic acid binding: the hyaluronic acid-coated glass slide and petri dish in the andrology and IVF laboratories. In: Nagy ZP, Varghese AC, Agarwal A (Eds). Practical Manual of In Vitro Fertilization: Advanced Methods and Novel Devices. New York: Springer; 2012. pp. 241-57.
46. Lazarevic J, Wikarczuk M, Somkuti SG, Barmat LI, Schinfeld JS, Smith SE. Hyaluronan binding assay (HBA) vs. sperm penetration assay (SPA): Can HBA replace the SPA test in male partner screening before in vitro fertilization? J Exp Clin Assist Reprod. 2010;7:2.
47. Worrilow KC, Eid S, Woodhouse D, Perloe M, Smith S, Witmyer J, et al. 2012. Use of hyaluronan in the selection of sperm for intracytoplasmic sperm injection (ICSI); significant improvement in clinical outcomes--multicenter, double-blinded and randomized trial. Hum Reprod. 2013; 28:306-14.
48. Nasr-Esfahani MH, Razavi S, Vahdati AA, Fathi F, Tavalaee M. Evaluation of sperm selection procedure based on hyaluronic acid binding ability on ICSI outcome. J. Assist Reprod Genet. 2008;25:197-203.
49. Razavi SH, Nasr-Esfahani MH, Deemeh MR, Shayesteh M, Tavalaee M. Evaluation of zeta and HA-binding methods for selection of spermatozoa with normal morphology, protamine content and DNA integrity. Andrologia. 2010; 42:13-9.
50. Parmegiani L, Cognigni GE, Bernardi S, Troilo E, Ciampaglia W, Filicori M. "Physiologic ICSI": hyaluronic acid (HA) favors selection of spermatozoa without DNA fragmentation and with normal nucleus, resulting in improvement of embryo quality. Fertil Steril. 2010;93:598-604.
51. Yagchi A, Murk W, Stronk J, Huszar G. Spermatozoa bound to solid state hyaluronic acid show chromatin structure with high DNA chain integrity: an acridine orange fluorescence study. J Androl. 2020;31:566-72.
52. Mongkolchaipak S, Vutyavanich T. No difference in high-magnification morphology and hyaluronic acid binding in the selection of euploid spermatozoa with intact DNA. Asian J Androl. 2013;15:421-4.
53. Huang MT, Kuo-Kuang Lee R, Lu CH, Chen YJ, Li SH, Hwu YM. The efficiency of conventional microscopic selection is comparable to the hyaluronic acid binding method in selecting spermatozoa for male infertility patients. Taiwan J Obstet Gynecol. 2015;54:48-53.
54. Erberelli RF, Salgado RM, Pereira DHM, Wolff P. Hyaluronan-binding system for sperm selection enhances pregnancy rates in ICSI cycles associated with male factor infertility. JBRA Reprod Assist. 2017;21:2-6.
55. Kim SJ, Kim H, Kim TH, Jeong J, Lee WS, Lyu SW. Effect of Sperm Selection Using Hyaluronan on Fertilization and Quality of Cleavage-Stage Embryos in Intracytoplasmic Sperm Injection (ICSI) Cycles of Couples with Severe Teratozoospermia. Gynecol Endocrinol. 2020;36:456-9.
56. Choe SA, Tae JC, Shin MY, Kim HJ, Kim CH, Lee JY, et al. Application of Sperm Selection Using Hyaluronic Acid Binding in Intracytoplasmic Sperm Injection Cycles: A Sibling Oocyte Study. J Korean Med Sci. 2012;27:1569-73.
57. Mokánszki A, Tóthné EV, Bodnár B, Tándor Z, Molnár Z, Jakab A, et al. Is sperm hyaluronic acid binding ability predictive for clinical success of intracytoplasmic sperm injection: PICSI vs. ICSI? Syst Biol Reprod Med. 2014;60:348-54.
58. Liu Y, Feenan K, Chapple V, Roberts P, Matson P. Intracytoplasmic Sperm Injection Using Hyaluronic Acid or Polyvinylpyrrolidone: A Time-Lapse Sibling Oocyte Study. Hum Fertil (Camb). 2019;22:39-45.
59. Beck-Fruchter R, Shalev E, Weiss A. Clinical benefit using sperm hyaluronic acid binding technique in ICSI cycles: a systematic review and meta-analysis. Reprod Biomed Online. 2016;32(3):286-98.
60. Lepine S, McDowell S, Searle LM, Kroon B, Glujovsky D, Yazdani A. Advanced sperm selection techniques for assisted reproduction. Cochrane Database Syst Rev. 2019; 7(7):CD010461.
61. Miller D, Pavitt S, Sharma V, Forbes G, Hooper R, Bhattacharya S, et al. Physiological, hyaluronan-selected intracytoplasmic sperm injection for infertility treatment (HABSelect): a parallel, two-group, randomised trial. Lancet. 2019;393:416-22.
62. Miki K, Clapham DE. Rheotaxis guides mammalian sperm. Curr Biol. 2013;23:443-52.
63. Bahat A, Caplan SR, Eisenbach M. Thermotaxis of human sperm cells in extraordinarily shallow temperature gradients over a wide range. PLoS One. 2012;7:e41915.
64. Berendsen JTW, Kruit SA, Atak N, Willink E, Segerink LI: Flow-free microfluidic device for quantifying chemotaxis in spermatozoa. Anal Chem. 2020;92:3302-6.
65. Xie L, Ma R, Han C, Su K, Zhang Q, Qiu T, et al. Integration of sperm motility and chemotaxis screening with a microchannel-based device. Clin Chem. 2010;56:1270-8.
66. Li Z, Liu W, Qiu T, Xie L, Chen W, Liu R, et al. The construction of an interfacial valve-based microfluidic chip for thermotaxis evaluation of human sperm. Biomicrofluidics. 2014;8:024102.
67. Zaferani M, Palermo GD, Abbaspourrad A. Strictures of a microchannel impose fierce competition to select for highly motile sperm. Sci Adv. 2019;5:eaav2111.
68. Elveflow. Microfluidics: A general overview of microfluidics. [online] Available from https://www.elveflow.com/microfluidic-reviews/general-microfluidics/a-general-overview-of-microfluidics/ [Last accessed April, 2024].
69. Feynman RP. There's plenty of room at the bottom. In: Hey A (Ed). Feynman and Computation. United States: CRC Press; 2018.
70. Kashaninejad N, Shiddiky MJA, Nguyen NT. Advances in microfluidics-based assisted reproductive technology: From sperm sorter to reproductive system-on-a-chip. Adv Biosyst. 2018;2:1700197.

71. Jebrail MJ, Bartsch MS, Patel KD. Digital microfluidics: a versatile tool for applications in chemistry, biology and medicine. Lab Chip. 2012;12:2452-63.
72. Suh RS, Phadke N, Ohl DA, Takayama S, Smith GD. Rethinking gamete/embryo isolation and culture with microfluidics. Hum. Reprod. Update. 2003;9:451-61.
73. Vaughan DA, Sakkas D. Sperm selection methods in the 21st century. Biol. Reprod. 2019;101:1076–82.
74. Huang HY, Huang PW, Yao DJ. Enhanced efficiency of sorting sperm motility utilizing a microfluidic chip. Microsyst Technol. 2017;23:305-12.
75. Huang HY, Lu CY, Wang IW, Yao DJ. Motility-driven Sperm-sorting Microfluidic Chip with Little Cell Damage for Oligozoospermia Patients. Sens Mater. 2020;32:2585-96.
76. Wu JK, Chen PC, Lin YN, Wang CW, Pan LC, Tseng FG. High-throughput flowing upstream sperm sorting in a retarding flow field for human semen analysis. Analyst. 2017;142:938-44.
77. Yalcinkaya Kalyan YE, Can Celik S, Okan O, Akdeniz G, Karabulut S, Caliskan E. Does a Microfluidic Chip for Sperm Sorting Have a Positive Add-on Effect on Laboratory and Clinical Outcomes of Intracytoplasmic Sperm Injection Cycles? A Sibling Oocyte Study. Andrologia. 2019;51:e13403.
78. Robles A, Reshef EA, Prosser RW, Forman EJ, Williams Z. Does microfluidic sperm sorting improve embryo development and euploidy rates in patients undergoing ICSI? Fertil Steril. 2021;116:e141.
79. Pujol A, García-Peiró A, Ribas-Maynou J, Lafuente R, Mataró D, Vassena R. A microfluidic sperm-sorting device reduces the proportion of sperm with double-stranded DNA fragmentation. Zygote. 2022;30(2):200-5.
80. Kocur OM, Xie P, Cheung S, Souness S, McKnight M, Rosenwaks Z, et al. Can a sperm selection technique improve embryo ploidy? Andrology. 2023;11(8):1605-12.
81. Yildiz K, Yuksel S. Use of Microfluidic Sperm Extraction Chips as an Alternative Method in Patients with Recurrent in Vitro Fertilisation Failure. J Assist Reprod Genet. 2019; 36:1423-9.
82. Ozcan P, Takmaz T, Yazici MGK, Alagoz OA, Yesiladali M, Sevket O, et al. Does the Use of Microfluidic Sperm Sorting for the Sperm Selection Improve In Vitro Fertilization Success Rates in Male Factor Infertility? J Obstet Gynaecol Res. 2021;47:382-8.
83. Yetkinel S, Kilicdag EB, Aytac PC, Haydardedeoglu B, Simsek E, Cok T. Effects of the Microfluidic Chip Technique in Sperm Selection for Intracytoplasmic Sperm Injection for Unexplained Infertility: A Prospective, Randomized Controlled Trial. J Assist Reprod Genet 2019:36:403-9.
84. Ferreira Aderaldo J, da Silva Maranhão K, Ferreira Lanza DC. Does microfluidic sperm selection improve clinical pregnancy and miscarriage outcomes in assisted reproductive treatments? A systematic review and meta-analysis. PLoS One. 2023;18(11):e0292891.
85. Romany L, Garrido N, Cobo A, Aparicio-Ruiz B, Serra V, Meseguer M. Obstetric and perinatal outcome of babies born from sperm selected by MACS from a randomized controlled trial. J Assist Reprod Genet. 2016;34:201-7.
86. Agarwal A, Barbăroşie C, Ambar R, Finelli R. The Impact of Single- and Double-Strand DNA Breaks in Human Spermatozoa on Assisted Reproduction. Int J Mol Sci. 2020; 21:3882.
87. Sakkas D, Seli E, Bizzaro D, Tarozzi N, Manicardi GC. Abnormal spermatozoa in the ejaculate: Abortive apoptosis and faulty nuclear remodelling during spermatogenesis. Reprod Biomed Online. 2003;7:428-32.
88. Smith TB, Cortez-Retamozo V, Grigoryeva LS, Hill E, Pittet MJ, Da Silva N. Mononuclear phagocytes rapidly clear apoptotic epithelial cells in the proximal epididymis. Andrology. 2014;2:755-62.
89. Sakkas D, Ramalingam M, Garrido N, Barratt CL. Sperm selection in natural conception: What can we learn from Mother Nature to improve assisted reproduction outcomes? Hum Reprod Update. 2015;21:711-26.
90. Lee TH, Liu CH, Shih YT, Tsao HM, Huang CC, Chen HH, et al. Magnetic-activated cell sorting for sperm preparation reduces spermatozoa with apoptotic markers and improves the acrosome reaction in couples with unexplained infertility. Hum Reprod. 2010;25:839-46.
91. Cakar Z, Cetinkaya B, Aras D, Koca B, Ozkavukcu S, Kaplanoglu İ, et al. Does combining magnetic-activated cell sorting with density gradient or swim-up improve sperm selection? J Assist Reprod Genet. 2016;33:1059-65.
92. Grunewald S, Paasch U. Sperm selection for ICSI using annexin V. Methods Mol Biol. 2013;927:257-62.
93. Miltenyi Biotec. Magnetic cell separation. [online] Available from https://www.miltenyibiotec.com/FR-en/resources/macs-handbook/macs-technologies/cell-separation/magnetic-cell-separation.html [Last accessed May, 2024].
94. Dirican EK, Ozgün OD, Akarsu S, Akin KO, Ercan O, Uğurlu M, et al. Clinical outcome of magnetic activated cell sorting of non-apoptotic spermatozoa before density gradient centrifugation for assisted reproduction. J Assist Reprod Genet. 2008;25:375-81.
95. Bucar S, Gonçalves A, Rocha E, Barros A, Sousa M, Sá R. DNA Fragmentation in Human Sperm after Magnetic-Activated Cell Sorting. J Assist Reprod Genet. 2015;32:147-54.
96. Delbes G, Herrero MB, Troeung ET, Chan PT. The Use of Complimentary Assays to Evaluate the Enrichment of Human Sperm Quality in Asthenoteratozoospermic and Teratozoospermic Samples Processed with Annexin-V Magnetic Activated Cell Sorting. Andrology. 2013;1:698-706.
97. Pacheco A, Blanco A, Bronet F, Cruz M, García-Fernández J, García-Velasco JA. Magnetic-Activated Cell Sorting (Macs): A Useful Sperm-Selection Technique in Cases of High Levels of Sperm DNA Fragmentation. J Clin Med. 2020; 9:3976.

98. Gil M, Sar-Shalom V, Melendez Sivira Y, Carreras R, Checa MA. Sperm Selection Using Magnetic Activated Cell Sorting (MACS) in Assisted Reproduction: A Systematic Review and Meta-Analysis. J Assist Reprod Genet. 2013;30:479-85.
99. Gil Juliá M, Hervas I, Navarro-Gomezlechon A, Mossetti L, Quintana F, Amoros D, et al. Semen processing using magnetic-activated cell sorting before ICSI is deemed safe for obstetric and perinatal outcomes: a retrospective multicentre study. Reprod Biomed Online. 2023;47: 103172
100. ESHRE Add-ons working group; Lundin K, Bentzen JG, Bozdag G, Ebner T, Harper J, Le Clef N, et al. Good practice recommendations on add-ons in reproductive medicine. Hum Reprod. 2023;38(11):2062-104.

Sperm DNA Fragmentation Index: Clinical Utility and Limitations

Ashish Kale, Ashwini Kale

INTRODUCTION

Sperm deoxyribonucleic acid (DNA) integrity is crucial for fertilization and development of healthy offspring. The sperm DNA plays a crucial role in communicating accurate genetic information from one generation to another. In order to prevent any harm, a haploid genome is often compressed and firmly wrapped with protamine inside the sperm nucleus. Nevertheless, a number of extrinsic and internal factors can compromise chromatin integrity, which can eventually result in damage to DNA and can affect both natural and assisted reproduction.[1] There are various predictable factors that may be accounted for sperm DNA damage, such as age, infections of the reproductive tract, systemic illnesses, pollution in the environment, and way of life. These variables may lead to sperm DNA fragmentation (SDF), which serves as a possible mediator for the development of infertility disorders in males.[2] A direct relationship has been found between sperm DNA damage and male infertility by many researchers. It has also been suggested that sperm DNA damage can be the culprit in many couples otherwise diagnosed with unexplained infertility. However, the relationship between sperm DFI (DNA fragmentation index) and primary or secondary infertility and unexplained miscarriage is still up for dispute in its implications for clinical settings.[1]

MECHANISM OF SPERM DNA FRAGMENTATION

Sperm DNA damage can be caused by many ways. A number of testicular and post-testicular factors can be implicated for the same. There are six major pathways that can cause both nuclear and mitochondrial DNA damage in spermatozoa. They may occur while the sperm cells are being produced or being transported. These include apoptosis during spermatogenesis, DNA strand breaks caused during spermiogenesis, post-testicular DNA fragmentation primarily caused by oxygen radicals, such as nitric oxide and the hydroxyl radical, during sperm transport through the seminiferous tubules and the epididymis, DNA fragmentation via endogenous caspases and endonucleases, and DNA damage from radiation, chemotherapy, and environmental toxicants.[3-5] While some DNA fragmentation is normal, excessive fragmentation can have a detrimental effect on reproduction, especially infertility in women, through a number of different processes.[6]

METHODS TO ASSESS SPERM DNA FRAGMENTATION

Sperm DNA fragmentation has become an intriguing area of research in the context of infertility, serving as a potential biomarker for diagnosing sperm-related infertility. Several approaches have been developed to assess SDF with direct clinical applications, although they exhibit varying sensitivity and specificity among the different assays. There are several methods to assess SDF **(Table 1)**:[4-6]

- *Sperm chromatin structure assay (SCSA):* This is a flow cytometry-based assay that measures the susceptibility of sperm DNA to acid-induced denaturation. It involves staining sperm cells with a DNA-binding dye and exposing them to acid. Damaged DNA strands denature more easily and bind less dye, leading to fluorescence changes that can be measured. The SCSA provides information on the extent of DNA fragmentation and the degree of susceptibility to denaturation. Because of its exceptional repeatability and independent capacity to forecast male fertility in vivo, SCSA is currently the advised approach.

TABLE 1: The summary of the assays to detect sperm DNA fragmentation along with the advantages and disadvantages associated with them.

Methods of assessment	*Type of damage detected single-stranded breaks (SSBs)/ double-stranded breaks (DSBs)*	*Advantages*	*Disadvantages*
TUNEL	SSB/DSB	• Both fluorescent microscopy and flow cytometry can be used for evaluation • High sensitivity and reliability • Minimal interobserver variability • Both fresh and frozen samples can be used for analysis	• Protocols not standardized • Trained personnel required and equipment is costly
Comet	SSB and/or DSB	• High sensitivity • Correlation with semen parameters • It can differentiate between SSB and DSB	• Poor repeatability and high variability • Time-consuming • Evaluation of a low number of cells • Variable protocols and thresholds • Imaging software required
SCSA	SSB/DSB	• Examination of a large number of cells altogether • Highly repeatability • Analysis of both frozen or fresh samples	• Commercial kits unavailable • Expensive equipment and trained personnel required
SCD or Halosperm test	SSB/DSB	• Commercial kits available • Repeatable and consistent results in 45 minutes • No expensive equipment required	• Interobserver variability

(TUNEL: terminal deoxynucleotidyl transferase dUTP nick end labeling; SCD: sperm chromatin dispersion; SCSA: sperm chromatin structure assay)

- *Terminal deoxynucleotidyl transferase dUTP nick end labeling (TUNEL) assay:* TUNEL is a technique that detects DNA fragmentation by labeling the free ends of broken DNA strands with a fluorescent marker. Sperm cells are fixed and then treated with an enzyme called terminal deoxynucleotidyl transferase (TdT), which adds labeled dUTP to the DNA ends. The labeled DNA fragments can be visualized and quantified under a fluorescence microscope.
- *Comet assay (single cell gel electrophoresis):* The comet assay assesses DNA damage at the level of individual sperm cells. Sperm cells are embedded in agarose on a microscope slide, lysed to release DNA, electrophoresed, and stained with a DNA-binding dye. Damaged DNA migrates farther from the nucleus and forms a "comet-like" tail, which can be quantified by image analysis. This method is sensitive to both single-strand and double-strand DNA breaks.
- *Sperm DNA fragmentation index:* The percentage of sperm cells in a semen sample that have fragmented DNA is measured by DFI. Often, methods like SCSA, TUNEL, or the Comet test are used to determine it. The proportion of sperm with damaged DNA is shown by DFI.
- *Halosperm test:* This is a commercial kit that assesses SDF by measuring the extent of DNA dispersion in an agarose gel. Sperm cells are mixed with agarose and electrophoresed, and the resulting halo pattern is analyzed to determine the level of DNA fragmentation.
- *Sperm chromatin dispersion (SCD) test:* Similar to the Halosperm test, the SCD test assesses DNA fragmentation by measuring the extent of DNA dispersion in a microscope slide. Sperm cells are mixed with a lysing solution, spread onto a slide, and stained with a DNA dye. A halo pattern around the sperm head is indicative of DNA fragmentation.
- *Acridine orange (AO) test:* This test uses a fluorescent dye (acridine orange) to differentiate between single-stranded and double-stranded DNA in sperm cells. Damaged DNA fluoresces differently, and the ratio of green to red fluorescence can be used to estimate DNA fragmentation.

These methods can help assess the level of SDF in a semen sample. High levels of DNA fragmentation may be associated with male infertility and can guide treatment options, such as assisted reproductive techniques or lifestyle changes to reduce DNA damage. It is important to consult with a healthcare professional or reproductive specialist for a thorough evaluation and interpretation of the results.

SPERM DNA FRAGMENTATION: EFFECTS ON FERTILITY

Despite not predicting sperm functional competence and reproductive potential, sperm concentration, count, and motility are classic characteristics traditionally used for evaluation of semen quality. Sperm DFI, which is independent of semen characteristics, is helpful for assessing sperm DNA integrity as a way to precisely determine male fertility.[1,2] Due to the high prevalence of sperm DFI in infertile men and miscarried couples, there is some evidence on the therapeutic usefulness of measuring sperm DFI in male infertility in addition to an advanced sperm function test to determine an individual's fertility.

Temperature, radiation, chemical pollution, aging, and other intra- and/or extratesticular harmful elements will all have an impact on sperm during their generation and maturation processes. Sperm DNA is harmed by reactive oxygen species (ROS) created under these circumstances, and when it reaches the cell nucleus, it fragments. Additionally, ROS negatively impact sperm motility. Consequently, there are more sperm DNA fragments and a progressive decline in motility.[7]

The SDF can affect female infertility by incapacitating sperm's ability to fertilize the egg. Damaged DNA may not function properly during fertilization, preventing successful fusion with the egg. Even if fertilization occurs, sperm with fragmented DNA can result in embryos with genetic abnormalities. These abnormalities can lead to miscarriages or failed implantation in the uterus, contributing to female infertility.[8] The damaged DNA in sperm can also affect gene expression patterns in the developing embryo. This can lead to abnormal development of the embryo and increased risk of infertility or birth defects and is also associated with a higher risk of pregnancy complications, such as preterm birth and preeclampsia. These complications can impact the health of the mother and the baby and can result in fertility challenges in the long term.[9] Additionally, couples undergoing assisted reproductive technologies (ARTs) such as in vitro fertilization (IVF) or intracytoplasmic sperm injection (ICSI) may experience reduced success rates when using sperm with high DNA fragmentation. This can lead to repeated failed IVF cycles, which can be emotionally and financially challenging for couples dealing with infertility.[10]

The assessment of the genetic integrity of sperm and its impact on the success of conception constitute the greater significance of sperm FDI. But although the majority of research on miscarriages that go unexplained, particularly recurring ones, has concentrated on maternal variables, there is mounting evidence that male factors also play a significant role. A number of meta-analyses have shown a strong correlation between sperm DNA damage levels and miscarriage. SDF analysis is useful in clinical settings because it can yield important insights on sperm quality and its possible effects on fertility and pregnancy outcomes.[11,12]

SPERM DNA FRAGMENTATION: INDICATIONS FOR TESTING

Do all male partners require SDF testing or are there any subset of patients in whom it is indicated? The answer to this question lies in the various meta-analyses.

A meta-analysis by Zini, which included three studies, revealed that high SDF, determined by the SCSA test, was associated with failure to achieve natural pregnancy with an odds ratio (OR) of 7.01.[13]

Various other meta-analyses have evaluated the impact of SDF on reproductive outcomes after IVF/ICSI including the pregnancy rates, miscarriage rates, and live birth rates. Four meta-analyses[13-16] reported that high SDF was associated with lower pregnancy rates with conventional IVF with an OR ranging between 0.68 and 1.7. With regards to ICSI, only Simon et al.[16] reported significantly lower pregnancy rates with high SDF, while the remaining three meta-analyses failed to find a significant association.[13-15]

A meta-analysis conducted by Wang et al. involving 12 studies revealed that varicocele was associated with significantly higher levels of SDF compared with controls with a mean difference (MD) of 9.84%. Varicocele treatment resulted in significant reduction of SDF levels when compared to control group.[17]

Tan et al. conducted a meta-analysis to understand the male contribution to recurrent pregnancy loss (RPL). The study revealed a significant association between RPL and SDF with an average MD of 11.98, which indicated that men with RPL had significantly higher SDF values than the control group.[18]

Unexplained male infertility is other group of patients in whom SDF testing is indicated. Oleszczuk et al. have shown that about one out of five men with unexplained infertility had a SDF level above 30%.[19]

Conditions which cause increase oxidative stress in male, like exposure to physical agents like radiation and heat; chemical agents, cigarette smoke, airborne pollutants, and chemotherapeutic drugs; biological factors like sexually transmitted infections, increasing male age, elevated body mass index (BMI); and medical conditions like diabetes lead to elevated levels of SDF.[5]

The following are the proposed indications for DFI testing:[20]

- Prolonged idiopathic infertility
- Low fertility rates or bad quality embryos in IVF
- Implantation failure following IVF
- Repeated abortions
- Prolonged exposure to toxic environmental conditions affecting fertility
- Conventional seminal parameters found below the reference ranges
- Advanced male partner age
- Varicocele patients
- Cancer patients.

American Society for Reproductive Medicine (ASRM) guidelines (2021) do not recommend routine SDF testing in the initial evaluation of the infertile couple but recommend testing of SDF in couples with RPL. ESHRE guidelines (2022) also recommend assessing SDF in couples with RPL for diagnostic purposes.

TREATMENT OF HIGH SPERM DNA FRAGMENTATION

A number of interventions including lifestyle modifications, varicocele surgery, shorter abstinence interval, use of testicular sperm, and advanced sperm selection techniques have been suggested for male patients with high SDF. **Flowchart 1** summarizes the algorithm for clinical management of males with high SDF.

Flowchart 1: Clinical algorithm to elucidate the applications of sperm DNA fragmentation (SDF) testing in clinical practice.

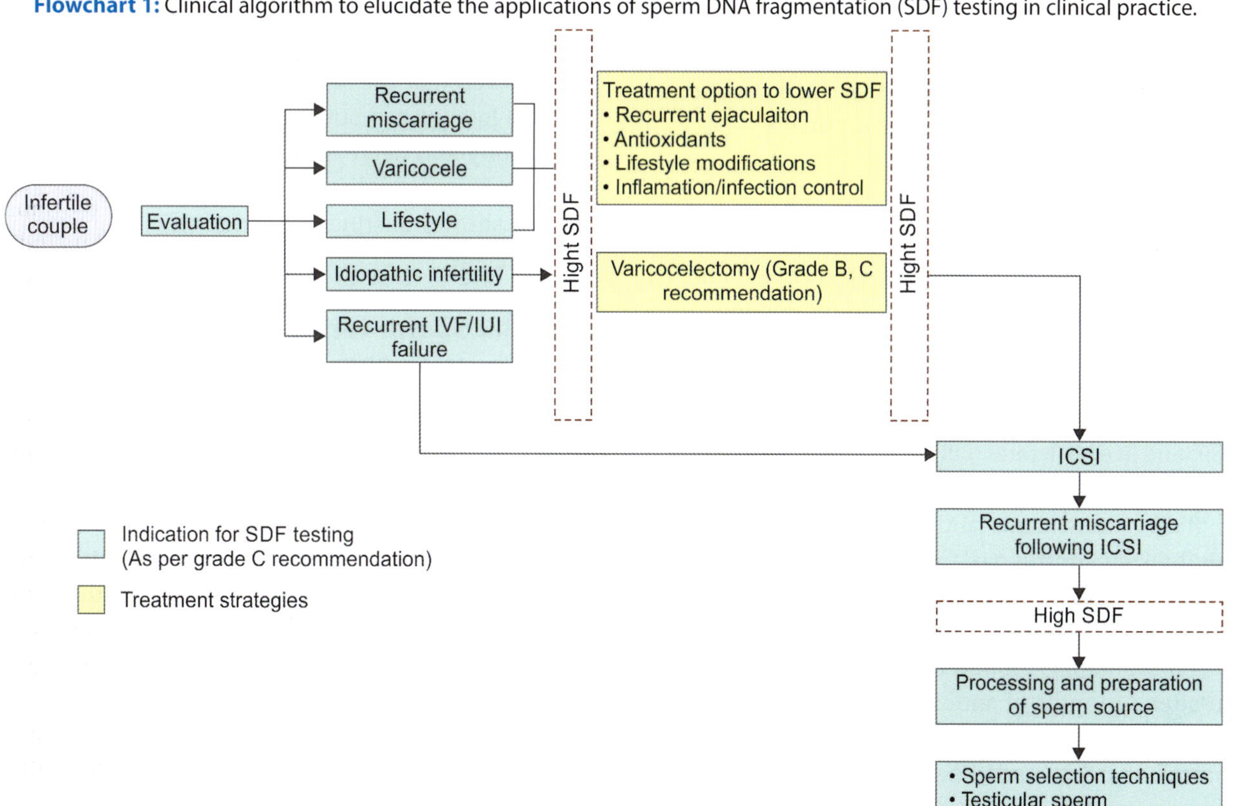

(ICSI: intracytoplasmic sperm injection; IUI: intrauterine insemination; IVF: in vitro fertilization)

Lifestyle Modifications

Various metabolic conditions, like diabetes, obesity, smoking, etc. are known to be associated with high SDF. Adopting a healthy lifestyle, which includes a balanced diet, regular exercise, and refraining from smoking, may help reduce or prevent high levels of SDF.[21] Cigarette smoking in particular has been strongly associated with high SDF. Higher levels of ROS and apoptotic caspases in smokers, gene variations induced by smoking and exposure to toxic polycyclic aromatic hydrocarbons present in cigarettes may play a role in increasing SDF.[22-24] A number of researches have emphasized that quitting smoking can prevent higher SDF levels and improve the reproductive outcomes.[25]

Varicocelectomy

Patients with clinical varicocele tend to have higher SDF due to heat and oxidative stress because of insufficient venous return.[26] A meta-analysis by Esteves et al. reported that varicocele repair significantly reduces SDF levels in patients with clinical varicocele.[27] Other studies have also reported that varicocele repair in patients with clinical varicocele and high SDF improve clinical pregnancy and live birth rates.[28,29] However, whether varicocele treatment should be offered to patients with otherwise normal semen parameters but high SDF is a matter of debate.[30]

Antioxidant Therapy

Antioxidants can scavenge the excess free radicals and therefore can mitigate the harmful effects of ROS in SDF. However, the actual effect of antioxidant therapy on the reproductive outcomes has been controversial. The latest Cochrane review observed that antioxidant therapy is beneficial in terms of increasing the clinical pregnancy (OR = 1.89) and live birth rates (OR = 1.43); however, the overall certainty of evidence was found to be low.[31] The MOXI trial (the Males, Antioxidants, and Infertility trial), which was a randomized control trial, demonstrated that baseline plasma antioxidant levels were not predictive of successful pregnancy or live birth.[32,33] Also, no significant change in sperm morphology, motility, or DNA fragmentation was seen after 3 months of antioxidant therapy (specifically vitamin E, selenium, and zinc). The trial was however criticized as it was ended before it reached the decent power size, and thus larger randomized controlled trials (RCTs) are needed to have clear conclusions on the subject. Overall, oral antioxidant therapy may be a cost-effective option for patients with elevated SDF; however, the selection of treatment should be guided by individual decisions made between the healthcare professional and the patient.

Short Ejaculatory Interval

Shorter abstinence interval can improve sperm parameters and SDF. In the absence of ejaculation, sperms accumulate in the epididymis and are exposed to ROS generated by abnormal sperms and granulocytes resulting in high SDF. Frequent ejaculations or shorter epididymal transit time can reduce the exposure to ROS reducing the sperm damage.[34,35] A recent meta-analysis by Sokol et al. observed that shorter abstinence was associated with better sperm motility and morphology and decreased SDF.[36]

Another study compared semen parameters from normozoospermic and oligoasthenoteratozoospermia (OAT) men after a 2- to 7-day abstinence period and a 1-hour abstinence period. The shorter abstinence period showed significant improvement in sperm morphology and a decrease in SDF in both the groups.[37] The OAT group also demonstrated an improvement in sperm motility with shorter abstinence. Another meta-analysis by Barbagallo et al. showed that the second ejaculate in patients with OATs has low volume but improved sperm concentration and motility and decreased SDF.[38] For ART procedures, where sperm quality is more important than the actual number, shorter abstinence period thus seems to be a useful strategy.

Testicular Sperm versus Ejaculate Sperm for High SDF

It has been observed that testicular sperm has low levels of oxidative damage and lower SDF compared to ejaculated sperm. A systematic review by Ambar et al.[39] and various other studies[40,41] observed that use of testicular sperm is associated with higher pregnancy and live birth rates in patients with high SDF. However, robust RCTs regarding this are still lacking. Retrieving testicular sperm required surgical intervention and SDF testing in testicular sperm lacks standardization. The recommendations regarding testicular sperm retrieval in males with high SDF are unresolved and European Association of Urology refrains from recommending testicular sperm retrieval for infertile patients with high SDF routinely.[42]

Advanced Sperm Selection Techniques

Various advanced sperm selection techniques have been explored to improve fertility outcomes in patients with high SDF.[43] These include physiological ICSI (PICSI) and magnetic-activated cell sorting (MACS). Where conventional ICSI relies on morphology and motility of sperm, PICSI involves placing the sperm on hyaluronan dots to mimic high DNA integrity binding, thereby selecting high integrity sperm. MACS separates apoptosed sperm cells from normal sperm cells by recognizing the phosphatidylserine residues.[44] Though these newer techniques appear promising, large multicentric trials are needed to evaluate their efficacy and find out the best sperm selection technique for patients with high SDF.

CONCLUSION

The impact of SDF can vary from one individual to another. The lifestyle factors, such as diet, smoking, and exposure to environmental toxins, can influence SDF levels. Couples experiencing fertility issues due to SDF should consult with a fertility specialist who can provide a thorough evaluation and discuss potential treatments or interventions, such as antioxidant therapy or sperm selection techniques, to improve their chances of achieving a successful pregnancy.

REFERENCES

1. Zhang F, Li J, Liang Z, Wu J, Li L, Chen C, et al. Sperm DNA fragmentation and male fertility: a retrospective study of 5114 men attending a reproductive center. J Assist Reprod Genet. 2021;38(5):1133-41.
2. Practice Committee of the American Society for Reproductive Medicine. Diagnostic evaluation of the infertile male: a committee opinion. Fertil Steril. 2015; 103(3):e18-25.
3. Andersen AG, Ziebe S, Jorgensen N, Petersen JH, Skakkebaek NE, Andersen AN. Time to pregnancy in relation to semen quality assessed by CASA before and after sperm separation. Hum Reprod. 2002;17(1):173-7.
4. Sakkas D, Alvarez JG. Sperm DNA fragmentation: mechanisms of origin, impact on reproductive outcome, and analysis. Fertil Steril. 2010;93(4):1027-36.
5. Agarwal A, Majzoub A, Baskaran S, Panner Selvam MK, Cho CL, Henkel R, et al. Sperm DNA Fragmentation: A New Guideline for Clinicians. World J Mens Health. 2020; 38(4):412-71.
6. Lopes S, Sun JG, Jurisicova A, Meriano J, Casper RF. Sperm deoxyribonucleic acid fragmentation is increased in poor-quality semen samples and correlates with failed fertilization in intracytoplasmic sperm injection. Fertil Steril. 1998;69(3):528-32.
7. Shoukir Y, Chardonnens D, Campana A, Sakkas D. Blastocyst development from supernumerary embryos after intracytoplasmic sperm injection: a paternal influence? Hum Reprod. 1998;13(6):1632-7.
8. Fatehi AN, Bevers MM, Schoevers E, Roelen BA, Colenbrander B, Gadella BM. DNA damage in bovine sperm does not block fertilization and early embryonic development but induces apoptosis after the first cleavages. J Androl. 2006;27(2):176-88.
9. Pratap H, Hottigoudar SY, Nichanahalli KS, Rajendran S, Bheemanathi HS. Sperm DNA Integrity in Leukocytospermia and Its Association with Seminal Adenosine Deaminase. J Hum Reprod Sci. 2019;12(3):182-88.
10. Tesarik J, Greco E, Mendoza C. Late, but not early, paternal effect on human embryo development is related to sperm DNA fragmentation. Hum Reprod. 2004;19(3):611-5.
11. Cayli S, Sakkas D, Vigue L, Demir R, Huszar G. Cellular maturity and apoptosis in human sperm: creatine kinase, caspase-3 and Bcl-XL levels in mature and diminished maturity sperm. Mol Hum Reprod. 2004;10(5):365-72.
12. Duran EH, Morshedi M, Taylor S, Oehninger S. Sperm DNA quality predicts intrauterine insemination outcome: a prospective cohort study. Hum Reprod. 2002;17(12):3122-8.
13. Zini A. Are sperm chromatin and DNA defects relevant in the clinic? Syst Biol Reprod Med. 2011;57:78-85.
14. Li Z, Wang L, Cai J, Huang H. Correlation of sperm DNA damage with IVF and ICSI outcomes: a systematic review and meta-analysis. J Assist Reprod Genet. 2006;23:367-76.
15. Zhao J, Zhang Q, Wang Y, Li Y. Whether sperm deoxyribonucleic acid fragmentation has an effect on pregnancy and miscarriage after in vitro fertilization/intracytoplasmic sperm injection: a systematic review and meta-analysis. Fertil Steril. 2014;102:998-1005.e8.
16. Simon L, Zini A, Dyachenko A, Ciampi A, Carrell DT. A systematic review and meta-analysis to determine the effect of sperm DNA damage on in vitro fertilization and intracytoplasmic sperm injection outcome. Asian J Androl. 2017;19:80-90.
17. Wang YJ, Zhang RQ, Lin YJ, Zhang RG, Zhang WL. Relationship between varicocele and sperm DNA damage and the effect of varicocele repair: a meta-analysis. Reprod Biomed Online. 2012;25:307-14.
18. Tan J, Taskin O, Albert A, Bedaiwy MA. Association between sperm DNA fragmentation and idiopathic recurrent pregnancy loss: a systematic review and meta-analysis. Reprod Biomed Online. 2019;38:951-60.
19. Oleszczuk K, Augustinsson L, Bayat N, Giwercman A, Bungum M. Prevalence of high DNA fragmentation index in male partners of unexplained infertile couples. Andrology. 2013;1:357-60.
20. Evgeni E, Charalabopoulos K, Asimakopoulos B. Human sperm DNA fragmentation and its correlation with

conventional semen parameters. J Reprod Infertil. 2014; 15(1):2-14.
21. Wright C, Milne S, Leeson H. Sperm DNA damage caused by oxidative stress: modifiable clinical, lifestyle and nutritional factors in male infertility. Reprod Biomed Online. 2014;28(6):684-703.
22. Humaidan P, Haahr T, Povlsen BB, Kofod L, Laursen RJ, Alsbjerg B, et al. The combined effect of lifestyle intervention and antioxidant therapy on sperm DNA fragmentation and seminal oxidative stress in IVF patients: a pilot study. Int Braz J Urol. 2022;48:131-56.
23. Axelsson J, Lindh CH, Giwercman A. Exposure to polycyclic aromatic hydrocarbons and nicotine, and associations with sperm DNA fragmentation. Andrology. 2022;10(4):740-8.
24. Amor H, Jankowski PM, Dahadhah FW, Al Zoubi MS, Hammadeh ME. Impact of tobacco smoking in association with H2BFWT, PRM1 and PRM2 genes variants on male infertility. Andrologia. 2022;54(11):e14611.
25. Esteves SC. Interventions to prevent sperm DNA damage effects on reproduction. Adv Exp Med Biol. 2019;1166: 119-48.
26. Zini A, Dohle G. Are varicoceles associated with increased deoxyribonucleic acid fragmentation? Fertil Steril. 2011; 96(6):1283-7.
27. Abdelbaki SA, Sabry JH, Al-Adl AM, Sabry HH. The impact of coexisting sperm DNA fragmentation and seminal oxidative stress on the outcome of varicocelectomy in infertile patients: a prospective controlled study. Arab J Urol. 2017;15(2):131-9.
28. Lira Neto FT, Roque M, Esteves SC. Effect of varicocelectomy on sperm deoxyribonucleic acid fragmentation rates in infertile men with clinical varicocele: a systematic review and meta-analysis. Fertil Steril. 2021;116(3):696-712.
29. Esteves SC, Roque M, Agarwal A. Outcome of assisted reproductive technology in men with treated and untreated varicocele: systematic review and meta-analysis. Asian J Androl. 2016;18(2):254–8.
30. Giagulli VA, Carbone MD. Varicocele correction for infertility: which patients to treat? Int J Androl. 2011;34(3): 236-41.
31. de Ligny W, Smits RM, Mackenzie-Proctor R, Jordan V, Fleischer K, de Bruin JP, et al. Antioxidants for male subfertility. Cochrane Database Syst Rev. 2022;5(5): CD007411.
32. Knudtson JF, Sun F, Coward RM, Hansen KR, Barnhart KT, Smith J, et al. The relationship of plasma antioxidant levels to semen parameters: the males, antioxidants, and infertility (MOXI) randomized clinical trial. J Assist Reprod Genet. 2021;38(11):3005-13.
33. Kuchakulla M, Ramasamy R. Re: the effect of antioxidants on male factor infertility: the males, antioxidants, and infertility (MOXI) randomized clinical trial. Eur Urol. 2021;79(1):159-60.
34. Agarwal A, Gupta S, Du Plessis S, Sharma R, Esteves SC, Cirenza C, et al. Abstinence time and its impact on basic and advanced semen parameters. Urology. 2016;94:102-10.
35. Bahadur G, Almossawi O, Zeirideen Zaid R, Ilahibuccus A, Al-Habib A, Muneer A, et al. Semen characteristics in consecutive ejaculates with short abstinence in subfertile males. Reprod Biomed Online. 2016;32(3):323-8.
36. Sokol P, Drakopoulos P, Polyzos NP. The effect of ejaculatory abstinence interval on sperm parameters and clinical outcome of ART. A systematic review of the literature. J Clin Med Res. 2021;10(15):3213.
37. Ayad BM, der Horst GV, Plessis SSD. Revisiting the relationship between the ejaculatory abstinence period and semen characteristics. Int J Fertil Steril. 2018;11(4): 238-46.
38. Barbagallo F, Cannarella R, Crafa A, Manna C, La Vignera S, Condorelli RA, et al. The impact of a very short abstinence period on conventional sperm parameters and sperm DNA fragmentation: a systematic review and meta-analysis. J Clin Med. 2022;11(24):7303.
39. Ambar RF, Agarwal A, Majzoub A, Vij S, Tadros NN, Cho CL, et al. The use of testicular sperm for intracytoplasmic sperm injection in patients with high sperm DNA damage: a systematic review. World J Mens Health. 2021;39(3):391-8.
40. Esteves SC, Coimbra I, Hallak J. Surgically retrieved spermatozoa for ICSI cycles in non-azoospermic males with high sperm DNA fragmentation in semen. Andrology. 2023;11(8):1613-34.
41. Zhang J, Xue H, Qiu F, Zhong J, Su J. Testicular spermatozoon is superior to ejaculated spermatozoon for intracytoplasmic sperm injection to achieve pregnancy in infertile males with high sperm DNA damage. Andrologia. 2019;51(2):e13175.
42. Tharakan T, Bettocchi C, Carvalho J, Corona G, Jones TH, Kadioglu A, et al. European Association of Urology guidelines panel on male sexual and reproductive health: a clinical consultation guide on the indications for performing sperm DNA fragmentation testing in men with infertility and testicular sperm extraction in nonazo-ospermic men. Eur Urol Focus. 2022;8(1):339-50.
43. Hozyen M, Hasanen E, Elqusi K, ElTanbouly S, Gamal S, Hussin AG, et al. Reproductive outcomes of different sperm selection techniques for ICSI patients with abnormal sperm DNA fragmentation: a randomized controlled trial. Reprod Sci. 2022;29(1):220-8.
44. González-Ravina C, Santamaría-López E, Pacheco A, Ramos J, Carranza F, Murria L, et al. Effect of sperm selection by magnetic-activated cell sorting in D-IUI: a randomized control trial. Cells. 2022;11(11):1794.

Chapter

Thin Endometrium: How Thin is Actually Thin?

Manish Banker, Jwal Banker, Parul Arora

INTRODUCTION

Implantation, a complex process involving interactions between the endometrium and the blastocyst, is necessary for establishing a viable pregnancy. To define the endometrium as a biosensor of embryo quality, the notions of endometrial receptivity and selectivity were introduced by Macklon and Brosens in 2014.[1] Endometrial receptivity is an indispensable part of implantation; however, a reliable and ideal marker of receptivity is not yet defined. Histological, biochemical, and genetic marker of receptivity lack validation have low predictive values and need invasive testing. Sonological assessment of endometrial thickness (EMT) remains to be the reliable, reproducible, cost-effective, and universally available noninvasive marker of endometrial receptivity.[2]

Endometrial thickness is easily quantified by transvaginal ultrasound (TVS). Studies that looked into the connection between EMT and in vitro fertilization (IVF) outcomes have yielded inconsistent results. According to some theories, thinner endometrium is linked to poorer IVF success rates. The fact that there is no precise definition of thin endometrium as determined by ultrasound may help to explain this lack of agreement.[3] As a result, it is impossible to draw a firm conclusion about the clinical importance of EMT for the likelihood of conceiving following IVF.

Despite all this, EMT evaluation has evolved into a useful tool of monitoring throughout IVF process. Clinicians and infertile couples may thus be forced to make the difficult decision of whether to move forward with a fresh IVF cycle or opt to cryopreserve the embryos for conceivably improved chances to conceive with an endometrium grown under natural circumstances in subsequent cycles.

IMPLANTATION PHYSIOLOGY AND IMPORTANCE OF ENDOMETRIUM

Human embryos are implanted through a series of stages that include apposition, adhesion, and invasion of an endometrium that has been hormonally prepped for receptivity. The EMT is supposed to be "surrogate marker for endometrial receptivity". The endometrial luminal epithelium develops pinopode-like projections that help the blastocyst adhere to the uterine lining and its invasion into the deeper endometrial stroma. The endometrium becomes decidualized and triggers the release of vascular factors which stimulate fetal vessels and remodeling of maternal uterine spiral arterioles to form fetomaternal circulatory connections.[4,5] Human implantation thus requires complicated molecular and physical interactions between the host endometrium and the embryo in a complex, well-coordinated, ongoing process.

With the successful endometrial preparation with exogenous hormones in a woman with premature ovarian failure and consequent live birth reported in 1984, importance has been given to optimal endometrial preparation in IVF leading to an optimal thickness.[6]

ASSESSMENT OF ENDOMETRIUM

Transvaginal sonography is an ideal noninvasive modality to evaluate the EMT. Endometrium is measured on an empty bladder with a transvaginal probe. This transducer is physically closer to the endometrium and uses a higher frequency (5–8 MHz) as compared to transabdominal assessment. This results in better visualization of the endometrium due to better resolution. Following are the markers used routinely for the endometrial assessment.[7]

- *Endometrial thickness:* It is measured from outside to outside in an anteroposterior view at the widest point.

It should be measured in the sagittal plane or the long axis. Measurement is of "thickest echogenic area from one stratum basalis endometrial interface to other". The definition and cutoff for "thin endometrium" differ but most of the studies use EMT <7–8 mm on the day of human chorionic gonadotropin (hCG) administration.

- *Endometrial pattern:* Apart from the EMT, another marker of an optimal endometrial preparation is the pattern of the endometrial stripe. An ideal endometrial pattern is trilaminar on the day of trigger (grade or type A).
  - *Type A:* Triple-line pattern consisting of central hyperechoic line surrounded by two hypoechoic layers.
  - *Type B:* An "intermediate isoechogenic pattern with the same reflectivity as surrounding myometrium and poorly defined central echogenic line".
  - *Type C:* "Homogeneous hyperechogenic endometrium"; likely nonreceptive
- Endometrial vascularity (measured by 3D color Doppler ultrasound). Vascularity in
  - *Zone 1:* 2 mm thick area surrounding the hyperechoic outer layer of endometrium
  - *Zone 2:* Hyperechoic outer layer of endometrium
  - *Zone 3:* Hypoechoic inner layer of endometrium
  - *Zone 4:* Endometrial cavity
- *Endometrial volume assessment using 3D ultrasonography:* Volume of <2.5 mL is predictive of low pregnancy rate or pregnancy loss, but it has low sensitivity.

THIN ENDOMETRIUM IN ASSISTED REPRODUCTIVE TECHNOLOGY

Over the last four decades, studies have noted the route of estrogen administration and the duration of estrogen to achieve the optimal thickness. The mode and dose of estrogen administration and duration of estrogen priming do not really matter as long as the EMT and the trilaminar pattern are adequately achieved.[8] A big proportion of embryo transfers are canceled because the endometrium is not optimal. However, what remains to be deciphered is what is the cutoff below which pregnancies are not possible or does architecture equally matter as the thickness in the endometrium.

Thin endometrium is often defined as EMT <7 mm or <8 mm. The incidence of thin endometrium in ovarian stimulated cycles can be as high as 38–66% while in IVF it is between 1 and 2.5%.[2,9] The true incidence of thin endometrium in assisted reproductive technology (ART) especially in frozen embryo transfer (FET) cycles cannot be reported as such cycles are canceled before reporting. The incidence of thin endometrium is higher in ovarian stimulation cycles and is also heterogeneous; depending upon the drug used in the cycle: clomiphene, letrozole, or gonadotropins.

FACTORS AFFECTING ENDOMETRIUM

The following are four crucial elements that have an impact on endometrial growth:

1. Levels of serum estradiol
2. Uterine blood flow
3. The condition of the endometrial tissue (any infections or prior injuries)
4. Age of the woman also influences the endometrium indirectly possibly due to reduced vascularity.

CAUSES OF THIN ENDOMETRIUM

- *Iatrogenic:* It can happen during D&C (dilation and curettage), myomectomy in which endometrial cavity is opened or, cesarean section in which uterine cavity has been curetted to remove placental bits, overzealous or repeated curettage, postabortal adhesions, polypectomy, etc.
- *Inflammatory:* In India, endometrial tuberculosis is a significant and frequent cause of thin and irreparably damaged endometrium. In addition, other conditions that can cause endometrial scarring permanently include chronic bacterial infections, sexually transmitted diseases (STDs), and pelvic inflammatory disease. Any infective trigger can lead to destruction of the basal layer and healing by fibrosis, adhesions, and shrinkage of the cavity.
- *Other causes:*
  - *Low estrogen levels:* Because the endometrium is an estrogen-dependent tissue, it will remain thin if estrogen stimulation is insufficient for any reason, as is the case in prepubertal girls, postmenopausal women, and hypogonadotropic hypogonadism instances.
  - *Excessive clomiphene use:* Clomiphene has an antiestrogenic impact on the endometrium and repeated use can result in the endometrial estrogen receptors being downregulated, which can cause the endometrium to remain thin for an extended period of time.

- *Prolonged usage of progesterone and combination contraceptive pills:* Endometrial lining becomes thin when oral contraceptive (OC) pills and progestins are used for an extended length of time.
- *Improper blood flow:* Blood flow to the uterus indirectly controls endometrial growth by improving vascular development of the endometrium. In 2010, Takasaki et al. demonstrated that a "thin endometrium was characterized by poor epithelial growth, decreased vascular endothelial growth factor (VEGF) expression, and poor vascular development. It is likely that endometrial growth partly depends on angiogenesis and uterine blood flow.[10]
- *Systemic causes:* Thin lining is thought to be more common in those who have certain illnesses, such as hypertension, diabetes mellitus, asthma, depression, and substance addiction like smoking.
- *Idiopathic:* Intrinsic properties of the endometrial architecture may cause it to be thin; unrelated to any pathology.

NATURAL VERSUS MEDICATED FROZEN EMBRYO TRANSFER

In natural cycle FET, endogenous estradiol secreted by dominant follicle is responsible for endometrial proliferation while in medicated FET, estrogen and progesterone are administered in sequential fashion to mimic the natural window of implantation.

Investigators have reported similar pregnancy rates and live birth rates (LBRs) between natural and medicated cycles.[11,12] Another systematic review also reported no advantage of any particular method of endometrial preparation in frozen transfer cycles with similar outcomes noted among modified natural and medicated FET.[13] A prospective cohort study of patients undergoing modified natural cycle FETs revealed no association between EMT and pregnancy outcomes and they reported that there is no minimal EMT below which pregnancy rates would be compromised.[14] A study conducted by Pan Y et al. 2020 showed that natural cycle protocol yielded thicker endometrium and higher implantation rate as compared to hormone replacement.[15]

EVIDENCE ON ENDOMETRIAL THICKNESS AND PREGNANCY RATES

Numerous studies have linked decreasing EMT at the time of both fresh embryo transfer and FET to a decreased likelihood of implantation and continued pregnancy. There is no EMT at which the chance of pregnancy and a subsequent live birth has been reported to be zero, despite the fact that the results appear to get worse as EMT drops to <7 mm or 8 mm.[16,17]

Perhaps the most important factor for positive perinatal outcomes is also the placenta, and placentation is likely to be affected by the underlying endometrium. According to several researches, thin endometrium (<8 mm) had low levels of VEGF, which caused poor endometrial vascularization and poor placentation. The risk of pregnancy loss, preeclampsia, preterm delivery, and placenta previa is also elevated in pregnancies conceived with thin endometrium, according to several studies.[18,19] Studies on obstetric and neonatal outcomes in intrauterine insemination (IUI) cycles with thin endometrium failed to identify a negative correlation between the two, hence the source of these findings is multifactorial.[20]

A systematic review by Kasius et al. did not find any difference in LBR and ongoing pregnancy rates for thin endometrium (≤7 mm), though the sample size was small. However, the clinical pregnancy rate (CPR) was significantly reduced with EMT ≤7 mm, with an odds ratio (OR) of 0.42 and a narrow confidence interval. They suggested that EMT alone cannot be used as a parameter for cycle cancelation, freezing embryos, or discontinuation of treatment. The review had studies with a mix of prospective and retrospective studies and selection bias.[18]

In a recent study, Liu et al. 2018 found that EMT of 8 mm at the end of the estrogen phase in >20,000 frozen-thawed embryo transfer (FET) cycles resulted in the best clinical and ongoing pregnancy rates following IVF. It was observed in the study that if EMT ≥8 mm, CPR was 43% while if endometrium is 7–7.9 mm, CPR was 34%. Thus, for every millimeter decrease in thickness below 8 mm for fresh embryo transfers and below 7 mm for FETs, the pregnancy rates decreased significantly. Numerous other studies on EMT have found results that are in agreement with the above. Therefore, it seems that the EMT of at least 8 mm and a trilaminar appearance on ultrasound would be the best for embryo implantation.[21]

As per Canadian guidelines 2019, in fresh IVF embryo transfer cycles, patient should be counseled that ET <8 mm may have deleterious impact on pregnancy and LBR while the cutoff for the same in frozen IVF embryo transfer cycles is <7 mm.[22]

In a similar study conducted by Banker et al. in 2021 on effect of EMT and IVF-ICSI (intracytoplasmic sperm injection) outcome, it was shown that a progressive improvement in LBR was noted with each millimeter increase in EMT starting from 6 mm after transfer of either single or double blastocyst.[23] A recent study on 96,000 autologous fresh and FET concluded that in cycles with a fresh embryo transfer, LBR increases significantly until an EMT of 10–12 mm, while in FET cycles LBR plateaus after 7–10 mm. However, an EMT <6 mm was associated clearly with a significant reduction in LBR in fresh and FET cycles.[24] Değer et al. recently concluded that each 1 mm increase in EMT resulted in a significant increase in CPR and LBR. The lowest CPR was detected at EMT <6 mm, while the EMT value with the highest CPR was 11–12 mm in both groups. Clinical pregnancy and LBRs are optimal if the EMT is between 11 and 12 mm in both fresh and frozen-thawed cycles.[25]

HOW THIN IS DELETERIOUS?

Despite the evidence positively correlating EMT thickness and pregnancy, EMTs as low as 4 mm have also led to pregnancies.[26-28] Mahutte et al. have reported a LBR of 22% in EMT of 6–7.9 mm in their study of 5,000 transfers below 8 mm. In EMT of 4–5.9 mm, the LBR was 15.8%. These results are only from those cases of thin endometrium where transfers were proceeded and appear reassuring.[24]

Women with thickness of below 8 mm in a fresh cycle can be counseled to choose between preceding with a fresh transfer or attempt a frozen cycle in a subsequent medicated cycle aiming for a higher EMT. In cases where the endometrium is <8 mm across repeated cycles despite different preparation methods, women should be counseled about the reduced but acceptable pregnancy rates and can proceed with transfer.

In contrast to IVF, thin endometrium has a less pronounced effect on pregnancy rates in controlled ovarian stimulation (COS) or IUI cycles.[20,29]

OBSTETRIC AND NEONATAL OUTCOMES

Despite the lower pregnancy and LBRs at thin EMTs, there is no EMT below which a pregnancy is not feasible. However, in any pregnancy, the placenta plays a pivotal role for obstetric and perinatal outcome by acting as a temporary organ. Placentation in pregnancy if influenced by the underlying endometrium as reported by Miwa et al. who found that VEGF was underexpressed in an endometrium <4 mm[30] causing impaired placentation. Several authors have reported increased risks of hypertensive disorders, pregnancy losses, preterm delivery, placenta previa, placenta accreta, etc., in cases with thin endometrium at conception. In addition, infants born to such mothers have additional risks of growth restriction, small for gestational age, and consequent neonatal risks. Such risks could be additional complicated by the medicated FET which itself has an additional risk due to absence of corpus luteum.

MANAGEMENT OF THIN ENDOMETRIUM

Identification of the optimal EMT for implantation and livebirth remains a challenge. For women with thin endometrium, both natural and medicated protocols have been proposed for better endometrial development. The choice of estradiol formulation in medicated FET cycles has been evaluated; but no differences have been found.

Estradiol adjustment: In majority of the cases, the thin EMT responds to simplest interventions. Sometimes, extended estrogen administration or increasing the estrogen dosage or changing the route of estrogen administration (oral, vaginal, and transdermal) helps in achieving the EMT in a different cycle. Vaginal administration of estradiol helps in achieving a higher blood level; however, implantation rates are not increased.[31,32] Another simple option is to extend the duration of estrogen exposure (14–82 days) to achieve the optimal EMT. Many authors opt for an extended oral estrogen regime with added vaginal estrogen. Some clinicians stop the endometrial preparation after 3 weeks if not optimal and start all over again in the next cycle with a different protocol or route after inducing menses. Sometimes, multiple hormone replacement therapy (HRT) cycles for endometrial preparation stimulate the regeneration of the endometrium.

In ovulatory women, natural cycle is another option for FET in cases with refractory thin EMT or the usage of low dose gonadotropins for a modified natural cycle.

Various adjuvants have been tried in the management of thin endometrium not responding to estrogen. Although few have shown promising results in small sample-sized observational studies, randomized controlled trials to validate their usage are lacking at present. The additional cost of such therapies and their experimental nature and nonvalidated results should always be discussed with the patient before they are tried in cases with thin EMT.

Adjuvants commonly used for management of thin endometrium:

- *Surgical intervention:* Hysteroscopy
- *Vascular approach to increase blood flow:* Aspirin, heparin, and vasodilators such as sildenafil and L-arginine
- Endometrial scratching/endometrial injury
- Endometrial receptivity analysis (ERA)
- *Reproductive immunology testing and potential therapies:*
    - Corticosteroids, intravenous immunoglobulin (IVIG), intralipid infusion, growth factor (GF) and granulocyte colony-stimulating factor (G-CSF)
    - Autologous platelet-rich plasma (PRP) therapy
    - Lymphocyte immune therapy and leukemia inhibitory factor
- Stem cell therapy
- *Uterine relaxants:* Piroxicam, atosiban, etc.

Some of the abovementioned adjuvants are explained in detail:

- *Hysteroscopy:* Routine use of diagnostic hysteroscopy before IVF to optimize the uterine thickness and receptivity is controversial; still it is practiced by some clinics. Routine use of hysteroscopy in asymptomatic women before the first IVF cycle is generally not recommended.[33] Role of hysteroscopy in refractory endometrium (failure to achieve EMT despite various attempts of endometrial preparation protocols) is justified to diagnose and correct undetected pathologies like adhesions or those with an abnormal sonological result pointing toward uterine pathology.[34]
- *Role of aspirin:*
    - *Mechanism:* By inhibition of *cyclooxygenase enzyme* in platelets and reduction of prostaglandin synthesis.
    - Causes shift from thromboxane A2 to prostacyclin
    - Inhibits platelet aggregation
    - Leads to vasodilatation and improves blood flow to implantation site.

  In 2017, Wang et al. conducted a meta-analysis that comprised 13 RCTs. The implantation rate, LBR, miscarriage rate, fertilization rate, and EMT did not differ significantly from each other, but it did show that aspirin treatment may marginally improve the CPR [risk ratio (RR): 1.16; 95% confidence interval (CI): 1.04–1.28] when compared to placebo or no treatment. Therefore, more high-quality studies are necessary to justify its empirical usage.[35]
- *Role of heparin:* It is postulated to act by
    - Improved blood flow at the implantation site by its antithrombotic effect
    - Promotes trophoblastic invasion
    - Modulation of inflammatory responses.

  Present evidence is weak such that its routine use in all women undergoing IVF treatment is not warranted.
- *Role of ERA:* Endometrial receptivity analysis is a molecular test to define the window of implantation by the analysis of receptivity genes. In a study by Mahajan et al. in women with EMT<6 mm, the ERA revealed a receptive ERA in 77% with a PR of 33.3%; suggesting that the proportion of receptive endometrium was not different from women with EMT >6 mm. ERA may be employed to personalize the timing in women with thin EMT after checking for receptivity.[2]
- *Endometrial scratching:* It is performed with a Pipelle during luteal phase prior to IVF cycle.
    - *Mechanism:*
        - Induction of endometrial decidualization
        - Wound-healing response, associated with a beneficial inflammatory response
        - Modulation of gene expression
        - An improved synchronicity

  Various studies have showed no significant increase in pregnancy rate or LBR with the use of scratching.[36,37]
- *Role of PRP:* It is a concentrate of autologous platelets in plasma collected from a peripheral vein.
    - *Mechanism:* Releases cytokines and growth factors [VEGF, transforming growth factor (TGF), platelet-derived growth factor (PDGF), and epidermal growth factor (EGF)] and exerts a regenerative effect on tissues and cells including the endometrial lining damaged secondary to a disease or procedure.
    - PRP is collected from autologous blood sample, so it is more accessible and cost-effective with minimal risks of transmission of infection and immunological reactions since it is made from autologous blood samples.
    - Few studies have shown promising results with the use of PRP in women with thin EMT with improvements in EMT and pregnancy rates;[38,39] however, its role in improvement of live births is still debatable in the absence of well-designed multicentric trials. There is still very limited evidence of its use,[38] so further larger well-designed multicentric RCTs are awaited before

recommending generalized usage of PRP for thin endometrium. Considering limited evidence, the additional cost, lack of standardized preparation protocols, the experimental nature of this intervention must be discussed with patients before offering it as a therapeutic modality.

- *Role of G-CSF:* It is a hematopoietic lineage-specific cytokine synthesized by stromal cells, bone marrow cells, endothelial cells, fibroblasts, lymphocytes, macrophages, endometrium, and human ovary.
    - *Mechanism:*
        - Suppresses immune response
        - Vascular modeling of the endometrium
        - Enhance cellular adhesion pathways
        - Improves endometrial receptivity
        - Embryonic development, implantation, and trophoblastic growth
            - *Dose:* Subcutaneous—300 μg G-CSF; Intrauterine—30 mIU/mL
            - *Route:* Subcutaneous—for recurrent implantation with normal EMT; Intrauterine—for thin endometrium (<7 mm).

  Few studies have shown improvement in EMT and endometrial regeneration after G-CSF instillation; however, these were poorly designed and had a small sample size. The Cochrane meta-analysis in 2020 for the usage of G-CSF in women with thin endometrium showed insufficient evidence for its use (Cochrane meta-analysis 2020; RR: 1.58, 95% CI: 0.95–2.63; 4 RCTs; low-quality evidence). These trials also did not address the safety of the procedure.[40]
- *Role of sildenafil:* Another adjuvant routinely used to improve the EMT in women with thin endometrium is sildenafil. It is a vasodilator which is theoretically beneficial to increase the endometrial prefusion and consequently improve EMT. Results from studies using sildenafil for endometrial improvement are mixed.[41] The Cochrane meta-analysis in 2018 found that although sildenafil did improve the EMT (0.80–3.57 mean difference higher) at the cost of adverse effects such as tachycardia and headache.[42]

CONCLUSION

Endometrial thickness is considered the indirect surrogate marker for endometrial receptivity. A rare but problematic occurrence in assisted reproduction is thin endometrium. Clinicians often try different protocols and wait across various menstrual cycles to achieve an optimal EMT before transfer as studies have consistently reported lower pregnancy outcomes with decreasing EMT. An endometrium >7 mm is acceptable by most authors as the cutoff for the optimal EMT. Studies have also shown that pregnancies have been reported below 6 mm when the pattern is trilaminar. Etiology of thin EMT also helps in prognosticating; endometrial damage secondary to inflammatory fibrosis may be more extensive than that due to idiopathic or architectural causes.

If a patient chooses to continue therapy despite having a thin endometrium or opts for alternative therapies, doctors must weigh the prognosis for that patient. Unfortunately, there is no agreement on what constitutes a thin endometrial lining; although studies have consistently indicated that decreased EMT is associated with a lower rate of implantation and pregnancy, yet successful pregnancies have been reported at so-called "thin endometrium" also. Therefore, a thin endometrial stripe is not always detrimental and pregnancies can be achieved. For patients with thin endometrium, there is currently little data to support any specific regimens or adjuvants that would significantly improve pregnancy outcomes. A change in dosage or route of estrogen or performing a diagnostic hysteroscopy may be simplest and the most rewarding intervention in majority of the cases. Adjuvants for increasing EMT should be individualized with the patients being counseled on their experimental nature, additional costs, and unproven results so far. Despite all interventions, if all measures fail to improve the EMT, patients should be counseled to proceed with transfer knowing the low results versus gestational surrogacy if feasible.

REFERENCES

1. Brosens JJ, Salker MS, Teklenburg G, Nautiyal J, Salter S, Lucas ES, et al. Uterine selection of human embryos at implantation. Sci Rep. 2014;4(1):3894.
2. Mahajan N, Sharma S. The endometrium in assisted reproductive technology: How thin is thin? J Hum Reprod Sci. 2016;9(1):3-8.
3. Senturk LM, Erel CT. Thin endometrium in assisted reproductive technology. Curr Opin Obstet Gynecol. 2008; 20(3):221-8.
4. Torry DS, Leavenworth J, Chang M, Maheshwari V, Groesch K, Ball ER, et al. Angiogenesis in implantation. J Assist Reprod Genet. 2007;24:303-15.
5. Bagheri A, Chianeh YR, Kumar P, Rao P. Angiogenic factors in relation to embryo implantation. Int J Reprod Contracept Obstet Gynecol. 2014;3(4):872-80.

6. Lutjen P, Trounson A, Leeton J, Findlay J, Wood C, Renou P. The establishment and maintenance of pregnancy using in vitro fertilization and embryo donation in a patient with primary ovarian failure. Nature. 1984;307:174-5.
7. Persadie RJ. Ultrasonographic assessment of endometrial thickness: a review. J Obstet Gynaecol Can. 2002;24(2):131-6.
8. Ghobara T, Gelbaya TA, Ayeleke RO. Cycle regimens for frozen-thawed embryo transfer. Cochrane Database Syst Rev. 2017;7(7):CD003414.
9. Bu Z, Sun Y. The impact of endometrial thickness on the day of human chorionic gonadotrophin (hCG) administration on ongoing pregnancy rate in patients with different ovarian response. PLoS One. 2015;10(12):e0145703.
10. Takasaki A, Tamura H, Miwa I, Taketani T, Shimamura K, Sugino N. Endometrial growth and uterine blood flow: a pilot study for improving endometrial thickness in the patients with a thin endometrium. Fertil Steril. 2010;93(6): 1851-8.
11. Labrosse J, Lobersztajn A, Pietin-Vialle C, Villette C, Dessapt AL, Jung C, et al. Comparison of stimulated versus modified natural cycles for endometrial preparation prior to frozen embryo transfer: a randomized controlled trial. Reprod Biomed Online. 2020;40:518-24.
12. Alur-Gupta S, Hopeman M, Berger DS, Gracia C, Barnhart KT, Coutifaris C, et al. Impact of method of endometrial preparation for frozen blastocyst transfer on pregnancy outcome: a retrospective cohort study. Fertil Steril. 2018; 110:680-6.
13. Yarali H, Polat M, Mumusoglu S, Yarali I, Bozdag G. Preparation of endometrium for frozen embryo replacement cycles: a systematic review and meta-analysis. J Assist Reprod Genet. 2016;33:1287-304.
14. Groenewoud ER, Cohlen BJ, Al-Oraiby A, Brinkhuis EA, Broekmans FJ, de Bruin JP, et al. A randomized controlled, non-inferiority trial of modified natural versus artificial cycle for cryo-thawed embryo transfer. Hum Reprod. 2016; 31:1483-92.
15. Pan Y, Li B, Wang Z, Wang Y, Gong X, Zhou W, et al. Hormone replacement versus natural cycle protocols of endometrial preparation for frozen embryo transfer. Front Endocrinol (Lausanne). 2020;11:546532.
16. Shaodi Z, Qiuyuan L, Yisha Y, Cuilian Z. The effect of endometrial thickness on pregnancy outcomes of frozen-thawed embryo transfer cycles which underwent hormone replacement therapy. PloS One. 2020;15(9): e0239120.
17. Moshkalova G, Karibayeva I, Kurmanova A, Mamedalieva N, Aimbetova A, Terlikbayeva A, et al. Endometrial thickness and live birth rates after IVF: a systematic review. Acta Biomed. 2023;94(3):e2023152.
18. Kasius A, Smit JG, Torrance HL, Eijkemans MJ, Mol BW, Opmeer BC, et al. Endometrial thickness and pregnancy rates after IVF: a systematic review and meta-analysis. Hum Reprod Update. 2014;20(4):530-41.
19. Lee JC, Badell ML, Kawwass JF. The impact of endometrial preparation for frozen embryo transfer on maternal and neonatal outcomes: a review. Reprod Biol Endocrinol. 2022;20:1-12.
20. Danhof NA, van Eekelen R, Repping S, Mol BW, van der Veen F, van Wely M, et al. Endometrial thickness as a biomarker for ongoing pregnancy in IUI for unexplained subfertility: a secondary analysis. Hum Reprod Open. 2020; 2020(1):hoz024.
21. Liu KE, Hartman M, Hartman A, Luo ZC, Mahutte N. The impact of a thin endometrial lining on fresh and frozen-thaw IVF outcomes: an analysis of over 40 000 embryo transfers. Hum Reprod. 2018;33(10):1883-8.
22. Liu KE, Hartman M, Hartman A. Management of thin endometrium in assisted reproduction: a clinical practice guideline from the Canadian Fertility and Andrology Society. Reprod Biomed Online. 2019;39(1):49-62.
23. Patel JA, Patel AJ, Banker JM, Shah SI, Banker M. Effect of endometrial thickness and duration of estrogen supplementation on in vitro fertilization-intracytoplasmic sperm injection outcomes in fresh ovum/embryo donation cycles. J Hum Reprod Sci. 2021;14(2):167-74.
24. Mahutte N, Hartman M, Meng L, Lanes A, Luo ZC, Liu KE. Optimal endometrial thickness in fresh and frozen-thaw in vitro fertilization cycles: an analysis of live birth rates from 96,000 autologous embryo transfers. Fertil Steril. 2022;117(4):792-800.
25. Değer U, Kalı Z, Çağıran F. Endometrial thickness is a good predictor of clinical pregnancy and live birth rates in fresh and frozen-thawed embryo transfer cycles. Eur Rev Med Pharmacol Sci. 2023;27(13):6351-8.
26. Kumbak B, Erden HF, Tosun S, Akbas H, Ulug U, Bahçeci M. Outcome of assisted reproduction treatment in patients with endometrial thickness less than 7 mm. Reprod Biomed Online. 2009;18:79-84.
27. Check JH, Cohen R. Live fetus following embryo transfer in a woman with diminished egg reserve whose maximal endometrial thickness was less than 4 mm. Clin Exp Obstet Gynecol. 2011;38:330-2.
28. Noyes N, Liu HC, Sultan K, Schattman G, Rosenwaks Z. Endometrial thickness appears to be a significant factor in embryo implantation in in-vitro fertilization. Hum Reprod. 1995;10:919-22.
29. Quaas AM, Gavrizi SZ, Peck JD, Diamond M, Legro R, Robinson R, et al. Endometrial thickness after ovarian stimulation with gonadotropin, clomiphene, or letrozole for unexplained infertility, and association with treatment outcomes. Fertil Steril. 2021;115:213-20.
30. Miwa I, Tamura H, Takasaki A, Yamagata Y, Shimamura K, Sugino N. Pathophysiologic features of "thin" endometrium. Fertil Steril. 2009;91:998-1004.
31. Tourgeman DE, Slater CC, Stanczyk FZ, Paulson RJ. Endocrine and clinical effects of micronized estradiol administered vaginally or orally. Fertil Steril. 2001;75:200-2.

32. Liao X, Li Z, Dong X, Zhang H. Comparison between oral and vaginal estrogen usage in inadequate endometrial patients for frozen-thawed blastocysts transfer. Int J Clin Exp Pathol. 2014;7:6992-7.
33. Eserol F, Göksever Çelik H, Aytan AN, Çelik A, Çelik E, Buyru F, et al. The effect of diagnostic hysteroscopy performed before fresh and frozen-thawed embryo transfer in IVF cycles on reproductive outcomes. J Turk Ger Gynecol Assoc. 2021;22(3):206-11.
34. El-Toukhy T, Campo R, Khalaf Y, Tabanelli C, Gianaroli L, Gordts SS, et al. Hysteroscopy in recurrent in-vitro fertilisation failure (TROPHY): a multicentre, randomised controlled trial. Lancet. 2016;387(10038):2614-21.
35. Wang L, Huang X, Li X, Lv F, He X, Pan Y, et al. Efficacy evaluation of low-dose aspirin in IVF/ICSI patients evidence from 13 RCTs: a systematic review and meta-analysis. Medicine (Baltimore). 2017;96(37):e7720.
36. Palomba S, Macklon N. Endometrial scratching: is it all over? Reprod Biomed Online. 2022;44(4):583-5.
37. Palomba S, Vitagliano A. Is the era of the endometrial scratching finished? Fertil Steril. 2022;118(3):603.
38. Dogra Y, Singh N, Vanamail P. Autologous platelet-rich plasma optimizes endometrial thickness and pregnancy outcomes in women with refractory thin endometrium of varied aetiology during fresh and frozen-thawed embryo transfer cycles. JBRA Assist Reprod. 2022;26(1):13-21.
39. Maged AM, El-Mazny A, Kamal N, Mahmoud SI, Fouad M, El-Nassery N, et al. The value of platelet-rich plasma in women with previous implantation failure: a systematic review and meta-analysis. J Assist Reprod Genet. 2023;40(5):969-83.
40. Kamath MS, Kirubakaran R, Sunkara SK. Granulocyte-colony stimulating factor administration for subfertile women undergoing assisted reproduction. Cochrane Database Syst Rev. 2020;1(1):CD013226.
41. Moini A, Zafarani F, Jahangiri N, Sadatmahalleh SJ, Sadeghi M, Chehrazi M, et al. The effect of vaginal sildenafil on the outcome of assisted reproductive technology cycles in patients with repeated implantation failures: a randomized placebo-controlled trial. Int J Fertil Steril. 2020;13:289-95.
42. Gutarra-Vilchez RB, Bonfill Cosp X, Glujovsky D, Viteri-García A, Runzer-Colmenares FM, Martinez-Zapata MJ. Vasodilators for women undergoing fertility treatment. Cochrane Database Syst Rev. 2018;10(10):CD010001.

Chapter

Endometrial Receptivity Array: Is it Beneficial?

Sulbha Arora, Jyoti Tripathi

INTRODUCTION

Assisted reproductive technologies (ARTs) have come a long way since the birth of the first in vitro fertilization (IVF) baby Louise Brown in 1978. Over the last forty years, success rates have dramatically improved and the incidence of unwanted complications has reduced. This has largely been due to the advent of simpler, more patient-friendly stimulation protocols, along with advances in the embryology laboratory such as more efficient culture media, advanced cryopreservation techniques, and the ability to culture embryos to the blastocyst stage. This has enabled the reduction of the number of embryos being transferred and the improvement in the implantation rate of each individual embryo produced. Yet, we seem to hit a glass ceiling beyond which the implantation rates cannot be further improved. The 2020 report published by SART (Society for Assisted Reproductive Technology) quotes a live birth rate of 54.5% for women <35 years of age.[1] This implies that the majority of the embryos transferred do not seem to implant.

Human embryo implantation involves a complex cross talk between the maternal endometrium and the developing embryo. The embryo needs to hatch out of its protective shell or zona pellucida. Simultaneously, the endometrium needs to open its window of implantation (WOI). Multiple pinopodes appear at this stage, which function to absorb uterine cavity fluid and bring the endometrium in close contact with the floating embryo. This is followed by the triad of apposition, adhesion, and invasion of the endometrium by the blastocyst, leading to successful implantation. Therefore, when the process of implantation fails, we are faced with the question—is it in the seed, or is it in the soil? Diagnosing the exact cause of implantation failure can be difficult.

RECURRENT IMPLANTATION FAILURE

For some women, the process of implantation may fail repeatedly. Recurrent implantation failure (RIF) is a challenging scenario in ART and several efforts are being made to improve and increase the success rates of IVF. There is no consensus to the number of attempts, or the number of transferred embryos required to qualify for a diagnosis of RIF. The difference of opinion stems from the number and stage of embryos being transferred. The 2005 ESHRE PGD Consortium defined RIF as failure to achieve a viable pregnancy, following "more than three embryo transfers with high quality embryos or the transfer of ≥10 embryos in multiple transfers; exact numbers to be determined by each center".[2] However in today's day and age where we are moving toward elective single embryo transfers at blastocyst stage, it is no longer practical to wait up to a failure of 10 such embryos before seeking answers. Orvieto et al. defined it as a failure to conceive after three transfers with good quality embryos.[3] Zeyneloglu's definition is similar, specifically adding two embryos of high quality.[4] Rinehart pointed out that maternal age and stage of embryos, whether cleavage or blastocyst, should be taken into consideration while defining RIF.[5] Coughlan et al. suggested a more working definition incorporating maternal age, the number of transfers, and the number of embryos.[6] As per their definition, *"Recurrent implantation failure refers to failure to achieve a clinical pregnancy after transfer of at least four good-quality embryos in a minimum of three fresh or frozen cycles in women under 40 years of age".*

Among the several definitions of RIF, the most accepted definition is failure to achieve pregnancy after three failed attempts of IVF in which one or two morphologically high-grade embryos were transferred.[7,8]

Multiple causes of RIF have been studied including both embryonic factors and maternal factors. The common causes of RIF include embryonic aneuploidies especially in advanced maternal age group;[9,10] hydrosalpinges;[11] pathological changes of the endometrial cavity, such as synechiae, endometritis, hyperplasia, submucous myomas, or endometrial polyps (which can be found in 18–27% of cases);[12] other causes, such lifestyle factors, thyroid dysfunction, and hereditary and acquired thrombophilias.[13]

Implantation still remains uncertain after correction of these pathological conditions and more challenging in cases where no identifiable cause has been discovered. Thus, in recent years, the focus of studies has shifted toward proposing the role of a dysfunctional endometrium as an important contributing factor for RIF. After all, the synchrony between a healthy embryo and a receptive endometrium is a well-established mandatory process that aids successful implantation.

ROLE OF THE ENDOMETRIAL RECEPTIVITY

The endometrium is a self-renewing dynamic tissue lining the uterine cavity. It undergoes continuous cyclic modifications, which are regulated by several endocrine and paracrine signals that control gene expression of the endometrial cells.[14] Morphologically, the endometrial lining is divided into functional and basal layers. The functional layer undergoes synchronized changes throughout the menstrual cycle to implant the embryo, while the basal layer helps to regenerate the functional layer postmenses. The endometrium is not receptive to the embryo at all times of the menstrual cycle. It acquires a functionally receptive phenotype under the influence of the ovarian steroid hormones for a very short period of time when it becomes favorable for implantation of the embryo. This period is known as the WOI. The WOI typically opens on day 19 or 20 of a regular 28-day cycle and remains open for just 4–5 days at the time when progesterone reaches peak serum concentrations.[15] To increase the outcome of simulated reproductive treatments like IVF it is imperative to identify this WOI more accurately, so the embryo transfer can be scheduled at the precise time when the window is open, and implantation is most likely. Histological, molecular, biochemical, and ultrasound markers of endometrial receptivity have low accuracy and low predictive value.[16] Search for an adequate marker of endometrial receptivity led to the development of a molecular diagnostic test—the endometrial receptivity array (ERA).

WHAT IS ENDOMETRIAL RECEPTIVITY ARRAY?

Endometrial receptivity array is a molecular diagnostic test of the endometrium, based on transcriptomics. Transcriptomics is considered the most established technology available for evaluation of the endometrial factor. After many years of research, decoding endometrial transcriptomics using next-generation sequencing (NGS) and thus objectively identifying the personalized window of implantation (pWOI) is now possible. The ERA test analyzes the expression of 238 genes in a biopsy sample of the endometrium, which are expressed differently at various stages of the endometrial cycle.[17] This test is patented by Igenomix in 2009. This gene expression result is coupled with computational analysis which predicts the personalized WOI of the given patient when the endometrium is receptive for implantation of the embryo.[17,18] The ERA results classify the given endometrial tissue sample as either "receptive" or "nonreceptive". Nonreceptive endometrium may again be either "prereceptive" or "postreceptive".[18]

PREPARATION OF ENDOMETRIUM AND SAMPLING FOR BIOPSY

The endometrial preparation for ERA can be done in three different ways: (1) endometrial biopsy in a natural cycle, (2) in a modified natural cycle, or (3) in a hormone replacement therapy (HRT) cycle. It is imperative to use the same method that will be used later during the actual embryo transfer. The medications used for endometrial preparation and luteal support including the dose, the route of administration, and method have to precisely mimic the protocol that will be used when the embryo transfer is planned. This ensures the reproducibility of the test results under the exact same circumstances.

Endometrial Biopsy in a Natural Cycle

It involves transvaginal ultrasound to track the follicular growth and the endometrial thickness in a natural cycle. Once the follicle has achieved dominance, it is important to monitor the luteinizing hormone (LH) surge. This can be done by urine test or blood test. The sample for ERA biopsy is taken 7 days after the LH surge (LH + 7).

Endometrial Preparation in a Modified Natural Cycle

The cycle monitoring is done by transvaginal ultrasound and injection human chorionic gonadotropin (hCG) is administered once the dominant follicle size is over 17–18 mm. The biopsy is done on hCG + 7.

ERA Test in a Hormone Replacement Therapy Cycle

Transvaginal ultrasound is done on day 2 of the menstrual cycle and estradiol tablets are started. Serial ultrasound scans are done from day 10 of the cycle onward. Once the endometrium is ready, which means it is at least 7 mm in thickness with a trilaminar appearance, a blood sample is drawn to assess the serum progesterone level, and the luteal phase support is started. The endometrial biopsy is taken on day P + 5 in an HRT cycle.

The endometrial biopsy is done under sterile conditions, using a Pipelle catheter from the uterine fundus. It is a minor, outpatient procedure, causing no to minimal discomfort and does not require anesthesia.

INTERPRETATION OF BIOPSY RESULTS

The ERA test results diagnoses the endometrial samples as receptive or nonreceptive.[19] A nonreceptive test signifies a displaced window of transfer. The ERA predictor also infers if it is prereceptive or postreceptive; and accordingly calculates and suggests a putative pWOI.

The gene profile analysis of a prereceptive ERA test indicates a delayed pWOI **(Fig. 1)** while a postreceptive

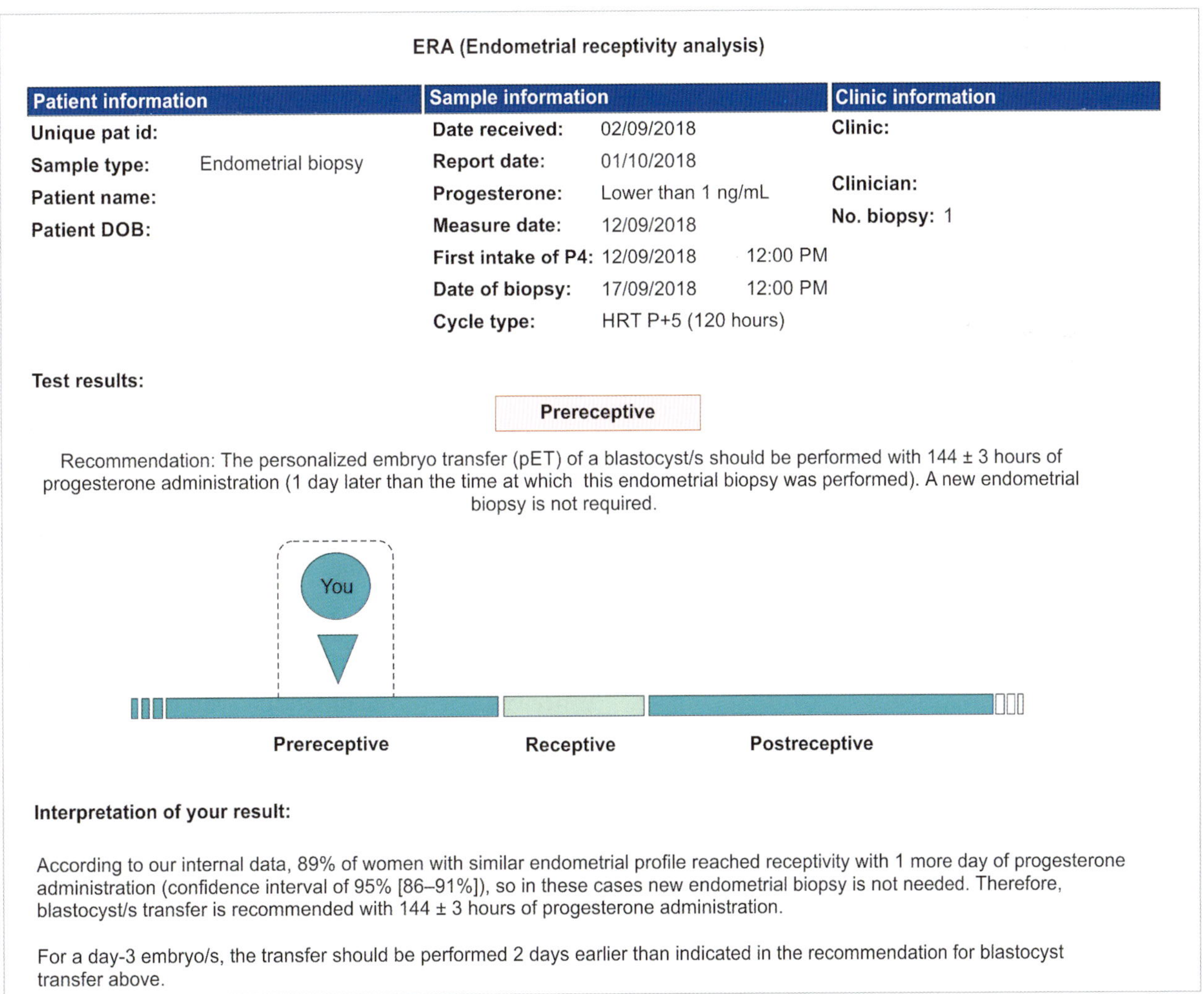

ERA (Endometrial receptivity analysis)

Patient information		Sample information			Clinic information
Unique pat id:		**Date received:**	02/09/2018		**Clinic:**
Sample type:	Endometrial biopsy	**Report date:**	01/10/2018		
Patient name:		**Progesterone:**	Lower than 1 ng/mL		**Clinician:**
Patient DOB:		**Measure date:**	12/09/2018		**No. biopsy:** 1
		First intake of P4:	12/09/2018	12:00 PM	
		Date of biopsy:	17/09/2018	12:00 PM	
		Cycle type:	HRT P+5 (120 hours)		

Test results:

Prereceptive

Recommendation: The personalized embryo transfer (pET) of a blastocyst/s should be performed with 144 ± 3 hours of progesterone administration (1 day later than the time at which this endometrial biopsy was performed). A new endometrial biopsy is not required.

You

Prereceptive **Receptive** **Postreceptive**

Interpretation of your result:

According to our internal data, 89% of women with similar endometrial profile reached receptivity with 1 more day of progesterone administration (confidence interval of 95% [86–91%]), so in these cases new endometrial biopsy is not needed. Therefore, blastocyst/s transfer is recommended with 144 ± 3 hours of progesterone administration.

For a day-3 embryo/s, the transfer should be performed 2 days earlier than indicated in the recommendation for blastocyst transfer above.

Fig. 1: The ERA result shows a prereceptive endometrium, and calculates the ideal time for transfer, in this instance, as 144 ± 3 hours of progesterone administration.

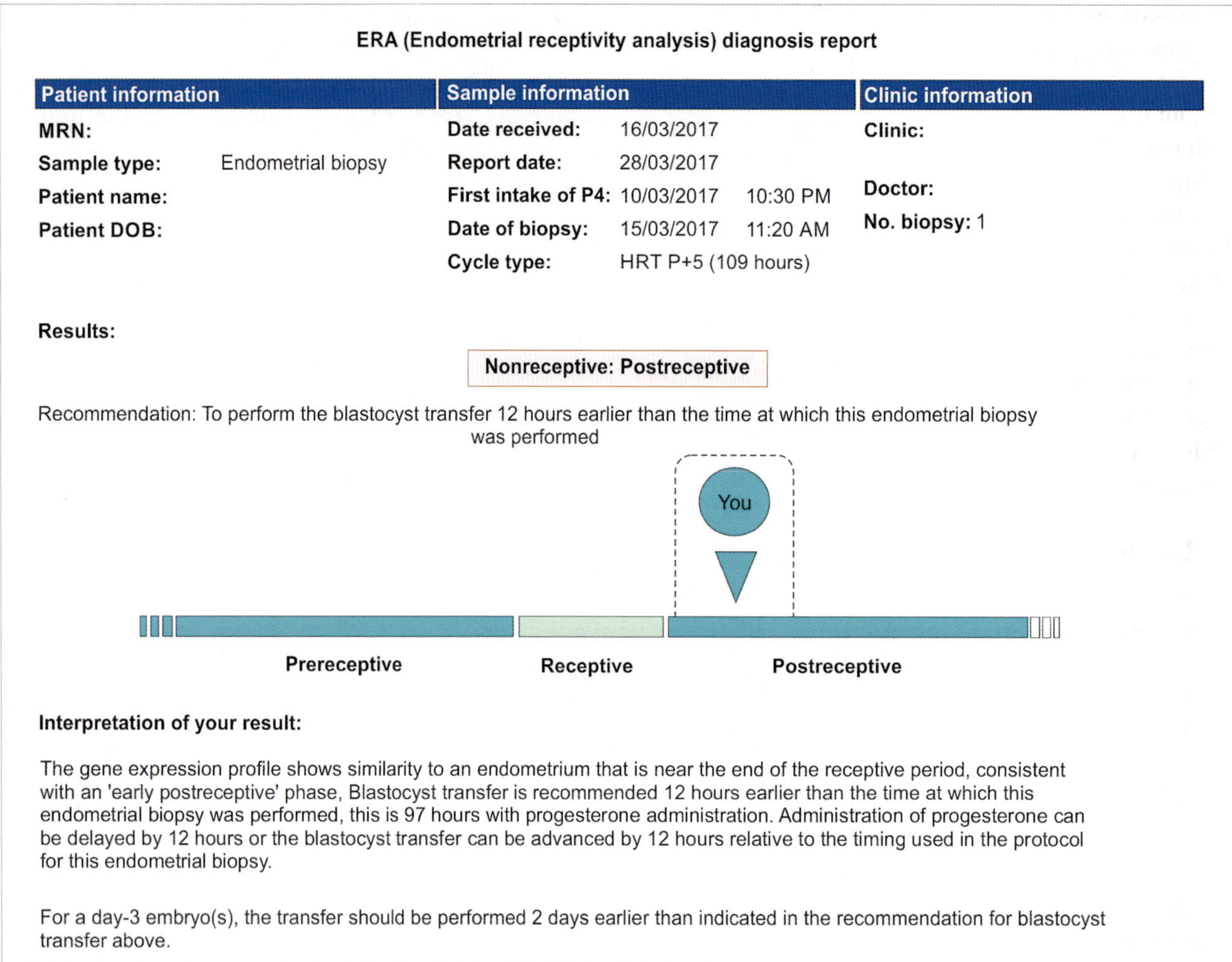

ERA (Endometrial receptivity analysis) diagnosis report

Patient information		Sample information			Clinic information
MRN:		Date received:	16/03/2017		Clinic:
Sample type:	Endometrial biopsy	Report date:	28/03/2017		
Patient name:		First intake of P4:	10/03/2017	10:30 PM	Doctor:
Patient DOB:		Date of biopsy:	15/03/2017	11:20 AM	No. biopsy: 1
		Cycle type:	HRT P+5 (109 hours)		

Results:

Nonreceptive: Postreceptive

Recommendation: To perform the blastocyst transfer 12 hours earlier than the time at which this endometrial biopsy was performed

Interpretation of your result:

The gene expression profile shows similarity to an endometrium that is near the end of the receptive period, consistent with an 'early postreceptive' phase, Blastocyst transfer is recommended 12 hours earlier than the time at which this endometrial biopsy was performed, this is 97 hours with progesterone administration. Administration of progesterone can be delayed by 12 hours or the blastocyst transfer can be advanced by 12 hours relative to the timing used in the protocol for this endometrial biopsy.

For a day-3 embryo(s), the transfer should be performed 2 days earlier than indicated in the recommendation for blastocyst transfer above.

Fig. 2: The ERA result shows a postreceptive endometrium, and calculates the ideal time for transfer, in this instance, as 12 hours earlier than the time when the biopsy was taken.

test indicates an advanced pWOI **(Fig. 2)**. In a few cases, a second endometrial biopsy is performed in order to validate the pWOI as per specific recommendation by the ERA classifier, although this is not usually required.

ACCURACY

The sensitivity and specificity of ERA test is 0.99758 and 0.8857, respectively.[17] The ERA test has been found superior compared to endometrial histology in past reports.[20] Importantly, the results of the test are highly reproducible for the same patient for up to 40 months from the time of the first biopsy and do not change significantly in-between the cycles.[18] In a study published by Ruiz Alonso M et al., 85 RIF and 25 controls underwent the ERA test. 88% of controls had a receptive report, whereas in RIF patients 74.1% had a receptive report. 15 RIF patients with a nonreceptive report subsequently had an embryo transfer done according to their pWOI, and 8 of them conceived.[19] A systematic review with meta-analysis was performed recently by Glujovsky et al. to assess whether a personalized embryo transfer (pET) guided by tests for endometrial receptivity increases the effectiveness of ART procedures.[21] Search terms included endometrial receptivity analysis, ERA, pET. CENTRAL, PubMed, Embase, reference lists, clinical trials registers, and conference proceedings (search date October 2022) were searched, with no language restrictions. They screened 2,136 studies and included 35 (85% used ERA and 15% used other receptivity tests). Two studies were randomized controlled trials (RCTs) comparing endometrial receptivity analysis (ERA)-guided pET versus standard embryo transfer (sET) in women with no history of RIF. In women without RIF, no important differences were found in live birth rates and clinical pregnancy rates (CPRs). They also performed a meta-analysis of four cohort studies that were adjusted for confounding. In agreement with the RCTs, no benefits were found in women without RIF. However, in women with RIF, low certainty of evidence suggests that pET might improve the CPR [odds ratio (OR): 2.50, 95% confidence interval (CI): 1.42–4.40]. They concluded that the use of receptivity testing-guided pET is not supported by current published evidence in women without RIF, while in women with RIF more research is needed to assess a potential benefit.

PLANNING OF EMBRYO TRANSFER

It is recommended to perform the blastocyst transfer as per the pWOI recommended by the ERA results. It is important to mimic the same cycle type with the same doses and routes of drugs used, if any, as was followed during the ERA cycle.

CONCLUSION

Recurrent implantation failure is one of the most challenging and frustrating situations in the field of ART. Our deeper understanding of the endometrium has led us to a stage where we have learnt that it is not just the morphology of the endometrium on ultrasound that is essential for implantation but also its functionality. Microarray studies have broadened our insight and have resulted in the development of gene expression diagnostic techniques that are aimed at translating findings into clinical applications. These studies can potentially improve implantation and pregnancy rates. The ERA test or the ERA is a tool that studies 238 endometrial genes responsible for receptivity in both natural and hormone replacement cycles. This array is more accurate than conventional histologic dating of the endometrium, and the test result for any given patient stays valid for up to 40 months after biopsy. This test was designed to detect a shifted WOI that may be either advanced or delayed, thus preventing implantation of a transferred embryo due to embryo-endometrial dyssynchronization. The endometrium is prepared using the identical protocol that is planned for the embryo transfer cycle. An endometrial biopsy is taken 5 days after starting luteal support when done in an HRT cycle and sent for the ERA analysis. The report is generated as either receptive or nonreceptive. A nonreceptive report indicates a shifted window which may be either pre- or postreceptive and is accompanied by a recommendation for the precise duration of luteal support required for embryo transfer. However, the safety, efficacy, and practicality of new emerging methods of diagnosis or treatment should be evaluated in prospective randomized clinical trials before being accepted into regular clinical practice.

REFERENCES

1. Society for Assisted Reproductive Technology, National Summary Report. (2021).
2. Thornhill AR, deDie-Smulders CE, Geraedts JP, Harper JC, Harton GL, Lavery SA, et al. Consortium, ESHRE PGD consortium 'Best practice guidelines for clinical preimplantation genetic diagnosis (PGD) and preimplantation genetic screening (PGS)'. Hum Reprod. 2005; 20:35-48.
3. Orvieto R, Brengauz M, Feldman B. A novel approach to normal responder patient with repeated implantation failures—a case report. Gynecol Endocrinol. 2015;31(6): 435-7.
4. Zeyneloglu HB, Onalan G. Remedies for recurrent implantation failure. Semin Reprod Med. 2014;32(4): 297-305.
5. Rinehart J. Recurrent implantation failure: definition. J Assist Reprod Genet. 2007;24(7):284-7.
6. Coughlan C, Ledger W, Wang Q, Liu F, Demirol A, Gurgan T, et al. Recurrent implantation failure: definition and management. Reprod Biomed Online. 2014;28(1):14-38.
7. Stephenson MD, Fluker MR. Treatment of repeated unexplained in vitro fertilization failure with intravenous immunoglobulin: a randomized, placebo-controlled Canadian trial. Fertil Steril. 2000;74:1108-13.
8. Simon A, Laufer N. Repeated implantation failure: clinical approach. Fertil Steril. 2012;97:1039-43.
9. Kung A, Munne S, Bankowski B, Coates A, Wells D. Validation of next- generation sequencing for comprehensive chromosome screening of embryos. Reprod Biomed Online. 2015;31:760-9.
10. Pehlivan T, Rubio C, Rodrigo L, Romero J, Remohi J, Simon C, et al. Impact of preimplantation genetic diagnosis on IVF outcome in implantation failure patients. Reprod Biomed Online. 2003;6:232-7.
11. Meyer WR, Castelbaum AJ, Somkuti S, Sagoskin AW, Doyle M, Harris JE, et al. Hydrosalpinges adversely affect markers of endometrial receptivity. Hum Reprod. 1997;12:1393-8.
12. Demirol A, Gurgan T. Effect of treatment of intrauterine pathologies with office hysteroscopy in patients with recurrent IVF failure. Reprod Biomed Online. 2004;8:590-4.

13. Penzias AS. Recurrent IVF failure: other factors. Fertil Steril. 2012;97:1033-8.
14. Ruiz-Alonso M, Blesa D, Simón C. The genomics of the human endometrium. Biochim Biophys Acta. 2012;1822: 1931-42.
15. Lessey BA. Assessment of endometrial receptivity. Fertil Steril. 2011;96:522-9.
16. Murray MJ, Meyer WR, Zaino RJ, Lessey BA, Novotny DB, Ireland K, et al. A critical analysis of the accuracy, reproducibility, and clinical utility of histologic endometrial dating in fertile women. Fertil Steril. 2004;8:1333-43.
17. Díaz-Gimeno P, Horcajadas JA, Martínez-Conejero JA, Esteban FJ, Alamá P, Pellicer A, et al. A genomic diagnostic tool for human endometrial receptivity based on the transcriptomic signature. Fertil Steril. 2011;95:50-60, 60.e1-15.
18. Garrido-Gómez T, Ruiz-Alonso M, Blesa D, Diaz-Gimeno P, Vilella F, Simón C. Profiling the gene signature of endometrial receptivity: Clinical results. Fertil Steril. 2013; 99:1078-85.
19. Ruiz-Alonso M, Blesa D, Díaz-Gimeno P, Gómez E, Fernández-Sánchez M, Carranza F, et al. The endometrial receptivity array for diagnosis and personalized embryo transfer as a treatment for patients with repeated implantation failure. Fertil Steril. 2013;100(3):818-24.
20. Díaz-Gimeno P, Ruiz-Alonso M, Blesa D, Bosch N, Martínez-Conejero JA, Alamá P, et al. The accuracy and reproducibility of the endometrial receptivity array is superior to histology as a diagnostic method for endometrial receptivity. Fertil Steril. 2013;99(2):508-17.
21. Glujovsky D, Lattes K, Miguens M, Pesce R, Ciapponi A. Personalized embryo transfer guided by endometrial receptivity analysis: a systematic review with meta-analysis. Hum Reprod. 2023;38(7):1305-17.

Intralipids and Intravenous Immunoglobulin in Infertility: Do They Actually Work?

Mohit Rajendra Saraogi

INTRODUCTION

The field of assisted reproductive technology (ART) and in vitro fertilization (IVF) has come a long way since its inception and the delivery of first IVF baby in 1978. Multiple new advances and breakthroughs have led to tremendous improvements in pregnancy and take-home baby rates. However, recurrent implantation failure (RIF) and recurrent pregnancy loss (RPL) still remain the most challenging and frustrating situations for both the clinician and the patient. The cause often remains unknown, leading to frustration and stress.

Repeated implantation failure has been observed in approximately 10% of women undergoing IVF.[1] Though there is no consensus for definition of RIF, it is generally defined as three or more failed treatment cycles as well as failure to achieve a clinical pregnancy after transfer of at least four good-quality embryos over three fresh or frozen embryo transfer (ET) cycles.[2]

Approximately 1–3% of women have RPL. According to the American Society for Reproductive Medicine (ASRM)[3] and the recent European Society of Human Reproduction and Embryology (ESHRE) guidelines,[4] RPL has been defined as two or more failed clinical pregnancies including biochemical pregnancy losses and/or resolved and treated pregnancies of unknown location after 6 weeks of gestation.

Immunological abnormalities are known to reduce endometrial receptivity, and impaired endometrial receptivity has been suggested as a major cause of RIF and RPL.[5]

Various immunotherapies have thus been explored to improve endometrial receptivity and increase the pregnancy rate in patients with RIF and RPL. These include intralipids, intravenous immunoglobulin (IVIG), leukocyte immunization, and low-molecular-weight heparin (LMWH).[6,7]

THE IMMUNE SYSTEM AND INFERTILITY

Immunological mechanisms have long been thought to play an important role in reproductive problems such as recurrent miscarriages and RIF.

Principally, for a successful pregnancy to occur, there needs to be an immunological maternal adaptation to the semi-allogeneic implanted embryo. Aspects of this immunological cross adaptation between the mother and the embryo still remain a mystery. How the uterus accepts a semi-allogeneic embryo without any immunological cross-reaction is incompletely understood, and it has been argued that alterations in this process may contribute to the failure to achieve a clinical pregnancy.

Statistically approximately 70% of spontaneous conceptions are lost prior to completion of the first trimester. Implantation failure and preclinical losses account for 85% of total pregnancy losses, and clinical miscarriage for 15%.[8] Recent advances in molecular biology have helped us better understand the fetomaternal cross-interaction during implantation. The atypical expression of major histocompatibility complex (MHC), the specific role of some hormones and cytokines, as well as the temporal and spatial distributions of uterine natural killer (NK) cells represent substantive parameters of fetomaternal immunotolerance during implantation.[5] RIF has been associated with elevated levels of antiphospholipid antibody (APA), elevated circulating levels of peripheral NK cells, and excess of T helper 1 (Th1)-type cytokines relative to Th2/3 cytokines.[9]

INTRALIPIDS IN INFERTILITY

Intralipid is a lipid emulsion made from soybean oil. Historically, it was used as a nutritional supplement for patients unable to eat orally due to its rich source of fat. Today in addition to its nutritional function, it has widespread use in immunotherapy as well. It has an immune-protective function, as its active component soybean oil is known to inhibit the cytotoxic activity of NK cells.

Mechanism of Action of Intralipids

Natural killer cytotoxicity has long been considered a leading reason for RIF and recurrent miscarriages.[10,11] The immune mechanism of intralipid has not been fully understood. However, it has been suggested that it has immunosuppressive properties. Its immunosuppressive properties act on inhibiting the cytotoxic activity of NK cells and reduce the production of certain cytokines, such as interleukin (IL) 6, tumor necrosis factor alpha, and IL 8, all of which are known to be proinflammatory cytokines.[12,13]

It has been shown that intralipids act on NK cells through their receptors such as the G protein-coupled receptor and peroxisome proliferator-activated receptor (PPAR). The fatty acids in intralipid and its metabolites act as ligands that bind and activate PPAR expressed in NK cells. It is this PPAR activation, which leads to reduced NK cell cytotoxicity and consequently increased implantation rates and viable pregnancy.[14-17] PPAR also contributes to implantation, invasion of cytotrophoblasts, embryo growth, and development of the placenta.[18,19]

Method of Administration

The method of intralipid administration varies from study to study. In most studies, 20% intralipid was given twice, intravenously. The first dose was given any day between day 4 and day 9 of controlled ovarian hyperstimulation or on the day of egg retrieval, or on the day of the ET. The second dose of intralipid was administered either on the day of ET or on the day of the pregnancy test, or within 1 week of a positive pregnancy test. The usual dose is 4 mL of 20% intralipid diluted in 250 mL of saline.

Intralipid is contraindicated in women with disturbances of normal fat metabolism such as pathologic hyperlipidemia, impaired kidney function, lipoid nephrosis, or acute pancreatitis if accompanied by hyperlipidemia.

Most studies of intralipids have shown no significant adverse effects on maternal or perinatal outcomes. Though there has been the occasional mention of congenital diaphragmatic hernia and congenital external ear abnormalities in the occasional case, none of them were statistically significant.

Intralipid Therapy and Reproductive Outcomes

The effectiveness of intralipid administration in cases of RIF and recurrent miscarriages is highly debatable and different studies seem to show conflicting results.

A study done by Martini et al. in women with RIF or recurrent spontaneous abortion (RSA) with elevated NK cells (>19%) failed to show any beneficial effect of intralipid therapy on clinical pregnancy or live birth rates (LBRs) when compared with baseline rates.[20] Contrary to this, Dakhly et al. used 250 mL of intralipid infusion on the day of oocyte retrieval in patients with RPL with elevated peripheral blood NK cells (>12%) and observed increased ongoing pregnancy and LBRs.[21]

A meta-analysis by Han et al., which included only randomized controlled trials (RCTs), concluded that in women with RIF and RPL, intralipid administration causes significant improvement in the clinical pregnancy rate, ongoing pregnancy rate, and LBR. No significant difference was seen on miscarriage rates.[11] Similar observations were reported in another meta-analysis by Asif et al.[22]

The findings of these meta-analysis suggest that use of intralipids is a promising intervention for women with RIF and RSA. However, the exact mechanisms and safety of intralipid and the optimal dose and protocol for its administration need to be explored in further studies.

INTRAVENOUS IMMUNOGLOBULINS IN INFERTILITY

Intravenous immunoglobulin is derived from plasma and contains polyclonal immunoglobulin G. It has been used widely to treat patients with humoral immune deficiency and autoimmune diseases. It acts as an immune modulator and reduces both innate and adaptive immune responses through multiple actions. It has also been found to be safe and well tolerated in pregnancy, even at high doses. However, as it is derived from blood, IVIG is expensive and must be used judiciously.

Anti-inflammatory and immune-modulating properties of IVIG have been considered as potential treatment for failed IVF and RPL, given the hypothesized role of inflammatory bias in these conditions. It has been suggested that patients with recurrent miscarriage and RIF have an excess of proinflammatory Th1-type cytokines relative to Th2/3 cytokines. IVIG has thus been proposed as a treatment modality for these patients.

Most fertility societies have been conflicted on their opinion on the use of IVIGs for fertility treatment. However, quite a few of them recommend the use of IVIG in women with RPL and/or repeated implantation failure. It has also been recommended in patients who show altered cellular immune factors, such as abnormal NK cell levels, elevated NK cell cytotoxicity, altered Th1/Th2 ratios, and altered Th17/regulatory T-cell ratios.

Intravenous Immunoglobulin: Mechanism of Action

Intravenous immunoglobulin has a multipronged action, mediated through the two different portions of the immunoglobulin **(Fig. 1)**.[23-26]

The F (ab) 2-dependent mechanisms include:

- Killing of target cells by antibody-dependent cytotoxicity
- Neutralization of cytokines and autoantibodies
- Blockade of cell-to-cell interactions mediated by cell surface receptors such as Fas and Fas ligand (CD95)
- Scavenging of anaphylatoxins such as C3a and C5a.

The Fc-dependent mechanisms include:

- The saturation of the neonatal Fc receptor
- The expansion of regulatory T-cell populations
- The blockade of immune complex binding to activating Fcγ receptors
- The modulation of dendritic cell activation via Fcγ receptor III.

Intravenous Immunoglobulin: Dosage and Administration

Intravenous immunoglobulin is derived and purified from the plasma of 3,000 or more donors and contains >95% unmodified immunoglobulin G. It is usually administered in a dose of 0.6–0.8 g/kg. The total dose is divided in two doses. The first dose is administered at least a week prior to the egg retrieval. An additional dose is given once pregnant. Once pregnancy is confirmed, it is administered in a dose of 400 mg/kg once in 3–4 weeks. There is no conclusion as to till what gestation it should be continued and the end point is usually at the clinician's discretion.

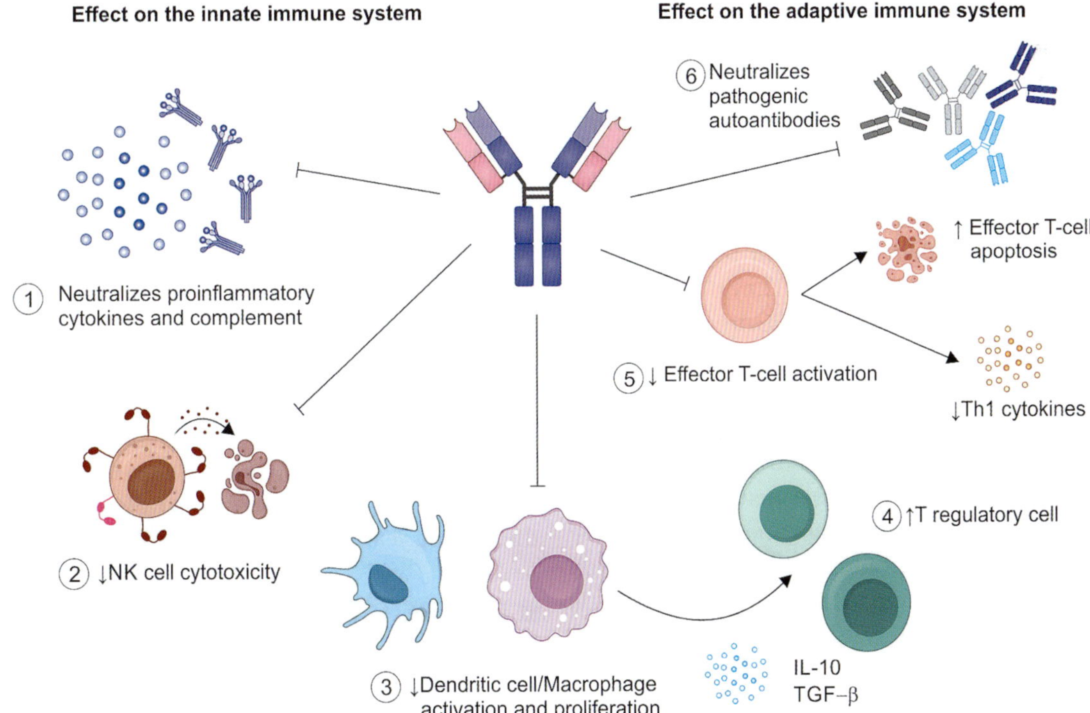

Fig. 1: Mechanism of action of intravenous immunoglobulin (IVIG).
(IL-10: interleukin 10; NK: natural killer; TGF-β: tumor necrosis factor beta)

Safety Profile of Intravenous Immunoglobulins

Intravenous immunoglobulin administration in prescribed doses is usually considered safe. There have been no serious teratogenic effects reported secondary to its administration. Mild maternal side effects include fever, malaise, myalgia, and headache. Serious side effects are rare and include renal failure, myocardial infarction, alopecia, and aseptic meningitis. It is advisable to check renal function test and the blood level of immunoglobulin A before starting the therapy.

Intravenous Immunoglobulin and Reproductive Outcomes

The results of IVIG treatment in women with RPL and RIF have been controversial. A review by Coulam et al. observed that IVIG enhances LBR in women with RPL and elevated NK cell levels.[27] However, two recent meta-analyses failed to see any improved results.[28,29]

Stephenson et al. conducted a prospective RCT in patients with ≥2 failed IVF-ET. The patients were randomized to receive IVIG 0.5 g/kg within 72 hours prior to ET or normal saline.[30] No significant difference in LBR was observed in both the groups. A meta-analysis by Li et al. concluded that IVIG is beneficial in women with RIF; however, these results must be interpreted with caution as study populations were heterogenous, and IVIG dose and timing of administration and administration with other immunomodulatory drugs differed between studies.[31] Abdolmohammadi-Vahid performed a systematic review to evaluate the effectiveness of IVIG in improving LBR in patients with ≥3 failed IVF-ET and high NK cells/cytotoxicity or high Th1/Th2 ratios. They observed that LBR was significantly higher in the IVIG-treated patients, however the study group was heterogeneous.[32] A recent review by Peero et al. concluded that IVIG administration increases the odds of live birth in patients with RIF, but more RCTs are required to confirm the observations.[33]

Overall, the available literature is heterogeneous and difficult to interpret. Also, there is no standardization of the dosage regimes, frequency of administration, and duration of therapy. The high cost and possibility of adverse effects are the other concerns with IVIG treatment. According to the latest ASRM guidelines, there is insufficient evidence to recommend IVIG administration to improve IVF outcomes.[34] Subpopulation that may benefit from IVIG may exist, but additional RCTs are required to exactly define these indications and explore the risks and benefits of IVIG. The good practice guidelines by ESHRE recommend against the routine use of immunomodulating agents in IVF.[35]

According to the Korean Society for Reproductive Immunology practice guidelines:[36]

- Empirical IVIG treatment in women with unexplained RPL is not recommended (evidence level A).
- IVIG treatment is recommended for women who have RPL with cellular immune abnormalities (evidence level A).
- In women with RPL with APA's the recommended first-line treatment is preferably low-dose aspirin (LDA) and LMWH. However IVIG can also be used.
- IVIG treatment in cases of unexplained RIF without immune evaluation is not recommended (evidence level A).
- In cases of RIF with cellular-immune abnormality, IVIG treatment can be considered (evidence level B).

CONCLUSION

The use of intralipids and IVIG in the cases of RIF, recurrent miscarriages, and unexplained infertility is being increasingly adopted by various fertility clinicians across the world. However, the available literature is not conclusive to make any definite recommendations. Evidence points to a definite beneficial role in patients with altered immunological factors and increase in NK cell activity with a debatable benefit. These tests are, however, not widely available, reproducible, or recommended. However, the relative safety of the administration of these drugs make them a popular choice of treatment, especially where all other options and resources are exhausted.

The use of intralipid is more economical and hence more popular as compared to the use of IVIG, which may be severalfold more expensive. However, the role of immunology in infertility still requires extensive study and research and is expected to grow by leaps and bounds in the coming years.

REFERENCES

1. Kumar P, Mahajan S. Preimplantation and postimplantation therapy for the treatment of reproductive failure. J Hum Reprod Sci. 2013;6:88-92.
2. Simon A, Laufer N. Repeated implantation failure: clinical approach. Fertil Steril. 2012;97:1039-43.

3. Practice Committee of the American Society for Reproductive Medicine. Evaluation and treatment of recurrent pregnancy loss: a committee opinion. Fertil Steril. 2012;98:1103-11.
4. ESHRE Early Pregnancy Guideline Development Group. (2023). Recurrent Pregnancy Loss.
5. Makrigiannakis A, Petsas G, Toth B, Relakis K, Jeschke U. Recent advances in understanding immunology of reproductive failure. J Reprod Immunol. 2011;90:96-104.
6. Kwak-Kim J, Han AR, Gilman-Sachs A, Fishel S, Leong M, Shoham Z. Current trends of reproductive immunology practices in in vitro fertilization (IVF): a first world survey using IVF-Worldwide.com. Am J Reprod Immunol. 2013; 69:12-20.
7. Penzias AS. Recurrent IVF failure: other factors. Fertil Steril. 2012;97:1033-8.
8. Tang AW, Alfirevic Z, Quenby S. Natural killer cells and pregnancy outcomes in women with recurrent miscarriage and infertility: a systematic review Hum Reprod. 2011;26(8): 1971-80.
9. Clark DA, Coulam CB, Stricker RB. Is intravenous immunoglobulins (IVIG) efficacious in early pregnancy failure? A critical review and meta-analysis for patients who fail in vitro fertilization and embryo transfer (IVF). J Assist Reprod Genet. 2006;23:1-13.
10. Meng L, Lin J, Chen L, Wang Z, Liu M, Liu Y, et al. Effectiveness and potential mechanisms of intralipid in treating unexplained recurrent spontaneous abortion. Arch Gynecol Obstet. 2016;294:29-39.
11. Han EJ, Lee HN, Kim MK, Lyu SW, Lee WS. Efficacy of intralipid administration to improve in vitro fertilization outcomes: a systematic review and meta-analysis. Clin Exp Reprod Med. 2021;48:203-10.
12. Granato D, Blum S, Rössle C, Le Boucher J, Malnoë A, Dutot G. Effects of parenteral lipid emulsions with different fatty acid composition on immune cell functions in vitro. JPEN J Parenter Enteral Nutr. 2000;24:113-8.
13. Mayer K, Meyer S, Reinholz-Muhly M, Maus U, Merfels M, Lohmeyer J, et al. Short-time infusion of fish oil-based lipid emulsions, approved for parenteral nutrition, reduces monocyte proinflammatory cytokine generation and adhesive interaction with endothelium in humans. J Immunol. 2003;171:4837-43.
14. Fournier T, Thérond P, Handschuh K, Tsatsaris V, Evain-Brion D. PPARgamma and early human placental development. Curr Med Chem. 2008;15:3011-24.
15. Leslie DS, Dascher CC, Cembrola K, Townes MA, Hava DL, Hugendubler LC, et al. Serum lipids regulate dendritic cell CD1 expression and function. Immunology. 2008;125:289-301.
16. Kostenis E. A glance at G-protein-coupled receptors for lipid mediators: a growing receptor family with remarkably diverse ligands. Pharmacol Ther. 2004;102:243-57.
17. Desmarais JA, Lopes FL, Zhang H, Das SK, Murphy BD. The peroxisome proliferator-activated receptor gamma regulates trophoblast cell differentiation in mink (Mustela vison). Biol Reprod. 2007;77:829-39.
18. Zhang X, Rodriguez-Galán MC, Subleski JJ, Ortaldo JR, Hodge DL, Wang JM, et al. Peroxisome proliferator-activated receptor-gamma and its ligands attenuate biologic functions of human natural killer cells. Blood. 2004;104:3276-84.
19. Delerive P, Fruchart JC, Staels B. Peroxisome proliferator-activated receptors in inflammation control. J Endocrinol. 2001;169:453-9.
20. Martini AE, Jasulaitis S, Fogg LF, Uhler ML, Hirshfeld-Cytron JE. Evaluating the utility of intralipid infusion to improve live birth rates in patients with recurrent pregnancy loss or recurrent implantation failure. J Hum Reprod Sci. 2018; 11:261-8.
21. Dakhly DM, Bayoumi YA, Sharkawy M, Gad Allah SH, Hassan MA, Gouda HM, et al. Intralipid supplementation in women with recurrent spontaneous abortion and elevated levels of natural killer cells. Int J Gynaecol Obstet. 2016;135:324-7.
22. Asif S, Alahwany H, Chittawar PB, Nigdelis M, Toulis KA, Goulis DG, et al. Immune therapies for women with history of unsuccessful implantation undergoing IVF/ICSI treatment: a Cochrane collaboration systematic review. Hum Reprod. 2018;33:85.
23. Morikawa M, Yamada H, Kato EH, Shimada S, Kishi T, Yamada T, et al. Massive intravenous immunoglobulin treatment in women with four or more recurrent spontaneous abortions of unexplained etiology: down-regulation of NK cell activity and subsets. Am J Reprod Immunol. 2001;46:399-404.
24. Gelfand EW. Intravenous immune globulin in autoimmune and inflammatory diseases. N Engl J Med. 2012;367:2015-25.
25. Kim DJ, Lee SK, Kim JY, Na BJ, Hur SE, Lee M, et al. Intravenous immunoglobulin G modulates peripheral blood Th17 and Foxp3(+) regulatory T cells in pregnant women with recurrent pregnancy loss. Am J Reprod Immunol. 2014;71:441-50.
26. Clark DA, Wong K, Banwatt D, Chen Z, Liu J, Lee L, et al. CD200-dependent and nonCD200-dependent pathways of NK cell suppression by human IVIG. J Assist Reprod Genet. 2008;25:67-72.
27. Coulam CB, Acacia B. Does immunotherapy for treatment of reproductive failure enhance live births? Am J Reprod Immunol. 2012;67:296-303.
28. Rasmark Roepke E, Hellgren M, Hjertberg R, Blomqvist L, Matthiesen L, Henic E, et al. Treatment efficacy for idiopathic recurrent pregnancy loss—a systematic review and meta-analyses. Acta Obstet Gynecol Scand. 2018;97: 921-41.
29. Egerup P, Lindschou J, Gludd C, Christiansen OB; ImmuReM IPD Study Group. The effects of intravenous immunoglobulin in women with recurrent miscarriages:

a systematic review of randomised trials with meta-analyses and trial sequential analyses including individual patient data. PLoS One. 2015;10:e0141588.
30. Stephenson MD, Fluker MR. Treatment of repeated unexplained in vitro fertilization failure with intravenous immunoglobulin: a randomized, placebo-controlled Canadian trial. Fertil Steril. 2000;74:1108-13.
31. Li J, Chen Y, Liu C, Hu Y, Li L. Intravenous immunoglobulin treatment for repeated IVF/ICSI failure and unexplained infertility: a systematic review and a meta-analysis. Am J Reprod Immunol. 2013;70:434-47.
32. Abdolmohammadi-Vahid S, Pashazadeh F, Pourmoghaddam Z, Aghebati-Maleki L, Abdollahi-Fard S, Yousefi M. The effectiveness of IVIG therapy in pregnancy and live birth rate of women with recurrent implantation failure (RIF): a systematic review and meta-analysis. J Reprod Immunol. 2019;134:28-33.
33. Peero EK, Banjar S, Khoudja R, Ton-Leclerc S, Beauchamp C, Benoit J, et al. Intravenous immunoglobulin for patients with unexplained recurrent implantation failure: a 6-year single center retrospective review of clinical outcomes. Sci Rep. 2024;14:3876.
34. Practice Committee of the American Society for Reproductive Medicine. The role of immunotherapy in in vitro fertilization: a guideline. Fertil Steril. 2018;110:387-400.
35. ESHRE Add-ons working group; Lundin K, Bentzen JG, Bozdag G, Ebner T, Harper J, Le Clef N, et al. Good practice recommendations on add-ons in reproductive medicine†. Hum Reprod. 2023;38:2062-104.
36. Sung N, Han AR, Park CW, Park DW, Park JC, Kim NY, et al. Intravenous Immunoglobulin G in women with reproductive failure: The Korean Society for Reproductive Immunology practice guidelines. Clin Exp Reprod Med. 2017;44:1-7.

Chapter

Recurrent Implantation Failure: Current Prospects

Manjiri Valsangkar, Mugdha Parasnis

INTRODUCTION

Recurrent implantation failure (RIF) is a frustrating clinical scenario in in vitro fertilization (IVF) practice for clinicians and an emotional turmoil for patient and her family. These may include patient with negative results as well as those landing up repeatedly with biochemical pregnancy. In IVF, around 10–15% of IVF patients undergo RIF.[1] There are several clinical and investigation dilemmas considering the unexplained nature of the problem, and this chapter deals with optimum diagnostic and management strategies in current scenario pertaining to RIF.

DEFINITION

Recurrent implantation failure is defined as failure to achieve a clinical pregnancy after the transfer of at least four good-quality embryos in minimum of three fresh or frozen embryo transfer (ET) cycles in a woman <40 years of age. European Society of Human Reproduction and Embryology (ESHRE) defined RIF as transfer of more than three good-quality embryos or ten embryos in multiple transfer cycles without achieving pregnancy.[2] Generally speaking, more than three cycles of good-quality embryo (day 3 >8 cells <10% fragmentation) or blastocyst >3BB failures is RIF.

ETIOLOGY

Implantation is a successful cross talk between embryo and endometrium mediated by cytokines and several immunological factors. RIF etiology is multifactorial including immunological causes, infective causes, thrombophilias, genetic, microbiome-related, mullerian dysgenesis/anatomical defects, embryo aneuploidy, severe oligoasthenoteratozoospermia (OATS), or high sperm DNA fragmentation. **Table 1** enlists the various causes of RIF. Once an RIF patient is assigned a tentative etiology, working toward it along with tender loving care is the key to treatment of RIF. **Box 1** enumerates the various risk factors, which increase the chances of RIF.

TABLE 1: Various factors associated with recurrent implantation failure (RIF).

	Treatment	
Risk factors	Body mass index	Low-energy diets, pharmacotherapy, and bariatric surgery
	Smoking	Stop smoking and avoid secondhand smoke
	Alcohol	Reduce alcohol intake to one or two units a week or abstinence from alcohol
	Stress	Healthy diet, regular exercise, psychological interventions
Maternal factors	Immunology	Glucocorticoids, intravenous immunoglobulin, tacrolimus, cyclosporine, intralipids
	Thrombophilias	Aspirin, low-molecular-weight heparin
	Endometrial receptivity	Frozen-thawed embryo transfer, peripheral blood mononuclear cells, platelet-rich plasma, granulocyte colony-stimulating factor, endometrial scratch, endometrial receptivity assay
	Microbiome	Antibiotics
	Anatomical abnormalities	Hysteroscopy and surgery
Male factors		Intracytoplasmic morphologically selected sperm injection
Embryo factor		Optimize ovarian stimulation protocol, assisted hatching, preimplantation genetic testing for aneuploidies

IMMUNOLOGY AND RECURRENT IMPLANTATION FAILURE

Successful implantation is a balance between helper and killer T cells or proinflammatory and anti-inflammatory cytokines. Blastocysts' invasion and adhesion trigger the maternal immune system to fetal cells, thereby activating local immune system at site of implantation too. Natural killer (NK) cells in decidual stroma express receptors mediating this process through release of human leukocyte antigen (HLA)-G-E. Apart from this, several angiogenic factors such as vascular endothelial growth factor (VEGF), placental growth factor (GF), angiopoietin, interferon-1 (IF-1), and transcriptions are mediators for implantation. Imbalance of T helper 1 (Th1)/Th2 lymphocytes results in RIF **(Fig. 1)**.[3]

BOX 1: Risk factors for recurrent implantation failure.

- Age >35 years
- Obesity; body mass index (BMI) >25
- Smoking
- Alcohol intake
- Stress

THROMBOPHILIA

Thrombophilia is involved in recurrent pregnancy loss (RPL) due to hypercoagulable state leading to microthrombosis but the clearcut association between thrombophilia and RIF is still doubtful. Thrombophilia are believed to affect implantation by impairing vascularization of the embryo and impaired decidual vascularity.[4]

Acquired Thrombophilia

The most prevalent acquired thrombophilia is the antiphospholipid syndrome. It is an autoimmune disorder due to antiphospholipid antibodies, such as anticardiolipin antibodies, lupus anticoagulant antibodies and anti-2-glycoprotein I antibodies. It mainly results in arterial or venous thrombosis resulting in pregnancy losses.[5]

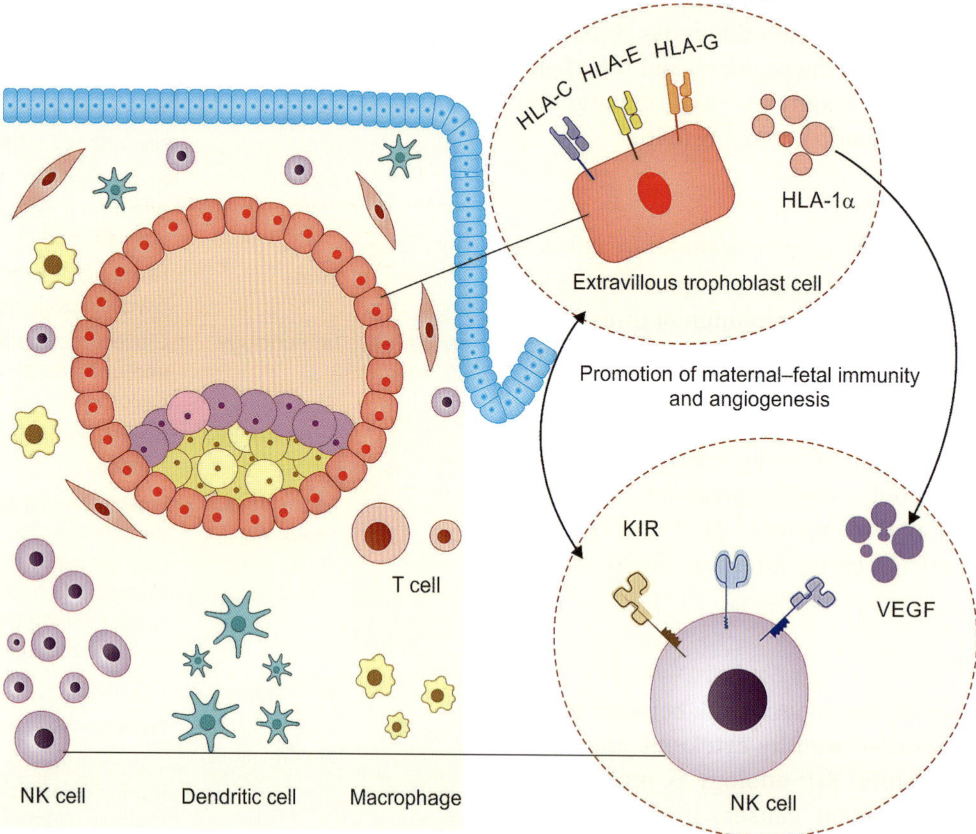

Fig. 1: Immunology of implantation. (HLA-C: human leukocyte antigen-C; KIR: killer immunoglobulin-like receptor; NK: natural killer; VEGF: vascular endothelial growth factor)

Source: Recurrent implantation failure: A comprehensive summary from etiology to treatment, Jnying Ma, Wengan Gaon, Da li. Front Endocrinol, 2023.

ENDOMETRITIS (MICROBIOME)

The reproductive system contains varied bacterial communities that form a continuous microbiota changing from the vagina to the ovaries. Any alterations in the vaginal flora are involved in female reproductive system diseases, such as bacterial vaginosis, urinary tract infections, RIF, and RPL. Hence, we can assume that microbiota might be involved in several steps of IVF-ET, including embryogenesis and implantation. Vaginal probiotic lactobacilli produce lactic acid and short-chain fatty acids, which maintain the acidic pH of the vagina. Infertile women display abnormal vaginal microbiota such as *Gardnerella vaginalis* and *Ureaplasma urealyticum*. Similar lactobacilli found in endometrium as well and infection with non-*Lactobacillus*-dominated microbiota, such as *Streptococcus*, during the implantation window results in implantation failures or losses. Microbiome testing is currently offered by many laboratories such as ALICE (Analysis of Infectious Chronic Endometritis) and EMMA (Endometrium Microbiome Metagenomic Analysis), which give a comprehensive array and suggested treatment.[6]

ANATOMICAL DEFECTS

Several types of uterine abnormalities can affect implantation rates including Mullerian duct abnormalities (MDA), which are congenital or acquired later, such as fibroids, polyps, Asherman's, adenomyosis, and hydrosalpinx.[7] Fibroids can be intramural, subserosal (that do not harm implantation), or submucous, which are known to cause RIF. Fibroids hinder implantation by excessive uterine myometrial contractions, abnormal vascularization, elevated cytokines and GFs.[8] Diagnosis is done by 3D sonography, magnetic resonance imaging (MRI), and confirmed by hysterolaparoscopy. Hysteroscopic myomectomy is advised in cases of RIF. Polyps are most common asymptomatic pathology, removal of which improves the RIF outcomes.[9] Mullerian duct anomalies are congenital occurrences confirmed by 3D ultrasound, MRI, or diagnostic hysterolaparoscopy. Mullerian abnormalities, such as septate and bicornuate uteri, should be considered in patients with RIF.[10] Compared with other congenital uterine anomalies, partial septate and septate uteri appear to have the poorest reproductive outcomes, such as reduced pregnancy rate and increased risk of RIF and RPL. Vascularity must be established by Doppler and preferred option is hysteroscopic septal resection. The major risks associated with bicornuate uterus are midtrimester abortion and preterm birth. Endometriosis and hydrosalpinx also potentially cause RIF due to cytokines, tumor necrosis factor alpha (TNF-α), and interleukin 1 (IL-1).[11] Asherman's syndrome and infections like genital tuberculosis (TB) can be suspected on 3D ultrasonography (USG), but are confirmed by hysteroscopy followed by adhesiolysis. Dilatation and curettage (D and C) too hampers functional layer of endometrium, thereby causing it to prevent implantation.

Paternal/Male Factor Causing Recurrent Implantation Failure

Sperm DNA damage is related to poor embryogenesis. American Society for Reproductive Medicine (ASRM), however, does not recommend DNA fragmentation as a routine study. Elevated sex chromosome disomies were seen in patients with recurrent RIF. Protamine 1/2 ratio when reversed has been linked to male causes of RIF.[12]

Embryo Factor as a Cause of Recurrent Implantation Failure

Abnormal embryos are a cause of concern in RIF. Chromosomal abnormalities such as aneuploidy attribute to 75% RIF, most common being translocations, inversions, mosaicism, and deletions. It is doubtful whether mosaicism in embryos can influence RIF. Those with whole chromosome aneuploidy detected by PGTA-PGD (preimplantation genetic testing for aneuploidies–preimplantation genetic diagnosis) display negligible implantation potential.[13]

INVESTIGATIONS

The following investigations are recommended for patients with RIF.

Hormonal tests such as anti-Müllerian hormone (AMH), antral follicle count (AFC), follicle-stimulating hormone (FSH), luteinizing hormone (LH), prolactin, thyroid, hemoglobin A1C (HbA1C), etc., must be done to rule out hormonal pathologies.

There is a positive correlation between the *sperm function tests* and RIF. Sperm DNA fragmentation is the simplest of the laboratory tests that can be offered to couples with RIF to rule out male etiology for RIF apart from the semen analysis.[14] DNA fragmentation >15% is unequivocal while >25% is abnormal and counseling needs to be done in view of repeated failures. Most common kits such as sperm chromatin dispersion and Comet Assays are available, and sensitive tests for estimation.[15]

Uterine factors can be congenital such as Mullerian duct anomalies or acquired such as fibroid and polyps. Various tests for diagnosis are available, simplest being USG. *Transvaginal (TVS) USG* forms the mainstay of diagnosis and with modalities such as 4D USG with Doppler studies, it gives a more comprehensive outlook. Obvious pathologies such as MDA, fibroids, and hydrosalpinx can be detected on outpatient basis. In suspected cases to rule out anatomical defects, congenital or acquired, hysteroscopy should be performed which can be both diagnostic and therapeutic. Endometrial receptivity assay helps to find the exact window of implantation in cases of RIF.

Hysterosalpingography or sonosalpingography has definitely found its foothold as it is cheap, effective, and diagnostic. For suspected cases of uterine defects or tubal blocks, diagnostic *hysteroscopy with laparoscopy* with a "SEE AND TREAT" approach is prudent.

Role of Pre-In Vitro Fertilization Hysteroscopy

There is a dilemma about the universal application of *pre-IVF hysteroscopy* to all IVF patients though some studies have shown better outcomes with it. Role of infertility counselor forms the mainstay of treatment in IVF to enable patient to make informed decisions based on current reports, as it is emotionally challenging for the couples.[16] Interestingly, literature suggests that around 25–50% of patients with normal USG might have abnormal findings on hysteroscopy and may need corrective measures such as hysteroscopic scratching, dilatation, and metroplasty. It must be repeated in patients if already done >1 year ago.

Laparoscopy

Laparoscopy is indicated in patients with MDA for confirmation of diagnosis. Laparoscopic myomectomy or endometriosis excision surgeries may be needed in acquired causes of RIF. Hydrosalpinx clipping or resection is advised to improve results.

Karyotyping

Though a controversial investigation, it must be offered to couples with RIF, as its known to be defective in more couples with RIF and RPL as compared to controls.

MANAGEMENT OF RECURRENT IMPLANTATION FAILURE

Treatment of RIF poses a major challenge for clinicians. Interventions, pharmacological treatment, along with lifestyle changes, de-addiction, and PGD can improve the situation. Lifestyle intervention and optimization of body mass index (BMI) must be done pre-IVF (BMI <19 and >30 kg/m^2).[17] Low-energy diets, exercise, yoga, meditation, and bariatric surgery, if necessary, can help the patients reduce weight and alleviate anxiety. Those eager to conceive should stop smoking, as it causes increased DNA fragmentation in sperms and poor-quality oocytes too.[18] Excessive alcohol intake harms gametes and hence patients must refrain from it.[19]

Ideally every RIF needs a multidisciplinary combined discussion and brain storming by infertility specialist, embryologist, and counselor considering its varied pathognomonic etiology. The couple who is emotionally distraught needs to be given extra time to discuss about further options, and reassurance, review of etiology, and investigations may be repeated if necessary and protocols may be changed if need be. Couple must be objectively counseled by independent counselor. Optimization of various factors is necessary before proceeding for the next cycle. Smoking in females shows positive correlation with excess gonadotropin ampoules, less fertilization, poor-quality oocytes, and poor blastulation rates. Excessive smoking in male partners is also known to increase DNA fragmentation index and lesser fertilization rates in IVF. Women with RIF must eliminate alcohol intake before next cycle.

Ovarian Stimulation Protocol

Stimulation protocols for controlled ovarian hyperstimulation (COH) must be tailor-made in each cycle especially in RIF based on age, BMI, previous response, presence of endometriosis, etc. If the response is deemed satisfactory, it is not necessary to change the stimulation protocol. However, in a small proportion of women who have low response to ovarian stimulation, the dose of gonadotropin may be increased or LH may be added.[20] In known cases of endometriosis, downregulation with gonadotropin-releasing hormone (GnRH) agonist prior to IVF or intracytoplasmic sperm injection (ICSI) may increase the pregnancy rate. Downregulated hormone replacement therapy (HRT) works better in these cases.

Embryo Assessment and Preimplantation Genetic Testing

It has been proven that euploid embryos tend to give better implantation and pregnancy rates. PGT-A to confirm chromosomal errors in embryos can help in selection of euploid embryos with better implantation potential. Choice of blastocyst transfers increases the rates by 10% per cycle.[21] A recent Cochrane review stated the rationale that blastocyst transfer improves implantation rates by enabling better selection of embryos and with better synchronicity between the embryo and endometrium. Detailed characterization of blastocyst cytogenetics using methods such as comparative genomic hybridization (CGH) and single-nucleotide polymorphism microarrays with a view to detecting and preferentially transferring euploid normal embryos is now preferred. Early studies suggest that an approach combining blastocyst biopsy and comprehensive chromosome screening using CGH or microarray CGH may represent the optimal approach for PGD.

Assisted Hatching

Hatching of the blastocyst plays an integral role in the implantation process. Failure to hatch mainly due to innate factors in either the blastocyst or zona pellucida is a possible cause of implantation failure. Assisted hatching involves the artificial thinning or breaching of the zona pellucida and has been proposed as one technique to improve implantation and pregnancy rates following IVF.[22] The Practice Committee guidelines of ASRM do not support the routine application of assisted hatching in all IVF cycles. However, it proposed that assisted hatching may be clinically useful in patients with a poor prognosis, including those with a history of two or more unsuccessful IVF cycles, poor embryo quality, and older women (>38 years of age).

Embryo Transfer Technique

Successful implantation with clinical pregnancy is based on embryo quality, endometrial receptivity, and transfer technique. Presence of stenosis at internal os, acutely anteverted or retroverted uteri, presence of blood or mucus on inner catheter, taking too long than usual, change of catheter during procedure, and too full or empty bladder are known to be detrimental to success in IVF-ET.[23] Use of *mock ET* is advocated prior to ET to eliminate these factors.

Role of Metabolomics in Embryos

Metabolomic testing in the spent culture of embryos (exometabolomics) helps to determine what the embryo consumes or secretes (e.g., amino acids, proteins, and oxygen consumption) and the parameters have been shown to correlate with embryo viability. Various genetic testing laboratories are now also offering noninvasive metabolomics testing.

Thin Endometrium

Recurrent implantation failure may sometimes be associated with a thin endometrium. Thin endometrium may be congenital and associated with Turner's syndrome or a T-shape uterus. It may also be acquired, as a result of previous D and C, radiotherapy, intrauterine surgery, or infections such as TB and chlamydia. Diagnosis by hysteroscopy is a must followed by following strategies to obtain an endometrium >7 mm in subsequent ET cycle. Various modalities to improve the endometrial thickness include:

- Downregulated HRT cycle with extended duration of estradiol valerate or hemihydrate.
- *Sildenafil citrate:* Sildenafil acts as a nitric oxide (NO) inhibitor and vasodilator improving the endometrial thickness and vascularity of endometrium. 25 mg daily to maximum QID dose can be administered. It has shown positive results in >25% of RIF cases.
- *Endometrial scratching/injury:* It is postulated that local injury of the endometrium in the cycle preceding IVF treatment increases the success rate of implantation.[24] Endometrial scratching can be ideally performed in luteal phase day 21/22 of previous cycle then followed by endometrial priming in subsequent cycle.
- *Granulocyte cell-stimulating factor (G-CSF):* G-CSF instillation is advised during endometrial priming a week before starting progesterone. It has shown promising results in patients with persistently thin endometrium as a cause of RIF.[25]
- *Endometrial platelet-rich plasma (PRP) injection/instillation:* PRP has shown promising results. Pre-cycle hysteroscopic injection of PRP can be done followed by priming after a month or so. Alternatively, PRP instillation has also been tried during the ET cycle.[26]
- *Endometrial receptivity array (ERA):* It is a personalized, sensitive, and objective dating method for ET based on 200 genes associated with receptivity and implantation by next-generation sequencing (NGS). It is precise, less

TABLE 2: Strategies to optimize in vitro fertilization (IVF) cycles in patients with recurrent implantation failure (RIF).

Protocols	• Agonist + hMG widens implantation window • Long-acting agonist can be used in endometriosis • Luteal phase single agonist a week after ET
Assisted hatching	• Zona thinning, drilling—laser or mechanical • Increases implantation but not pregnancy rates
Embryo transfer (ET)	• Blastocyst better than cleavage stage • Embryo glue (controversial) • Frozen better than fresh ET for implantation rates
Immunotherapy	• Lymphocyte immunization therapy (LIT) (ESHRE does not recommend routinely except in proven cases) • IVIG/intralipids • Immunomodulating agents such as tacrolimus, steroids, cyclosporine not routinely recommended but may be helpful in RIF
Anticoagulants	Aspirin, LMWH
Intrauterine infusions	hCG infusions post ET, PBMC infusions, platelet-rich plasma (PRP), G-CSF infusions pre ET
Endometrial scratching	Releases endokines and pro-inflammatory mediators for implantation
ERA test	Endometrial receptivity array genetic test personalized ET
PGTA	Aneuploidy and mosaicism detection helps in preventing RIF

(ERA: endometrial receptivity array; ESHRE: European Society of Human Reproduction and Embryology; G-CSF: granulocyte-cell stimulating factor; hCG: human chorionic gonadotropin; hMG: human menopausal gonadotropin; IVIG: intravenous immunoglobulin; LMWH: low-molecular-weight heparin; PBMC: peripheral blood mononuclear cells)

invasive, effective, and reduces need for prolonged Rx cycles. It gives exact window of implantation based on molecular diagnostic array.[27]

Low-molecular-weight Heparin

The Practice Committee of ASRM advises that regular use of low-molecular-weight heparin (LMWH) among couples undergoing IVF is not justified on the basis of existing data. However, it has been found effective in patients with immunological disorders [antiphospholipid antibodies (APLA), lupus antocoagulant (LA), etc.], especially for the role of immunomodulation.[28]

Gamete Donation or Surrogacy

Third-party reproduction options stand as a last alternative to RIF patients and must be discussed after three failures. Altruistic donation and surrogacy is the current legal mandate for treatment as per Assisted Reproductive Technology (ART) law 2021.

CONCLUSION

Recurrent implantation failure is defined as the failure to achieve a clinical pregnancy after transfer of at least four good-quality embryos in a minimum of three fresh or frozen cycles in a woman under the age of 40 years. Detailed and appropriate investigations to rule out an underlying cause for the repeated failure is necessary. Optimization of male and female gametes, embryo assessment, genetic testing, hysteroscopy, and use of advanced technologies like ERA can be resorted to improvise outcomes in RIF. Coexisting conditions such as Asherman's syndrome, septum, fibroids, endometriosis, and hydrosalpinx, which may be the cause for implantation failures must be evaluated and treated pre-cycle. Most importantly, counseling the couple by infertility counselor, giving them tender loving care and positive approach is vital while dealing with RIF cases. RIF still remains a Pandora's box, hence identifying the right etiology and individualizing the treatment is the key to success in RIF. **Table 2** summarizes the various strategies to optimize the IVF cycles in patients with RIF.

REFERENCES

1. Enders AC, Nelson DM. Pinocytotic activity of the uterus of the rat. Am J Anat. 1973;138:277-99.
2. Thornhill AR, deDie-Smulders CE, Geraedts JP, Harper JC, Harton GL, Lavery SA, et al.; ESHRE PGD Consortium. 'Best practice guidelines for clinical preimplantation genetic diagnosis (PGD) and preimplantation genetic screening (PGS)'. Hum Reprod. 2005;20:35-48.

3. Li D, Zheng L, Zhao D, Xu Y, Wang Y. The role of immune cells in recurrent spontaneous abortion. Reprod Sci. 2021; 28:3303-15.
4. Simon A, Laufer N. Assessment and treatment of repeated implantation failure (RIF). J Assist Reprod Genet. 2012;29: 1227-39.
5. Martinelli I, Taioli E, Ragni G, Levi-Setti P, Passamonti SM, Battaglioli T, et al. Embryo implantation after assisted reproductive procedures and maternal thrombophilia. Haematologica. 2003;88:789-93.
6. Hyman RW, Fukushima M, Jiang H, Fung E, Rand L, Johnson B, et al. Diversity of the vaginal microbiome correlates with preterm birth. Reprod Sci. 2014;21:32-40.
7. Hosseini MA, Ebrahimi N, Mahdavi A, Aleyasin A, Safdarian L, Fallahi P, et al. Hysteroscopy in patients with repeated implantation failure improves the outcome of assisted reproductive technology in fresh and frozen cycles. J Obstet Gynaecol Res. 2014;40:1324-30.
8. Franasiak JM, Alecsandru D, Forman EJ, Gemmell LC, Goldberg JM, Llarena N, et al. A review of the patho-physiology of recurrent implantation failure. Fertil Steril. 2021;116:1436-48.
9. Richlin SS, Ramachandran S, Shanti A, Murphy AA, Parthasarathy S. Glycodelin levels in uterine flushings and in plasma of patients with leiomyomas and polyps: implications for implantation. Hum Reprod. 2002;17: 2742-7.
10. Chan YY, Jayaprakasan K, Tan A, Thornton JG, Coomarasamy A, Raine-Fenning NJ. Reproductive outcomes in women with congenital uterine anomalies: a systematic review. Ultrasound Obstet Gynecol. 2011;37:371.
11. Practice Committee of American Society for Reproductive Medicine in collaboration with Society of Reproductive Surgeons. Salpingectomy for hydrosalpinx prior to in vitro fertilization. Fertil Steril. 2008;90:S66-8.
12. Caseiro AL, Regalo A, Pereira E, Esteves T, Fernandes F, Carvalho J. Implication of sperm chromosomal abnor-malities in recurrent abortion and multiple implantation failure. Reprod Biomed Online. 2015;31:481-5.
13. Taylor TH, Gitlin SA, Patrick JL, Crain JL, Wilson JM, Griffin DK. The origin, mechanisms, incidence and clinical consequences of chromosomal mosaicism in humans. Hum Reprod Update. 2014;20:571-81.
14. Carrell DT, Emery BR, Hammoud S. Altered protamine expression and diminished spermatogenesis: what is the link? Hum Reprod Update. 2007;13:213-27.
15. Lo Monte G, Murisier F, Piva I, Germond M, Marci R. Focus on intracytoplasmic morphologically selected sperm injection (IMSI): a mini-review. Asian J Androl. 2013;15: 608-15.
16. El-Toukhy T, Campo R, Khalaf Y, Tabanelli C, Gianaroli L, Gordts SS, et al. Hysteroscopy in recurrent in-vitro fertilisation failure (TROPHY): a multicentre, randomised controlled trial. Lancet. 2016;387:2614-20.
17. Legro RS, Dodson WC, Kunselman AR, Stetter CM, Kris-Etherton PM, Williams NI, et al. Benefit of delayed fertility therapy with preconception weight loss over immediate therapy in obese women with PCOS. J Clin Endocrinol Metab. 2016;10:2658-66.
18. Budani MC, Tiboni GM. Ovotoxicity of cigarette smoke: A systematic review of the literature. Reprod Toxicol. 2017; 72: 64-81.
19. Frederiksen Y, Farver-Vestergaard I, Skovgård NG, Ingerslev HJ, Zachariae R. Efficacy of psychosocial interventions for psychological and pregnancy outcomes in infertile women and men: a systematic review and meta-analysis. BMJ Open. 2015;5:e006592.
20. Tur-Kaspa I, Confino E, Dudkiewicz AB, Myers SA, Friberg J, Gleicher N. Ovarian stimulation protocol for *in vitro* fertilization with gonadotropin-releasing hormone agonist widens the implantation window. Fertil Steril. 1990;53: 859-64.
21. Pantou A, Mitrakos A, Kokkali G, Petroutsou K, Tounta G, Lazaros L, et al. The impact of preimplantation genetic testing for aneuploidies (PGT-a) on clinical outcomes in high risk patients. J Assist Reprod Genet. 2022;39:1341.
22. Gabrielsen A, Agerholm I, Toft B, Hald F, Petersen K, Aagaard J, et al. Assisted hatching improves implantation rates on cryopreserved-thawed embryos. A randomized prospective study. Hum Reprod. 2004;19:2258.
23. Zhang J, Wang C, Zhang H, Zhou Y. Sequential cleavage and blastocyst embryo transfer and IVF outcomes: a systematic review. Reprod Biol Endocrinol. 2021;19:142.
24. Nastri CO, Lensen SF, Gibreel A, Raine-Fenning N, Ferriani RA, Bhattacharya S, et al. Endometrial injury in women undergoing assisted reproductive techniques. Cochrane Database Syst Rev. 2015;CD009517.
25. Scarpellini F, Klinger FG, Rossi G, Sbracia M. Immuno-histochemical study on the expression of G-CSF, G-CSFR, VEGF, VEGFR-1, Foxp3 in first trimester trophoblast of recurrent pregnancy loss in pregnancies treated with G-CSF and controls. Int J Mol Sci. 2019;21:285.
26. Kim MK, Yoon JA, Yoon SY, Park M, Lee WS, Lyu SW, et al. Human platelet-rich plasma facilitates angiogenesis to restore impaired uterine environments with Asherman's syndrome for embryo implantation and following pregnancy in mice. Cells. 2022;11:1549.
27. Ruiz-Alonso M, Blesa D, Díaz-Gimeno P, Gómez E, Fernández-Sánchez M, Carranza F, et al. The endometrial receptivity array for diagnosis and personalized embryo transfer as a treatment for patients with repeated implantation failure. Fertil Steril. 2013;100:818-24.
28. Nelson SM, Greer IA. The potential role of heparin in assisted conception. Hum Reprod Update. 2008;14:623-45.

Chapter

How to Choose the Best Embryo: Conventional versus Future Strategies

Akanksha Mishra, Divya Bansal

INTRODUCTION

In vitro fertilization (IVF) has revolutionized the landscape of assisted reproductive technologies, offering hope to individuals struggling with infertility. According to the World Health Organization (WHO), the percentage of population suffering from infertility or subfertility is 17.5%, which translates to about every one in six people struggling to conceive naturally. The *International Committee for Monitoring Assisted Reproductive Technologies* (*ICMART*) has recently reported that since the birth of Louis Brown in 1978, approximately 12 million children have been born worldwide via assisted conception. About two and a half million treatment cycles are performed every year and the figure is expected to rise by 6.7% every year.

With the increasing demand for assisted reproduction treatments (ART) and inability of a significant number of couples to conceive naturally, there has been tremendous advancement in reproductive research to achieve the best possible treatment outcome. According to the data collected in the United States of America (USA) since 1985, self-egg pregnancy rates went up from 15% initially to 40% by 2002. Similarly, donor egg embryos have resulted in 40% positive pregnancies as compared to 25% in the early years.[1]

Presently, with the advent of better incubators and culture systems, better laboratory air quality, cryopreservation, and such techniques, there has been a dramatic rise in clinical pregnancy rates and live birth rates.

Though success of an IVF cycle depends on many factors, embryo selection proves to be one of the major contributors for getting a successful pregnancy. Knowledgeful monitoring of growth of embryos and subsequent accurate grading helps selecting the embryos with higher implantation potential.

One distinct disadvantage of ART procedures is multiple gestation. The purpose of transferring multiple embryos altogether is to increase the chances of a positive treatment outcome, but this also increases the chances of more than one embryo implanting in the uterus. Multiple gestation is relatively uncommon in natural conception. The chances of multiple pregnancy in nature versus ART is 6% and 26%, respectively.[2]

Multiple gestation is associated with a gamut of complications including medical and financial. Since the chances of multiple conception is directly proportional to the number of embryos transferred, the ART world is now moving toward single-embryo transfer (SET). The aim is to select a single embryo that has the best implantation potential of its cohort, so that there can be a reduction in the chances of multiple pregnancy while having good chances of positive result.

The chapter attempts to shed light on various techniques, conventional and futuristic, that can assist an embryologist to select that one embryo that will not compromise the treatment outcome as well as help prevent chances of multiple gestation.

HISTORICAL PERSPECTIVE: PAST TECHNIQUES

Observational Assessment

In the early stages of IVF, embryo selection was primarily reliant on visual observations or morphological evaluation of the embryo. Embryologists examined embryos under a microscope, assessing parameters such as cell number, symmetry, and fragmentation. While this subjective approach served as the foundation for subsequent techniques, its reliability was limited due to the lack of standardized criteria and variability among embryologists.

Grading Systems

To mitigate the subjectivity in embryo selection, grading systems were introduced. These systems involved categorizing embryos based on visible characteristics such as cell division rate, quality of blastomeres, and the presence of fragmentation. Embryo development is a dynamic process with the embryo changing its morphological characteristics every few hours. The embryo needs to be observed at specific time points and assessed based on the key characteristics associated with that particular developmental stage. Specific criteria observed are morphology of pronuclei and nucleoli, number and size of blastomeres, and percentage of fragmentation. In the later stage of development, blastocyst expansion, quality of inner cell mass (ICM) and trophoectoderm (TE) are taken into consideration.[3] Various grading systems have been devised with the aim to categorize embryos based on morphology that may provide an insight into the embryo's viability and implantation potential. While these grading systems provided a more standardized approach, their reliance on observable criteria made them less reliable for predicting implantation potential and live birth rates.

Depicted in **Figure 1** are the key features associated with a viable embryo at various stages of its development. However, different embryos develop differently in a cohort, and their assessment is based on their cleavage based on the timeline, uniformity in number and shape of blastomeres, and fragmentation. In further culture up to blastocyst stage, the key morphological features observed are compaction, cavitation, followed by number and spacing of the TE, and the size and compaction of ICM.

An embryologist can observe these various stages at a specified time but cannot continually monitor the sequence of events that lead to that stage of embryo development. It is difficult to manually assess the exact time of syngamy, cleavage, compaction, cavitation, or expansion. That coupled with the subjectivity of human interpretation and bias, manual observation makes for an inexpensive but relatively unreliable tool for embryo selection.

ADVANCEMENTS AND PRESENT TECHNIQUES

Time-lapse Imaging

One of the most groundbreaking advancements in embryo selection is the incorporation of time-lapse imaging. Although this technology was introduced by Payne et al. in as early as 1997,[5] it found its place in mainstream human embryo observation in only 2010.[6] Embryos traditionally need to be morphologically assessed at various time points to assess their developmental milestones. However, constant handling of embryos exposes them to changes in temperature, pH, and humidity, compromising their further growth and implantation potential.[7] With the advent of time-lapse imaging, it has been possible to increase the number of observations, which has helped in dynamically assessing embryo development. Furthermore, time lapse enables uninterrupted embryo culture and no fluctuation in the culture environment. An additional benefit of time-lapse technique is to observe the events such as direct cleavage and reverse cleavage, which again helps us mark the embryos with abnormal division which would not have been possible without the constant monitoring.

A time-lapse system typically comprises two systems: The culture dishes and camera can be placed either as a separate system inside a regular box incubator (open system), or be completely integrated into a small, benchtop incubator (closed system). Algorithms have been developed taking into account the Known Implantation data (KIDscore) that claims to predict with high accuracy, the implantation potential of the developing embryo. The aspects of embryo development taken into account for the algorithm are primarily, time taken to reach the development milestones, movement of pronuclei within the cytoplasm, and fading of nucleolar envelop,[8] cleavage pattern, and morphology. The synchrony of cleavage, especially during blastulation, may allow identification of most viable embryos. This is a completely noninvasive method of the assessing embryo potential; however, this technology is very expensive, and it requires expertise and training. Also, this might result in deselection of viable embryos capable of implantation as it has certain limitations like it does not allow the rotation in visualizing the embryos, which can miss the overlapping blastomeres. It should be noted that although time lapse allows continuous monitoring of embryo development, assessment and selection of embryos is still a manual event performed by the embryologist. The annotation time and interpretation of events are subject to human error and might result in difference of score.[9] In fact, there have been randomized controlled trials that suggest that there is no difference in cumulative pregnancy rates between embryos selected traditionally and those selected by time lapse.[10]

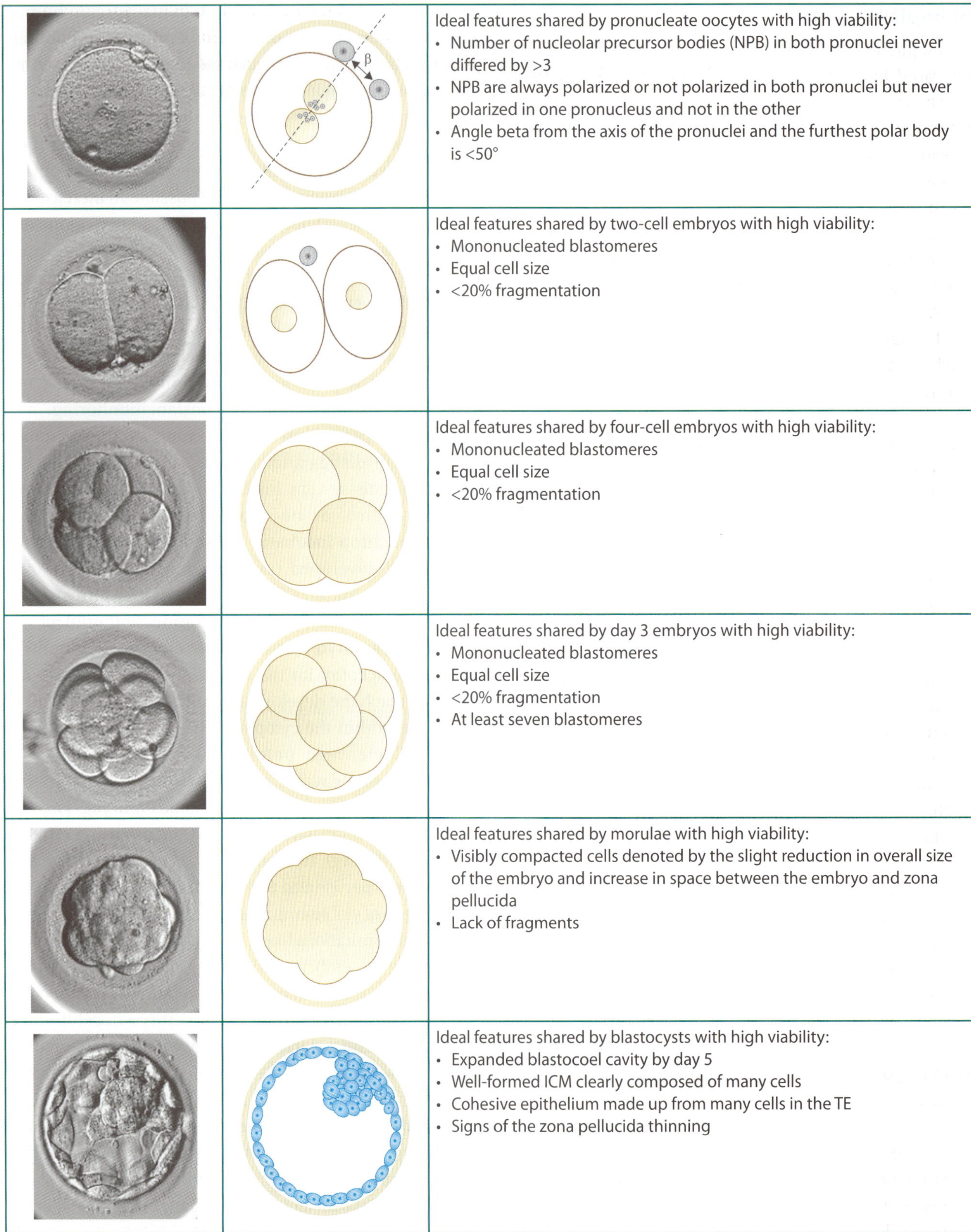

Fig. 1: Key morphological features of human embryos with high viability. (ICM: inner cell mass; TE: trophectoderm)[4]

Preimplantation Genetic Testing

The majority of human oocytes harvested, and embryos generated have compromised developmental potential mainly due to genetic abnormalities of gamete or embryonic origin. Preimplantation genetic testing (PGT) is a way of genetically analyzing the embryos to select the normal ones to be used for implantation. PGT has been in experiments with animals since the late nineteenth century. In 1976, Edwards and Gardner managed to stain rabbit blastocyst sex chromatin.[11] This experiment provided a template for future PGT studies, and many experiments were conducted on animal models. The first human experiment was recorded by Verlinsky et al. wherein they attempted to analyze the polar body of unfertilized oocytes to check for a maternal unaffected gene.[12] Today several advanced technologies are available to us such as single-nucleotide polymorphism (SNP) testing, Quantitative real-time polymerase chain reaction (QT-PCR), and next-generation sequencing (NGS). Chromosomal aneuploidies are responsible for over 70% of spontaneous miscarriages. Aneuploidy detection via PGT can help ascertain transfer of a euploid embryo, thereby reducing time taken to pregnancy or a healthy live birth.

Preimplantation genetic testing does have its limitations. Certain conditions such as subtelomeric deletions, microdeletions, microduplications, and small structural rearrangements may be difficult to detect. However, the advent of array comparative genomic hybridization (CGH) and NGS has been able to address subchromosomal abnormalities.[13]

One of the newer techniques of genetic evaluation is mitochondrial DNA (mtDNA). It has been proposed that higher copies of mtDNA in a blastocyst are associated with lower implantation potential.[14] There have been conflicting studies to prove or disprove the hypothesis. More data and a meta-analysis are required before this assessment finds a place in the mainstream.

Since embryo biopsy is an invasive procedure and requires extreme skill to be performed without harming the embryo, efforts are being made in the direction of noninvasive genetic testing. This involves isolation of cell-free DNA from the spent culture medium. An attempt is then made to amplify the whole genome and accurately assess aneuploidy. This approach is still in its infancy and the results are yet nowhere as accurate as biopsied cells. The most significant hurdles in noninvasive preimplantation genetic testing (niPGT) are insufficient DNA, maternal DNA contamination, and embryonic mosaicism. The challenge is to generate enough copies of DNA to be able to accurately determine not only aneuploidies but segmental anomalies and mosaicism as well. Perhaps with better cell-free DNA amplification techniques and more sensitive assays, it will be possible to harness the potential of cell-free DNA for routine clinical use.

Genetic mosaicism is known to occur when embryos have two or more cell lines, wherein one cell line is normal while others are abnormal. Although it gets difficult to decide which cell line truly represents the genetic state of the embryo, transfer of mosaic embryos have led to healthy live births. It was proposed by Munné et al. in 2017 that transferring embryos with low mosaicism has better clinical outcomes as compared to when embryos with complex or higher degree of mosaicism were transferred.[15] This outcome was, however, challenged by Kushnir et al. in 2018, who maintained that although transferring euploid embryos resulted in better pregnancy rates as compared to mosaic, the degree of mosaicism had no effect on cycle outcome and that TE cell mosaicism was not a true indicator of the embryo's ploidy status.[16]

A recent meta-analysis determined that PGT-A in women below 35 years of age plays no role in increasing the cumulative pregnancy rate. However, it does help in better outcomes for women over 35 years of age.[17] However, the authors conceded that more data is required before accurately assessing the role of PGT in reproductive outcomes.

In conclusion, PGT can help improve treatment outcomes in women of advanced age, reduce time taken to pregnancy, and help prevent hereditary genetic disorders. That said, it is prudent to understand the pitfalls of this technology and integrate it into clinical practice judiciously.

Multiomics Method

Implantation is not an isolated event. It is a highly coordinated process that has a very brief restricted period to establish itself. Maternal–embryo cross talk is a two-way dialogue between the endometrium and the embryo that encourages changes in both entities that in turn facilitate implantation. Whether it is a friendly dialogue or a fight where only the best embryo is allowed to implant, the embryo has to cross three hurdles to be successful. The steps, in that order, are: (1) Apposition (orienting the ICM toward the epithelium), (2) adhesion (interaction between TE and endometrial epithelial cells), and finally

(3) invasion (TE cells undergo differentiation and penetrate the epithelium to reach the maternal vasculature).[18]

In recent times, there has been an emergence of various "omics" approaches. These are high-throughput techniques that simultaneously analyze a multitude of molecules affording an in-depth analysis of biological processes, like implantation. The various types of omics are:[19]

- *Proteomics:* Identification and quantification of proteins that are translated by specific segments of the genome and are influenced by external and internal situational changes.
- *Proteinomics:* Analysis of protein structures and protein-protein interactions.
- *Metabolomics:* Identification of the complete set of small-molecule metabolites that are the final downstream products of gene expression, thereby providing information about both genotype-phenotype and genotype-environment interaction.
- *Exomics:* Analysis of exons.
- *Epigenomics:* Assessment of epigenetic modifications.
- *Secretomics:* Analysis of secreted products.
- *Lipidomics:* Large-scale analysis of the whole lipid species and finally.
- *Interactomics:* Assessment of the complete set of molecular interactions in a particular biological system to be able to study the process as a whole rather than its individual components.

Simultaneous analysis of multiple molecules as offered by the integration of various omics might provide a deeper understanding of complex biological interactions like implantation and improve patient management by helping the embryologist predict the embryo with the best implantation potential. Omics have revealed new potential biomarkers of a viable embryo and a receptive endometrium. However, more prospective, robust, well-designed, and multicentric studies need to be performed to fully elucidate the contribution that development of omics might make toward understanding embryo implantation fully.

ARTIFICIAL INTELLIGENCE

The two main reasons for application of artificial intelligence (AI) in any field is to increase productivity and eliminate subjectivity or human error/bias. AI is a niche area as far as embryo selection is concerned but has shown great promise in predicting embryo viability.[20] A recent systematic review incorporating data and publications over various platforms over a period of almost 17 years has reached a conclusion that AI predicts embryo viability and implantation potential at least 4% better as compared to embryologists. Most of the studies took into account a combination of clinical information and embryo images as a prediction tool for embryo viability. Overall, the ability of AI to study multiple sets of images in great detail per second makes it an important tool of assessment. However, the setback is the requirement of a huge dataset for computational training of the AI for it to make accurate judgement. The advent of 3D continuous imaging may further facilitate AI learning of embryo quality.

While AI might be able to predict embryo potential, ART requires a personalized, tailor-made approach toward every individual patient depending on their clinical history.

Embryologists usually make conservative judgements to mitigate risks associated with clinical treatments. At present, AI is not capable of incorporating clinical history into its prediction model.

Artificial intelligence is, currently, at best, a very good decision-support tool to the embryologist in selecting the ideal embryo. Its high cost is a prohibitive factor in its widespread application. However, there is no denying the fact that extensive research is going on in the field of AI in ART, and we might soon witness its integration in mainstream ART laboratories.

CURRENT BEST PRACTICES AND CHALLENGES

While these advanced techniques have significantly improved the accuracy of embryo selection, the challenges remain. The cost associated with implementing these technologies can be a barrier for some individuals seeking IVF. Moreover, despite the advances, no method guarantees absolute accuracy in predicting success of an embryo. Each technique has its limitations and may not capture the entire spectrum of embryo viability. Furthermore, the ethical considerations in genetic testing and the need for continual research to refine and standardize these methods for broader applicability and accuracy are ongoing challenges in the field of IVF.

EMERGING TECHNOLOGIES AND FUTURE PROSPECTS

Researchers continue to explore new frontiers in technology to enhance viable embryo selection. AI and machine learning are being increasingly integrated into embryo selection process. These technologies have the potential to analyze vast amounts of data, identifying patterns and markers that could further refine the selection process, enhancing predictive models and improving success rates in ART.

Additionally ongoing research in other areas, such as single-cell sequencing and noninvasive embryo assessment, holds promise for advanced embryo selection techniques in the future.

CONCLUSION

A good embryo is the key to successful IVF cycle. Conventional methods of embryo grading have poor predicability in terms of success. The newer techniques like PGT, niPGT, time-lapse imaging and AI can help in better selection of embryos with improved success rates.

REFERENCES

1. Toner JP. Progress we can be proud of: U.S. trends in assisted reproduction over the first 20 years. Fertil Steril. 2002;78(5):943-50.
2. Reimundo P, Gutiérrez Romero JM, Rodríguez Pérez T, Veiga E. et al. Single-embryo transfer: a key strategy to reduce the risk for multiple pregnancy in assisted human reproduction. Adv Lab Med. 2021;2(2):179-88.
3. Scott L. The biological basis of non-invasive strategies for selection of human oocytes and embryos. Hum Reprod Update. 2003;9:237-49.
4. Gardner DK, Balaban B. Assessment of human embryo development using morphological criteria in an era of time-lapse, algorithms and 'OMICS': is looking good still important. Mol Hum Reprod. 2016;22(10):704-18.
5. Payne D, Flaherty SP, Barry MF, Matthews CD. Preliminary observations on polar body extrusion and pronuclear formation in human oocytes using time-lapse video cinematography. Hum Reprod. 1997;12:532-41.
6. Wong CC, Loewke KE, Bossert NL, Behr B, De Jonge CJ, Baer TM, et al. Non-invasive imaging of human embryos before embryonic genome activation predicts development to the blastocyst stage. Nat Biotechnol. 2010;28:1115-21.
7. Aparicio B, Cruz M, Meseguer M. Is morphokinetic analysis the answer? Reprod Biomed Online. 2013;27(6):654-63.
8. Athayde Wirka K, Chen AA, Conaghan J, Ivani K, Gvakharia M, Behr B, et al. Atypical embryo phenotypes identified by time-lapse microscopy: high prevalence and association with embryo development. Fertil Steril. 2014;101:1637-48.e1-5.
9. Sundvall L, Ingerslev HJ, Breth Knudsen U, Kirkegaard K. Inter- and intra-observer variability of time-lapse annotations. Hum Reprod. 2013;28(12):3215-21.
10. Wu YG, Lazzaroni-Tealdi E, Wang Q, Zhang L, Barad DH, Kushnir VA, et al. Different effectiveness of closed embryo culture system with time-lapse imaging (Embryo Scope (TM)) in comparison to standard manual embryology in good and poor prognosis patients: a prospectively randomized pilot study. Reprod Biol Endocrinol. 2016; 14(1):49.
11. Edwards RG, Gardner RL. Sexing of live rabbit blastocysts. Nature. 1967;214:576-7.
12. Verlinsky Y, Ginsberg N, Lifchez A, Valle J, Moise J, Strom CM. Analysis of the first polar body: Preconception genetic diagnosis. Hum Reprod. 1990;5:826-9.
13. Wells D, Alfarawati S, Fragouli E. Use of comprehensive chromosomal screening for embryo assessment: Micro-arrays and CGH. Mol Hum Reprod. 2008;14:703-10.
14. Diez-Juan A, Rubio C, Marin C, Martinez S, Al-Asmar N, Riboldi M, et al. Mitochondrial DNA content as a viability score in human euploid embryos: Less is better. Fertil Steril. 2015;104:534-41.e1.
15. Munné S, Blazek J, Large M, Martinez-Ortiz PA, Nisson H, Liu E, et al. Detailed investigation into the cytogenetic constitution and pregnancy outcome of replacing mosaic blastocysts detected with the use of high-resolution next-generation sequencing. Fertil Steril. 2017;108:62-71.e8.
16. Kushnir VA, Darmon SK, Barad DH, Gleicher N. Degree of mosaicism in trophectoderm does not predict pregnancy potential: A corrected analysis of pregnancy outcomes following transfer of mosaic embryos. Reprod Biol Endocrinol. 2018;16:6.
17. Simopoulou M, Sfakianoudis K, Maziotis E, Tsioulou P, Grigoriadis S, Rapani A, et al. PGT-A: who and when? A systematic review and network meta-analysis of RCTs. J Assist Reprod Genet. 2021;38(8):1939-57.
18. Makrigiannakis A, Minas V. Mechanisms of implantation. Reprod Biomed Online. 2007;14(1):102-9.
19. Altmäe S, Reimand J, Hovatta O, Zhang P, Kere J, Laisk T, et al. Research resource: interactome of human embryo implantation: identification of gene expression pathways, regulation, and integrated regulatory networks. Mol Endocrinol. 2012;1:203-17
20. VerMilyea M, Hall JMM, Diakiw SM, Johnston A, Nguyen T, Perugini D, et al. Development of an artificial intelligence-based assessment model for prediction of embryo viability using static images captured by optical light microscopy during IVF. Hum Reprod. 2020;35(4):770-84.

Chapter

Tubal Tales Deciphered: Which Tubal Patency Test is the Best?

Shalini Gainder, Rakshya Parajuli

INTRODUCTION

The evaluation of tubal patency is a critical step in the evaluation of cause of infertility in the female partner, offering insights into the functionality of the fallopian tubes. In this chapter, we explore various diagnostic tests employed to assess tubal patency, each with its unique advantages and considerations.

VARIOUS TUBAL PATENCY TESTS

Hysterosalpingography (Figs. 1 and 2)

Hysterosalpingography, a widely utilized radiologic procedure, takes center stage in our day-to-day practice. It is the primary diagnostic method for assessing the status of the fallopian tubes in women experiencing infertility. It is radiographic evaluation of the fallopian tubes that is performed by injecting radiocontrast of either oil-based or water-soluble media into the uterine cavity via the cervix. For optimal uterine visibility and to avoid the possibility of disturbing early pregnancy, it is done during the early follicular period.[1] Pain, vasovagal episode, pelvic inflammatory disease (PID), and dye intravasation are a few of the often reported side effects of this test. Older studies have shown post-HSG infection can occur in 0.3–3.1% of cases, particularly in the presence of abnormal tubes.[2] However, newer studies show lesser PID occurred in 0.3% of the HSGs performed with oil-based contrast versus 0.4% with water-based contrast and PID occurred in 0.3% of the HSGs in clinics using antibiotic prophylaxis and 0.2% in clinics not using antibiotic prophylaxis.[3] Contraindications to this test are contrast allergy, pregnancy, and active pelvic infection.

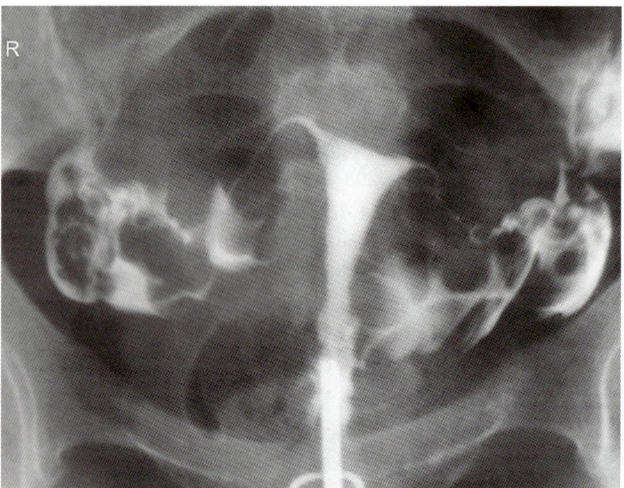

Fig. 1: Normal hysterosalpingography (HSG).

Method: The patient is placed in the lithotomy position on the fluoroscopy table during the procedure. For cervical stabilization and uterine positioning, a tenaculum may be placed with or without local anesthesia following cervical preparation, which is often done with povidone-iodine solution. The Leech-Wilkinson cannula or Foley catheter (usually 8 Fr or 10 Fr) is introduced into the endocervix, through which oil- or water-based contrast medium is inserted into the uterine cavity. Intermittent radiographs are taken to capture the filling of the uterine cavity and fallopian tubes. An antispasmodic and an anti-inflammatory agent should be given 30 minutes before the procedure.

In a Cochrane review meta-analysis, pregnancy rates (PRs) varied from 17 to 23% after using water-soluble contrast media and 24 to 38% after using oil-soluble contrast media, compared with a PR of 8–21% without the HSG procedure. A Cochrane review has shown evidence of effectiveness of tubal flushing with oil-soluble contrast media in increasing the odds of pregnancy and

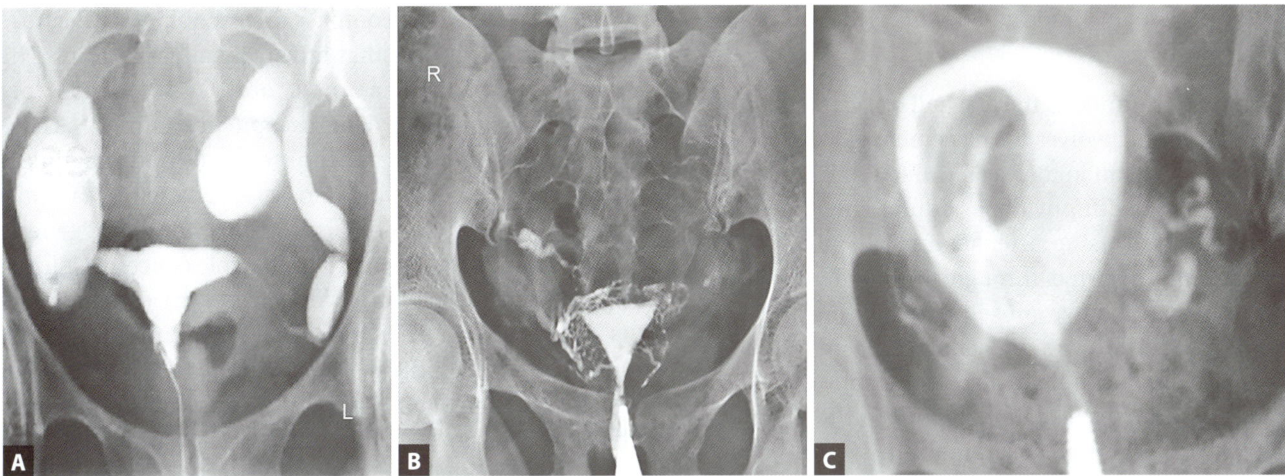

Figs. 2A to C: Abnormal hysterosalpingography (HSG) showing: (A) Hydrosalpinx, (B) Intravasation of dye with bilateral tubal block, and (C) Distended uterine cavity with filling defects.

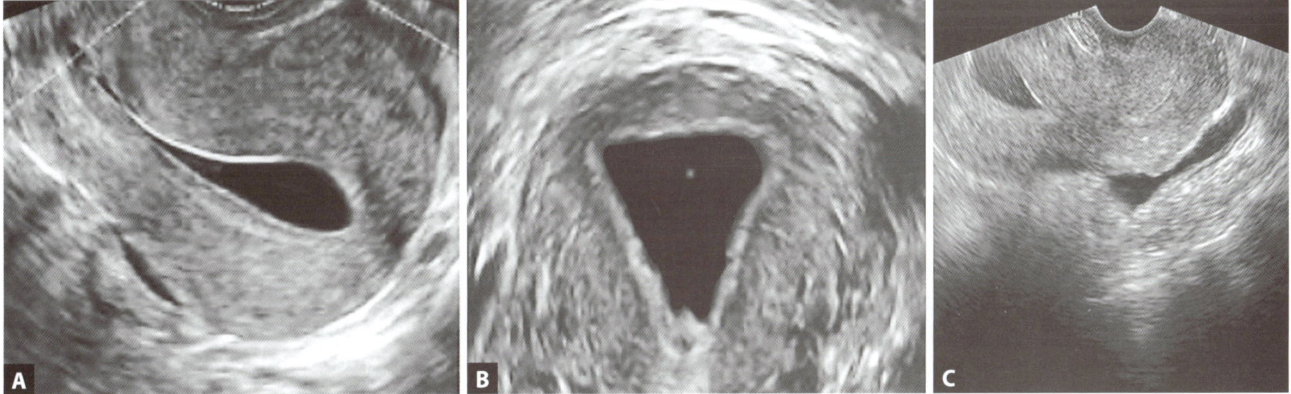

Figs. 3A to C: Normal sonohysterography (SHG).

live birth versus no intervention.[4] Couples experiencing unexplained infertility can benefit from oil-based contrast media flushing, but it works especially well for endometriosis patients with healthy ovaries and fallopian tubes.[5]

Hysterosalpingography has a reasonable specificity (83%) but a low sensitivity (65%) to document patency of the fallopian tubes.[6] Also, it has been shown that HSG is insufficient for predicting tubal patency for some patients with risk of pelvic adhesions, with a sensitivity between 0.01 and 83% and specificity between 50 and 90%.[7]

Sonohysterography or Saline Infusion Sonography (Figs. 3 and 4)

The emergence of this test involving saline injection during transvaginal ultrasound offers a noninvasive alternative. This versatile test, initially designed for uterine

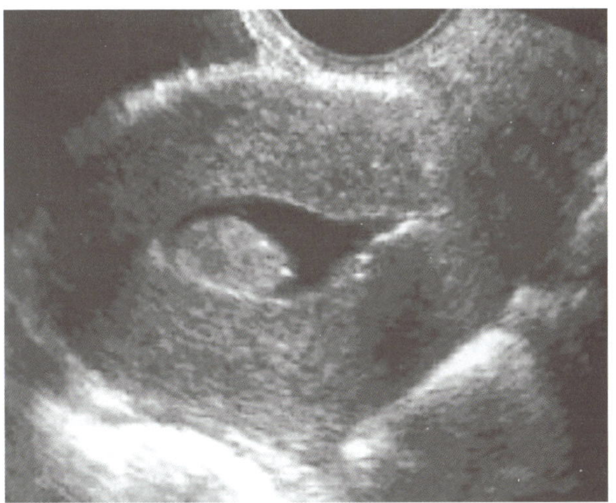

Fig. 4: Abnormal sonohysterography (SHG) showing lesion protruding into the uterine cavity.

cavity assessment, finds its place in discussion as a test for tubal patency.

Method: Performed in the first half of the menstrual cycle, the procedure involves the placement of a Cusco's bivalve vaginal speculum in the vagina, followed by the cleansing of the cervix with povidone-iodine. The upper cervical lip is secured using a tenaculum, and Foley catheter is carefully inserted through the cervical os into the endometrial cavity, subsequently filling the balloon with saline. Afterward, the tenaculum and speculum are removed, and the transvaginal sonography (TVS) probe is reinserted into the posterior vaginal vault. Simultaneously, an ultrasonographic examination is conducted, and 5–15 mL of physiologic saline solution is slowly infused to expand the endometrial cavity. Throughout and at the conclusion of the distension, the cavity is assessed, focusing on the contour, dimensions, thickness, and regularity of the endometrium, as well as the presence of polypoid lesions (polyps or myomas) or adhesions. With the balloon in position, a comprehensive examination of the endometrial cavity is carried out in both longitudinal and coronal planes. The inflated balloon prevents retrograde saline flow through the cervix, enabling an extended examination. Following the examination, the balloon is deflated, and the catheter is removed.

Identification of fallopian tubes on ultrasound is possible only in the presence of fluid in the tubal lumen or outside the tubes. This implies that tubes can be visualized on ultrasound when there is hydrosalpinx, free fluid in the pelvis, or when fluid is introduced into the tubal lumen or pelvic region.[8] The disadvantage of this test compared to HSG is that it lacks documentation and is observer dependent and films cannot be reproduced.

Although sonohysterosalpingography (sono-HSG) avoids the risks of allergy and ionizing radiation associated with iodinated contrast and fluoroscopic guidance of HSG, it has greater sensitivity and specificity for the detection of intrauterine pathologies, such as fibromas, polyps, and synechiae, in subfertile patients than tubal pathology.[9]

Laparoscopy

Our journey through tubal patency assessment would be incomplete without acknowledging laparoscopy combined with chromopertubation, regarded as the gold standard. As an invasive surgical procedure, laparoscopy provides direct visualization of pelvic organs, allowing unparalleled insights into tubal health.

Its advantages encompass the capability to diagnose and treat conditions that adversely affect fertility. The incidence of complications is observed to be 0.84 per 1,000 cases for minor laparoscopic procedures.[10] These findings underscore the assertion that diagnostic laparoscopy is not devoid of risks, emphasizing that while the risk of complications is lower compared to general laparoscopic surgery, it is still a tangible concern. Utilizing laparoscopy exclusively for investigating cases of infertility is not advised.[11] However, if laparoscopy is already being performed, the demonstration of tubal patency or documentation of proximal or distal tubal obstruction can be achieved through chromopertubation using a diluted solution of methylene blue or indigo carmine introduced via the cervix.

Obstruction in the interstitial part of the fallopian tube is observed in 15% of HSGs.[12] The diagnostic approach for tubal occlusion should avoid introducing instruments into the tube, as this could result in false-negative outcomes and impact our understanding of proximal tubal occlusion (PTO) therapies. Tubal catheterization, with or without wire-guide cannulation, is the preferred management when PTO is present without distal tubal disease. In cases where apparent PTO is identified, over 90% of patients could potentially undergo successful tube recanalization, leading to a pregnancy rate of 24%, with 12% of pregnancies being ectopic. It is important to note that PTO may reoccur after transuterine recanalization, emphasizing the importance of follow-up HSG for monitoring.[13]

It must be mentioned that in evaluation of women with unexplained infertility or minimal or mild endometriosis although laparoscopy has lost its role as the tubal patency is documented by less invasive tests; however, evaluating the cost factor and based on clinical judgement especially where the HSG suggests loculation of dye or the doubtful evidence of patency, it would be worthwhile to offer laparoscopy to confirm the correct tubo-ovarian relationship or perform adhesiolysis leading to correction of this relationship which may in future lead to a natural pregnancy without any intervention.

Performing laparoscopy in a woman with doubt of hydrosalpinx must have a counseling and consent for salpingectomy and in presence of one during surgery be performed simultaneously if so consented.

Method of hysteroscopic technique of tubal cannulation: A 5.5 F Teflon cannula equipped with a metal obturator is inserted through the operating channel of the

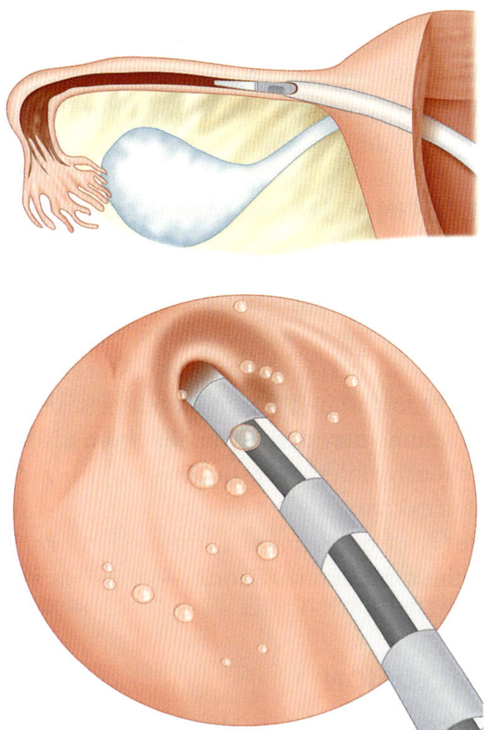

Fig. 5: Schematic diagram showing tubal cannulation.
Source: Jones HW, Rock JA. Te Linde's Operative Gynecology, 11th edition. Philadelphia, PA: Lippincott Williams and Wilkins; 2015. p. 325.

hysteroscopic sheath. Following removal of the obturator, a 3 F catheter with a guide cannula wire is threaded into the 5.5 F cannula using a Y-adapter attached to the end of the cannula. The catheter is carefully maneuvered into the tubal ostium and gently advanced into the tube. If there is resistance or negotiation of the cornual portion of the tube, the guide wire is retracted, and indigo carmine dye is introduced through the 3-F catheter. Concurrent laparoscopy enables the observation of dye exiting the fimbrial end of the tube, confirming its patency **(Fig. 5)**.[14]

Hysterosalpingo-contrast-sonography

A cutting-edge combination of hysterosonography and contrast agents, hysterosalpingo-contrast-sonography (HyCoSy) takes the spotlight. We explore its real-time imaging capabilities and the advantages it holds as a less invasive alternative to laparoscopy.

Hysterosalpingo-contrast-sonography with Air-saline

Method: Combine a small quantity of saline with an equal volume of air, for example, 10 mL saline and 10 mL air in a 20 mL syringe. Administer small increments of air alternating with saline (in 1–3 mL portions) into the uterine cavity. Periodically invert the syringe to facilitate the movement of air (or saline) to the top of the syringe lumen, thereby controlling the injection into the endometrial cavity. Utilize real-time cine imaging to track the passage of air from the endometrial cavity through the fallopian tube segments to the ovary. Repeat the injection on the contralateral side. For simultaneous evaluation of the interstitial fallopian tubes, position the transvaginal probe in the transverse plane to visualize both uterine cornua, inject the air and saline mixture, and observe for swift forward movement of the echogenic air-saline from the fundal endometrial cavity through the interstitial fallopian tubes. Direct signs of tubal patency include high-contrast echoes in the interstitial fallopian tube and new air adjacent to the ipsilateral ovary. The presence of new or increasing fluid in the cul-de-sac serves as an indirect sign of patency of at least one fallopian tube.

The reasons for inaccuracies in assessment can be summarized as follows: the absence of anatomical details of the fallopian tube, particularly the overflow of the contrast agent from the fimbrial part, owing to factors like the trajectory of the fallopian tube, an inexperienced operator, equipment limitations, or inappropriate pre-setting's. Additionally, pseudo-obstruction of the proximal part of the fallopian tube may occur due to various factors including tubal spasm, intrauterine lesions, and improper catheter placement. It is a well-tolerated and inexpensive test with sensitivity of 76.1% and specificity of 79.4%.[15]

Hysterosalpingo-contrast-sonography with microbubble: For this examination, a diluted microbubble ultrasound contrast solution and specialized software for contrast-enhanced ultrasound are required.

The presence of free contrast material in the adnexa and cul-de-sac is indicative of the patency of at least one fallopian tube.

Hysterosalpingo-foam Sonography

By utilizing the concepts of contrast-enhanced imaging, hysterosalpingo-foam sonography (HyFoSy) involves carefully inserting contrast foam into the uterus, followed by real-time ultrasound visualization to examine the tubal patency.

Method: It employs the intrauterine injection of air polymer-type A foam alongside standard gray-scale ultrasound. The foam is generated by vigorously blending 5 mL of sterile purified water with 5 mL of a gel containing hydroxyethyl cellulose and glycerol. This foam is nonembryotoxic and holds Food and Drug Administration (FDA) approval in the United States for evaluating fallopian tube patency. The initial dose involves 2–3 mL administered via intrauterine infusion, and this can be repeated in 2–3 mL increments, with a maximum dose capped at 10 mL. The sonographically visible foam persists for a minimum of 5 minutes. Assessment of fallopian tubes can be conducted individually or simultaneously, following the methodology outlined in the HyCoSy section. A patent fallopian tube is identified when the foam moves from the tube into the peritoneal cavity, with the tube's lumen appearing as a thin, high-contrast line. This test is said to have sensitivity of 87.5% and specificity 100%, with a possible fertility enhancing effect. HyCoSy and HyFoSy (sono-HSG) are potentially more cost-effective and efficient option than HSG.[15]

Magnetic Resonance Hysterosalpingography

This technique allows for the simultaneous evaluation of tubal patency and the identification of intra- and extrauterine pathologic conditions. It offers superior contrast resolution and heightened sensitivity to the spillage of even small amounts of contrast material when compared to traditional HSG methods. However, the use of magnetic resonance hysterosalpingography (MR HSG) comes with certain drawbacks. It tends to be expensive, is motion-dependent, and catheter repositioning may not always be feasible during the procedure, potentially affecting its accuracy. Additionally, the process tends to be longer in duration compared to conventional methods. The advantages of enhanced contrast resolution and sensitivity should be weighed against these limitations when considering the use of MR HSG in clinical settings.

Virtual Computed Tomography Hysterosalpingography

The modality offers the ability to simultaneously assess tubal patency and intra- and extrauterine pathologic conditions, albeit with limitations when compared to magnetic resonance imaging (MRI). The associated radiation dose varies within the range of 0.3–3 mSv, underscoring the importance of considering potential radiation exposure concerns. Moreover, it is essential to acknowledge the higher cost associated with procedures utilizing this method. While the technique provides valuable diagnostic insights, careful consideration of the balance between diagnostic benefits and potential drawbacks, including radiation exposure and financial considerations, is imperative for informed decision-making by healthcare professionals and patients alike.

SELECTING THE SUITABLE TEST FOR FALLOPIAN TUBE PATENCY CUSTOMIZED FOR THE PATIENT

It depends on the cost, availability, expertise, and risk factors associated. Low-risk individuals lacking preexisting conditions including PID, endometriosis, or congenital malformations may derive benefits from a singular and comprehensive infertility assessment utilizing ultrasound. In instances characterized by adhesions, preexisting tubal pathology, or adenomyosis, the preference may lean toward the application of fluoroscopic HSG as a diagnostic modality.

CONCLUSION

The choice of the most suitable tubal patency test depends on various factors including cost, availability, expertise, and the presence of specific risk factors. For low-risk individuals without preexisting conditions, such as PID, endometriosis, or congenital malformations, a one-stop comprehensive infertility evaluation utilizing ultrasound may be sufficient.

In cases where adhesions, preexisting tubal pathology, or adenomyosis are suspected, fluoroscopic HSG could be considered as a preferred diagnostic modality. HSG, while having reasonable specificity, does have limitations in terms of sensitivity, particularly in predicting tubal patency for patients with a risk of pelvic adhesions.

For a more noninvasive option, sonohysterography (SHG) or saline infusion sonography (SIS) may be considered, offering versatility and effective detection of intrauterine pathologies.

Laparoscopy combined with chromopertubation is acknowledged as the gold standard, providing direct visualization of pelvic organs and the ability to diagnose and treat conditions affecting fertility. However, it is an invasive surgical procedure with associated risks.

Hysterosalpingo-contrast-sonography and HyFoSy emerge as potentially more cost-effective and efficient options than traditional HSG, with good sensitivity and specificity. HyFoSy, in particular, shows promising results with a high sensitivity and near perfect specificity.

Ultimately, the selection of the best tubal patency test should be personalized based on the individual's clinical profile, preferences, and the specific diagnostic requirements of the infertility evaluation. Each method has its unique advantages and considerations, and the choice should align with the patient's needs and the clinical context.

REFERENCES

1. Roux I, Ronn R, Chan PT, Tulandi T, Holzer HE. Initial investigation of the infertile couple. In: Gardner DK, Weissman A, Howles CM, Shoham Z (Eds). Assisted Reproductive Techniques, 5th edition. Florida: CRC Press; 2018. pp. 475-86
2. Stumpf PG, March CM. Febrile morbidity following hysterosalpingography: identification of risk factors and recommendations for prophylaxis. Fertil Steril. 1980; 33(5): 487-92.
3. Roest I, van Welie N, Mijatovic V, Dreyer K, Bongers M, Koks C, et al. Complications after hysterosalpingography with oil- or water-based contrast: results of a nationwide survey. Hum Reprod Open. 2020;2020(1):hoz045.
4. Luttjeboer F, Harada T, Hughes E, Johnson N, Lilford R, Mol BW. Tubal flushing for subfertility. Cochrane Database Syst Rev. 2007;(3):CD003718.
5. Johnson NP, Farquhar CM, Hadden WE, Suckling J, Yu Y, Sadler L. The FLUSH trial—flushing with lipiodol for unexplained (and endometriosis-related) subfertility by hysterosalpingography: a randomized trial. Hum Reprod. 2004;19(9):2043-51.
6. Swart P, Mol BW, van der Veen F, van Beurden M, Redekop WK, Bossuyt PM. The accuracy of hysterosalpingography in the diagnosis of tubal pathology: a meta-analysis. Fertil Steril. 1995;64(3):486-91.
7. Montoya JM, Bernal A, Borrero C. Diagnostics in assisted human reproduction. Reprod Biomed Online. 2002;5(2): 198-210.
8. Panchal S, Nagori C. Imaging techniques for assessment of tubal status. J Hum Reprod Sci. 2014;7(1):2-12.
9. Soares SR, Barbosa dos Reis MM, Camargos AF. Diagnostic accuracy of sonohysterography, transvaginal sonography, and hysterosalpingography in patients with uterine cavity diseases. Fertil Steril. 2000;73(2):406-11.
10. Chapron C, Querleu D, Bruhat MA, Madelenat P, Fernandez H, Pierre F, et al. Surgical complications of diagnostic and operative gynaecological laparoscopy: a series of 29,966 cases. Hum Reprod. 1998;13(4):867-72.
11. Practice Committee of the American Society for Reproductive Medicine. Fertility evaluation of infertile women: a committee opinion. Fertil Steril. 2021;116(5): 1255-65.
12. Novy MJ, Thurmond AS, Patton P, Uchida BT, Rosch J. Diagnosis of cornual obstruction by transcervical fallopian tube cannulation. Fertil Steril. 1988;50(3):434-40.
13. Woolcott R. Proximal tubal occlusion: a practical approach. Hum Reprod. 1996;11(9):1831-3.
14. Jones HW, Rock JA. Te Linde's Operative Gynecology, 11th edition. Philadelphia, PA: Lippincott Williams and Wilkins; 2015. p. 325.
15. Grigovich M, Kacharia VS, Bharwani N, Hemingway A, Mijatovic V, Rodgers SK. Evaluating Fallopian Tube Patency: What the Radiologist Needs to Know. Radiographics. 2021; 41(6):1876-18961.

26

Chapter

Changing Perspectives of Ovarian Stimulation

Manisha Takhtani Kundnani, Pritimala Gangurde

INTRODUCTION

Controlled ovarian stimulation (COS) is one of the fundamental steps in in vitro fertilization (IVF) treatment. Exogenous gonadotropins are administered to overcome the process of dominant selection and enable multiple follicular recruitment.[1] The aim is to retrieve many oocytes and have multiple embryos to improve the success rates. Conventionally, the stimulation is started in the follicular phase as it was believed that there is one wave of follicular growth which starts early in the follicular phase. However, it has now been proposed that there are multiple waves of follicular growth in a menstrual cycle.[2] This theory of multiple waves of follicular recruitment forms the basis of newer stimulation protocols, such as random start, luteal phase, and dual stimulation. The protocols can be especially beneficial in certain category of patients like cancer patients undergoing fertility preservation who can be at any stage of menstrual cycle and waiting for follicular phase can cause significant delay in cancer treatment. Dual stimulation can be beneficial for women undergoing fertility preservation for nononcology reasons and also for women with poor ovarian reserve/response (POR) as it helps in collecting maximum number of oocytes and embryos in limited time period. Progesterone-primed ovarian stimulation (PPOS) is another novel concept to prevent premature luteinizing hormone (LH) surge during ovarian stimulation. The chapter discusses the evolution of new forms of ovarian stimulation due to expanding knowledge of ovarian physiology and discusses the implications of this strategy in clinical practice.

FOLLICULOGENESIS: NEW CONCEPTS

Folliculogenesis is an ongoing process in which multiple follicles are in the process of development. Traditionally, it was believed that the antral follicles are recruited in each ovary only once, in late luteal phase of preceding menstrual cycle, and this formed the basis of starting ovarian stimulation in the early follicular phase.[3] However, there is increasing evidence now to support that there are multiple waves of follicular recruitment in the same menstrual cycle, challenging the traditional concept of single follicular wave.[4,5]

Three theories of antral follicle recruitment have been suggested—continuous recruitment, single recruitment, and the wave theory **(Figs. 1A to C)**.[3] According to the "continuous recruitment" theory, small antral follicles are continuously growing and regressing throughout the inter-ovulatory interval. Selection of dominant follicle happens by chance from the pool following luteal regression. According to the "single recruitment theory", the dominant follicle is selected from a single follicular cohort that emerges after luteolysis. The third "wave theory" of follicle recruitment suggests that two or more cohorts of antral follicles are recruited during the same ovarian cycle. The dominant follicle that develops in the final wave of the interovulatory interval ovulates while preceding waves are anovulatory.

The understanding of these new theories of follicular recruitment have revolutionized the concept of ovarian stimulation and has paved path for the development of newer stimulation protocols, such as random start, luteal phase, and dual stimulation. However, it still needs to be determined if synchronization of the emergence of follicular waves with ovarian stimulation enhances the efficiency of assisted reproductive technology and produces more competent oocytes and healthier embryos.[6]

Newer Stimulation Protocols

The understanding of the new theory of follicular recruitment led to the development of the newer ovarian

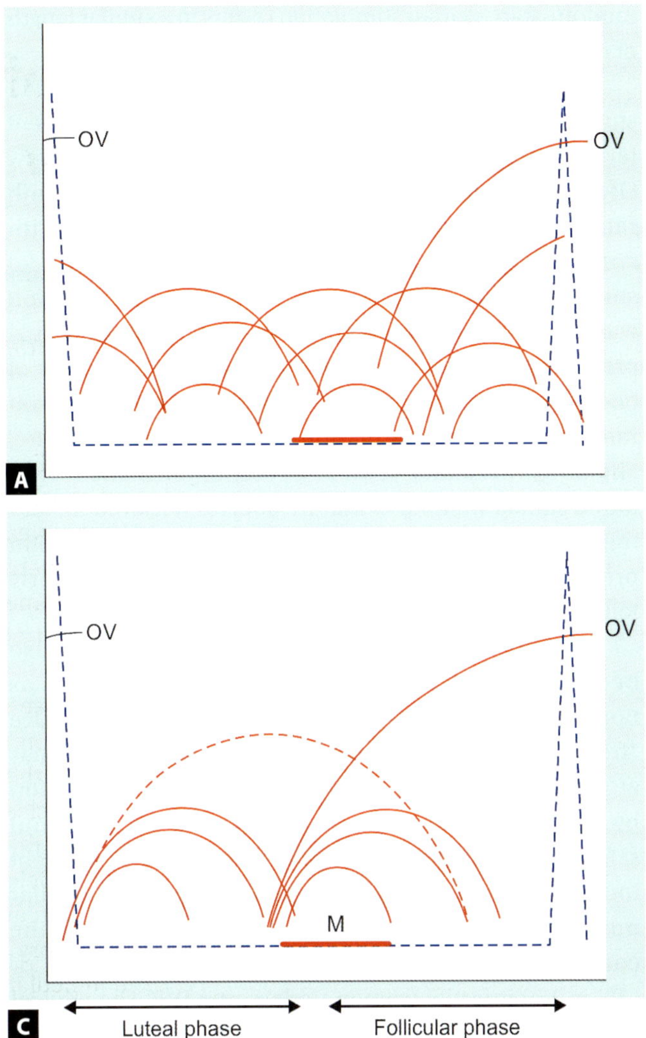

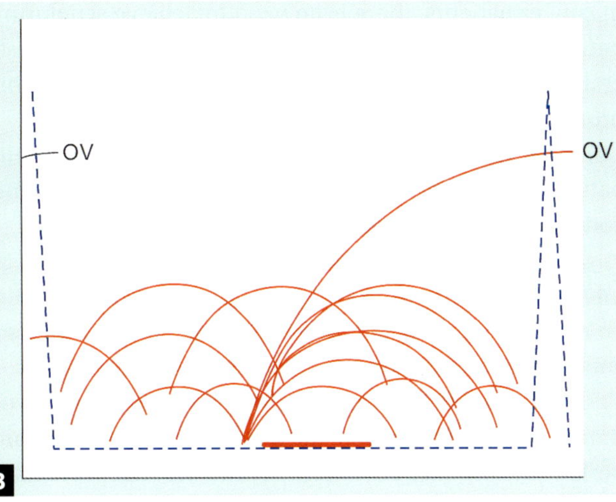

Figs. 1A to C: Theories of follicular recruitment. The theory of continuous recruitment (A) suggests that small antral follicles grow and regress constantly throughout the interovulatory interval (IOI) and the dominant ovulatory follicle is selected, by chance, from the pool following luteal regression. The theory of a single recruitment episode (B) suggests that an ovulatory follicle is selected from a single follicular cohort that emerges following luteal regression. The wave theory of follicle recruitment (C) suggests that two or more cohorts (i.e., waves) of antra follicles are recruited (i.e., emerge) during the ovarian cycle. The dominant follicle that develops in the final wave of the IOI ovulates while preceding waves are anovulatory; dominant follicles develop in a minority of anovulatory waves (dotted line). (M: menses)

stimulation protocols. These are especially beneficial in cancer patients, women with poor ovarian reserve, or those undergoing fertility preservation. These include random-start protocol, luteal phase stimulation (LPS), dual stimulation, and PPOS.

Random-start Ovarian Stimulation Protocol

Random-start ovarian stimulation protocol means to start ovarian stimulation immediately irrespective of the phase of menstrual cycle. The increasing need for shortening the duration required for IVF cycles had led to the emergence of this protocol. Multiple wave theory of folliculogenesis forms the basis of this protocol. According to this theory, follicle-stimulating hormone (FSH)-sensitive follicles are existing at any stage of the cycle which gives an opportunity to start the stimulation in late follicular phase as well as luteal phase.

Indications of random-start ovarian stimulation: The most common indication is fertility preservation in cancer patients. The women in reproductive age group detected with malignancy and desirous of fertility preservation are the candidates for random-start ovarian stimulation. This allows them to undergo ovarian stimulation with gonadotropins and cryopreservation of oocytes or embryos immediately without wasting time. Such patients are in need of either surgery, radiotherapy, or chemotherapy for treatment of the malignancies. Waiting for the onset of menses to start conventional follicular phase stimulation (FPS) can lead to significant delay in cancer treatment which may be detrimental to the patient.

In cancer patients, there is no need to achieve synchrony between ovaries and endometrium as there is no fresh embryo transfer, thus allowing random-start stimulation protocols.

Other indications include *social egg freezing* wherein patient is elderly with poor ovarian reserve or with time constraint because of hectic unplanned work schedule.

Patients who are detected with entities like *absence of uterus [Mayer-Rokitansky-Küster-Hauser (MRKH)]* who do not have any idea about the phase of the cycle are also good candidates to take the benefit of this protocol.

International patients who come for a short period of time and want to complete the process in the limited time period can also take advantage of random-start protocol.

Random-start Protocol

The concept of multiple waves in the process of folliculogenesis forms the basis for random-start stimulation protocols. The stimulation is started any day irrespective of the day of the cycle. Age of the woman and anti-Müllerian hormone (AMH) value are taken as markers for deciding the doses of gonadotropins along with other ultrasound markers. Once the leading follicle is around 14 mm or day 6 of stimulation gonadotropin-releasing hormone (GnRH) antagonist can be added to achieve synchronous growth as well as to prevent premature luteinization of the follicles. When majority of follicles are >17 mm in size, the trigger injection is planned. Serum estradiol levels along with number of follicles are a good guide to decide for the trigger.

Random-start Ovarian Stimulation: Available Evidence

Multiple studies and case reports are published evaluating the random stimulation for variable indications. The available literature confirms its safety and efficacy and has shown comparable outcomes in terms of number and quality of oocytes or embryos. Hakan Cakemak et al. analyzed the relevant reports and published a review article mentioning the advantages of random-start ovarian stimulation over conventional protocol in reducing total time for the IVF cycle. According to the author, random protocols are a boon in cases of emergency. It provides flexibility of starting ovarian stimulation at a random cycle date for the purpose of preservation of fertility without compromising the outcome in the form of number of oocytes as well as the maturity.[7] It was also observed that random-start ovarian stimulation results in a similar length of ovarian stimulation and in similar gonadotropin use.

A meta-analysis done by Sonmerez et al. included 11 studies and a total of 1,764 cancer patients who underwent fertility preservation before the gonadotoxic therapy. Of the 1,764 patients, 688 patients were treated with random-start protocol and 1,076 were treated with conventional stimulation protocol. The duration of stimulation and cumulative gonadotropin consumption was higher in random-start protocol than conventional protocol. But, the outcome in the form of total number of oocytes, number of metaphase II (MII) oocytes, fertilization rates, and embryo formation rates were comparable.[8] Similarly, Alexander et al. in a recent systematic review found similar number of mature oocytes retrieved in both the groups of women treated with random stimulation protocol and conventional protocol started in early follicular phase.[9]

The random-start ovarian stimulation has also been evaluated in other clinical setting, such as normoresponders, egg donors, and in clinics that practice "freeze all". A recently published case report by Kumar et al. concluded that oocyte or embryo cryopreservation by random-start ovarian stimulation is effective and safe and can be offered to young women under different indications.[10] In another study by Qin et al., a similar number of mature oocytes were obtained after the conventional follicular phase, late follicular phase, or LPS in 150 infertile women undergoing IVF. The clinical pregnancy rates (CPRs) and the implantation rates were also similar between the three groups.[11]

Guerrero et al. recently evaluated the efficacy of random-start protocols in oocyte donors. The authors concluded that the number of oocytes retrieved in oocyte donation cycles and live birth rates (LBRs) in recipients was similar after conventional and random-start ovarian stimulation and that the random-start ovarian stimulation protocols in oocyte donation cycles do not negatively affect oocyte yield or clinical outcomes in recipients compared with conventional protocols.[12]

Luteal Phase Stimulation

Luteal phase ovarian stimulation is based on the concept that at least two or more waves of follicular recruitment are there in one menstrual cycle. Though initially LPS was reserved for women with cancer patients undergoing fertility preservation,[13-15] it is now being used in women with

POR also,[16] to obtain sufficient number of competent oocytes. A typical LPS starts 2–7 days after ovulation or oocyte retrieval (in case of dual stimulation—discussed).

Wang et al. evaluated the efficacy of LPS in normoresponders.[17] They compared short agonist with minimal and LPS. The numbers of mature oocytes retrieved, and top-quality embryos obtained per ovum pick-up (OPU) cycle were significantly increased in the LPS group compared with the mild treatment group or the short-term group. The authors also observed that implantation rates were comparable in luteal stimulation and mild stimulation, but significantly lower with the standard short agonist protocol. Neonatal outcomes in the LPS group were similar to the other two groups. The similar group of researchers in another study compared FPS to luteal stimulation in poor responders.[18] The authors observed that LPS was associated with significantly higher number of oocytes and top quality embryos compared to conventional stimulation. The stimulation however lasted longer, and a higher total dose of gonadotropins was required.

Chen et al. compared live birth defects after luteal phase ovarian stimulation versus conventional ovarian stimulation for IVF and vitrified embryo transfer cycles.[19] No significant difference in gestational age, birth weight, length, congenital defects, and neonatal death was found between the two groups.

A systematic review and meta-analysis done by Lu et al. concluded that LPS group could achieve pregnancy outcomes noninferior to those in the FPS. However, because of current debate over freeze-all policy and the limited data about LBR, the universal use of LPS is considered controversial.[20]

Dual Stimulation

The new understanding of ovarian folliculogenesis, feasibility of LPS, and the availability of cryopreservation facilities with disarticulation of ovarian stimulation and embryo transfer led to the possibility of performing consecutive ovarian stimulation in the same cycle in order to increase the number of oocytes available (and possibly embryos) per patient in one given cycle.

Dual stimulation means two successive ovarian stimulations in the follicular and ensuing luteal phase with two oocyte retrievals in the same menstrual cycle. The protocol allows maximum exploitation of the ovarian reserve in a limited time period especially in poor prognosis patients when time is an essence. The protocol is especially suited for women with poor ovarian reserve—advanced age/low AMH, patients with no oocytes/no competent embryos after conventional FPS, or cancer patients for fertility preservation.

Dual stimulation was first performed by Kuang et al. in women with POR. The protocol used by them became popular as Shanghai protocol **(Fig. 2)**.[21] They observed that total number of MII oocytes obtained were higher after LPS. The fertilization rate, cleavage rate, and the mean number of viable embryos were similar after FPS or LPS. No difference was observed in embryo survival rate, CPR, ongoing pregnancy rate, or miscarriage rate between FPS and LPS. The authors concluded that double stimulation provides opportunities for retrieving more

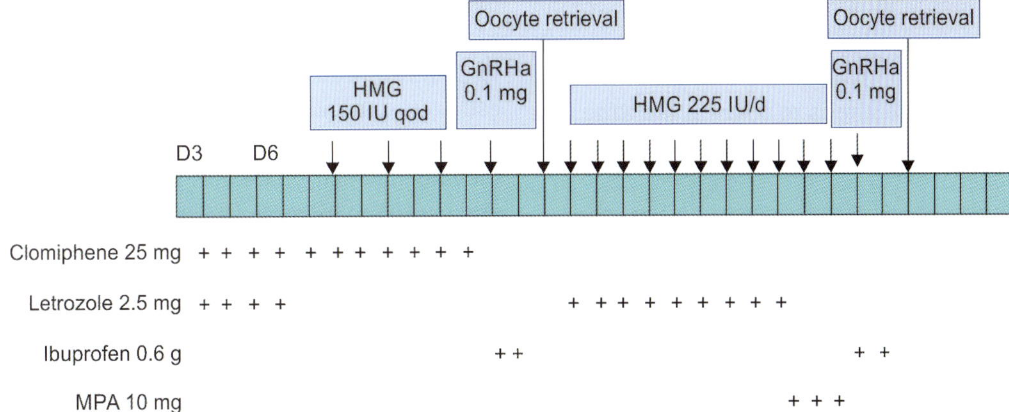

Fig. 2: Shanghai protocol for dual stimulation.
(HMG: human menopausal gonadotropin; MPA: medroxyprogesterone acetate)
Source: Kuang Y, Chen Q, Hong Q, Lyu Q, Ai A, Fu Y, et al. Double stimulations during the follicular and luteal phases of poor responders in IVF/ICSI programmes (Shanghai protocol). Reprod Biomed Online. 2014;29(6):684-91.

oocytes and to have more viable embryos in the same cycle, avoids cycle cancellation, and increases the possibility of pregnancy.

Similar findings were observed subsequently by many researchers in individual studies.[22-25] A comparative study by Polat M et al. in 2021 compared dual stimulation with conventional ovarian stimulation in POR patients.[26] They reported significantly less cycle cancellation rates and significantly higher number of MII oocytes, blastocysts, and cryopreserved/available embryos with dual stimulation.

A SWOT (Strengths, Weaknesses, Opportunities, and Threats) analysis on dual stimulation concluded that it helps retrieve higher number of oocytes and embryos in shorter time period in women with poor ovarian reserve, and is better tolerated than consecutive FPS, thereby reducing the dropout rates. The oocytes obtained after LPS or FPS are observed to be equally competent. However, freeze-all approach is mandatory, cost-effective analysis is not available, and the studies comparing efficacy of dual stimulation to two consecutive follicular phase stimulation are scarce.[27]

BISTIM was a multicenter, open-labeled RCT, performed in four IVF centers from September 2018 to March 2021.[28] The aim was to compare the dual stimulation to two consecutive antagonist cycles in women with poor ovarian response. The primary outcome of the study was the number of oocytes retrieved. The authors observed that there was no significant difference in the number of oocytes, mature oocytes, or number of embryos in the two groups. The cumulative LBR also was comparable between the two groups. The authors concluded that based on the number of total and mature oocytes retrieved in women with poor ovarian response (POR), there is no benefit of DuoStim versus two consecutive antagonist cycles. The only benefit of DuoStim is to shorten the time to a second retrieval by 2 weeks if accumulation of oocytes/embryos is needed.

Dual Stimulation: The Protocol

The follicular stimulation is usually started on day 2/3 of the menstrual cycle. GnRH antagonist is administered once the leading follicle reaches 13–14 mm in diameter and continued until the day of trigger of ovulation. Trigger is given when at least two follicles had reached 17–18 mm in diameter and oocyte retrieval is scheduled 34–35 hours later. The second stimulation is usually started 5 days after the first oocyte retrieval and similar antagonist protocol is followed. Many clinicians prefer adding oral progesterone after the first retrieval to avoid occurrence of menses during the second retrieval.

Certain problems with double-ovarian stimulation (DOS) remain unsolved: Firstly, it is not known which is the best day to start the second stimulation. Most studies reported an interval of 1–5 days without significant difference in terms of length of stimulation and number of oocytes retrieved. There is no scientific basis to choose the duration of interval between first pick-up and the start of the second ovarian stimulation. It is also not known what the ideal drug is for triggering. Some authors have reported successful pick-up with the use of human chorionic gonadotropin (hCG) even in the first stimulation while the majority used GnRH agonist triggering. The utility of using a higher dose of gonadotropin in the second stimulation or an LH activity drug is still unclear.

Progesterone-primed Ovarian Stimulation

Oral progesterone has recently surfaced an efficient substitute for pituitary suppression and prevention of premature LH surge during ovarian stimulation in IVF cycles. Kuang et al., in 2015, were the first to evaluate this new PPOS protocol for prevention of LH surges during COS.[29] And since then multiple studies have been conducted evaluating the efficacy of progesterone in prevention of LH surge in IVF cycles.

Progesterone-primed Ovarian Stimulation: Mechanism of Action

Progesterone is known to play a key role in the follicular dynamics. Though the exact mechanism of action of progesterone is unclear, it is known that the effect of progesterone can be synergistic or antagonistic to estrogen depending on the concentration and time of exposure.[30] The mildly elevated levels of progesterone in the late follicular phase acts synergistically with estrogen and cause the increase in GnRH pulse frequency and LH surge. However, persistently elevated progesterone level as is seen in luteal phase, pregnancy, or as seen with progestin contraceptives, is observed to have an inhibitory effect on the action of estrogen, blunting the GnRH pulse frequencies, and blocking the LH surge and ovulation.[31,32] The persistent high levels of progesterone desensitize its own as well as GnRH receptors. This inhibitory effect of high levels of progesterone on the LH surge forms the basis of PPOS protocols.

Progesterone-primed Ovarian Stimulation: Protocols

Two types of PPOS protocols have been used by different researchers: (1) the fixed and (2) the flexible protocol.

In the fixed PPOS protocol, progestin is started from day 2/3 of the cycles along with gonadotropins, and is continued till the day of trigger **(Fig. 3)**.[33] In the flexible protocol, progestin is started either on day 7 or when the leading

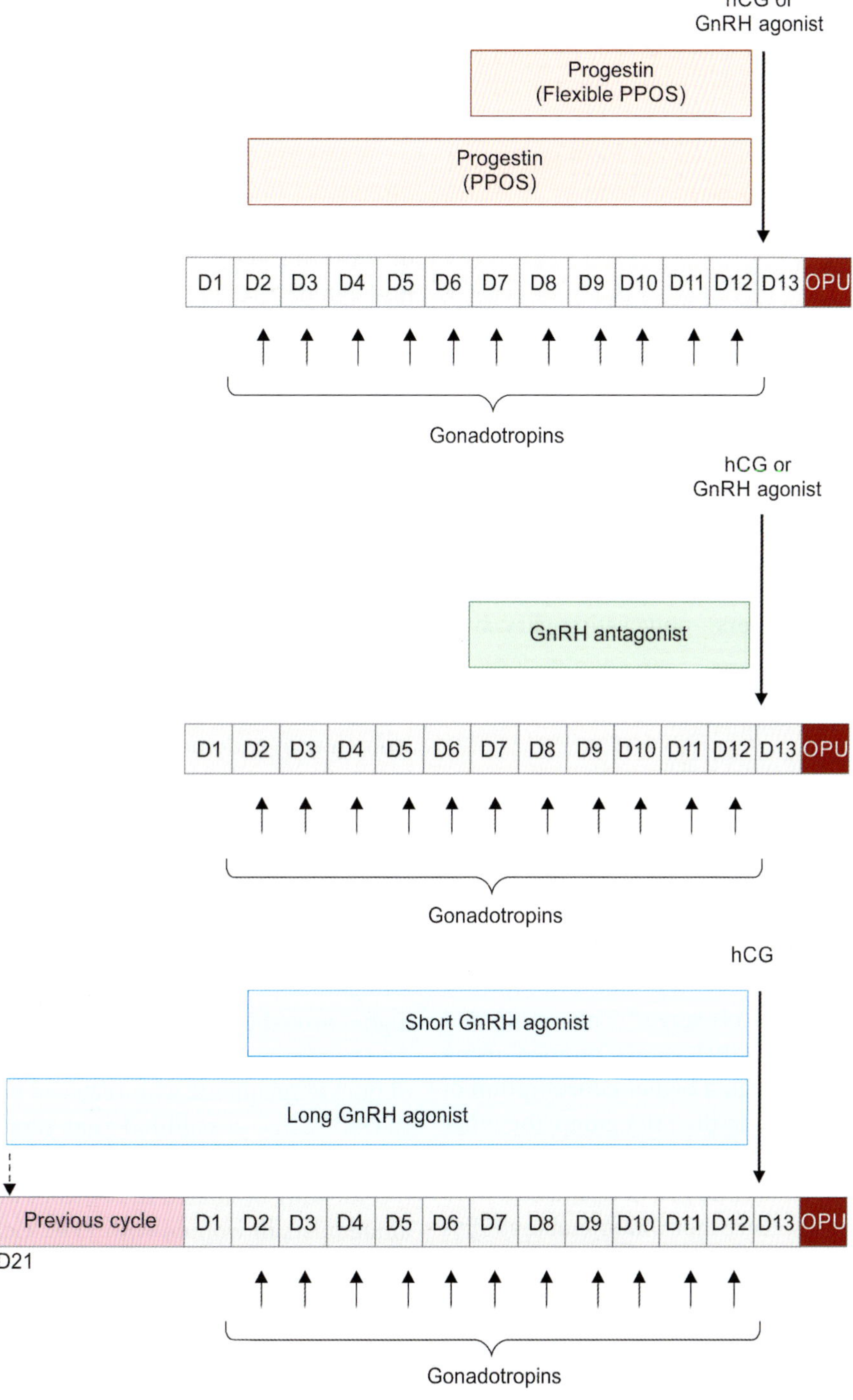

Fig. 3: Commonly used ovarian stimulation protocols and PPOS protocol.
(GnRH: gonadotropin-releasing hormone; hCG: human chorionic gonadotropin; OPU: ovum pick-up; PPOS: progesterone-primed ovarian stimulation)

follicle reaches 14 mm, and is then continued till the day of trigger. Both the protocols have been found to be equally efficacious in terms of prevention of LH surge, number of mature oocytes retrieved, and pregnancy outcomes.

The progestin most commonly used for PPOS is medroxyprogesterone acetate (MPA) in a dose of 10 mg/day. The advantage of MPA is that it does not interfere with intrinsic progesterone measurements. The other commonly used progestins are dydrogesterone 20 mg/day and micronized progesterone 200 mg/day.

Ideal Candidates for Progesterone-primed Ovarian Stimulation

As PPOS involves administration of progesterone from the early follicular phase, endometrium is exposed to high doses of progesterone from the beginning and so is not suitable for fresh transfer. As a result, freezing of all embryos becomes mandatory in PPOS. Therefore, the ideal candidates for PPOS are those in whom no transfer is planned in the same cycle. These include:

- Patients undergoing fertility preservation
- Donor egg cycles
- Predicted hyperresponders—polycystic ovary syndrome (PCOS)
- Nonconventional protocols—random start, luteal stimulation, and dual stimulation
- Poor responder and advanced age
- Preimplantation genetic testing (PGT) for aneuploidies or monogenic diseases.

Efficacy of PPOS Protocol Compared to GnRH Analogs

Kuang et al., in 2015, were the first to evaluate the efficacy of progestins to suppress the LH surge.[29] They compared MPA 10 mg/day with short GnRH agonist protocol using triptorelin 0.1 mg/day. Though a higher consumption of gonadotropins was observed in the MPA group, the other outcomes including prevention of LH surge, number of oocytes retrieved, number of embryos, CPR, and LBR were similar in both the groups. Since then innumerable studies have been done comparing the efficacy of the novel PPOS with conventional GnRH agonists and antagonist protocols. In another study conducted by Chen et al., MPA 10 mg/day was compared with GnRH antagonists.[34] The incidence of premature LH surge and premature ovulation was significantly low in MPA group compared to antagonist group (0 vs. 5.88%, $p < 0.05$).

A meta-analysis conducted by Ata et al. comparing the efficacy of progestins and GnRH analogs for prevention of LH surge observed that the duration of stimulation, gonadotropin consumption, and oocyte yield were similar with progestins and GnRH analogs.[35] The clinical pregnancy, ongoing pregnancy, and LBRs were also similar with progestins and analogs. However, in women with PCOS, short GnRH agonist protocol showed higher CPRs, though the quality of evidence was low.

A few researchers have evaluated the efficacy of progestins for LH suppression in women undergoing fertility preservation. Huang et al. evaluated the efficacy of random-start progestin stimulation in women undergoing fertility preservation.[36] The authors observed that in random-start protocols, progestins were similar to antagonist in the number of days of stimulation, total dose of gonadotropin preparation, and the number of mature oocytes obtained and blastocysts formed. The number of hospital visits for monitoring was significantly lower in the PPOS and the incidence of start of menstruation before oocyte collection was also significantly less in the PPOS group. Mathieu d'Argent E et al. evaluated the efficacy of PPOS for fertility preservation in women with endometriosis.[37] They observed that number of mature oocytes obtained were similar in both groups. However, contrary to the above study, Yang et al. evaluated PPOS in women with endometrioma and observed that PPOS had inferior reproductive outcomes in terms of biochemical pregnancy, clinical pregnancy, and live birth than ultra-long GnRH antagonist protocol. No significant difference however was observed between PPOS and GnRH antagonist protocol.[38] The authors concluded that in women with endometrioma the ultra-long GnRH antagonist protocol was associated with a significant higher probability of live birth than PPOS protocol.

Devesa et al. evaluated the reproductive outcomes of oocyte recipients who received vitrified oocytes after PPOS.[39] They concluded that reproductive outcomes were not affected by donor PPOS stimulation. Another recent study evaluated the efficacy of PPOS compared to antagonists in women with POR. Compared with PPOS, GnRH antagonist protocol had higher risk of premature LH surges for POR.[40] However, it did not affect the overall pregnancy rates. Du et al. observed that for low-prognosis patients diagnosed as per the POSEIDON (Patient-Oriented Strategies Encompassing Individualized Oocyte Number) criteria, the cumulative live birth rate (CLBR) of PPOS protocols is comparable to that of GnRH antagonist protocols.[41] However, in the POSEIDON group 1 population, the GnRH antagonist protocols resulted in a shorter time to live birth.

Effect on Oocyte Development and Embryo Euploidy with PPOS

With PPOS protocols, there had been concerns that high level of progesterone on the day of trigger can significantly reduce the formation rate of good quality blastocysts, as was observed in some animal studies. However, as embryo quality assessment is subjective, a more objective proof of embryo quality is the euploidy status. La Marca et al. compared the euploidy rates of blastocysts formed after PPOS and conventional stimulation.[42] PGT was offered because of different indications, such as advanced age, recurrent miscarriages, and repeated implantation failures. The authors observed that the euploid blastocyst rate was similar in both groups, which was 21%. Also, the total number of euploid blastocysts per patient was also similar. Similar results were observed in a recent study done by Yang et al.[43] Zolfaroli et al. observed the impact of PPOS on newborn outcome and concluded that newborns born after PPOS are not at increased risk of congenital abnormality or low birth weight (LBW) compared from those born after GnRH analogs protocols.[44] They in fact observed a decreasing trend of preterm birth in PPOS group.

Is PPOS cost-effective?

Progesterone-primed ovarian stimulation is assumed to be cost-effective compared to conventional analog protocol as progestins are orally administered and are cheaper than GnRH analogs. However, PPOS involves the additional cost of freezing and thawing of embryos and monitoring of thaw embryo transfer cycle, which in turn increases the cost. A study by Evans et al. observed a higher cost per live birth in PPOS compared to analog cycles which were completed with fresh ET.[45] These protocols are however cost-effective only when freeze-all is the plan otherwise or for donor egg cycles. A study conducted by Khurana et al. observed that use of PPOS in egg donor cycles actually reduces the cost of per donor oocyte retrieved by half thus making it a cost-effective.[46]

Progesterone-primed Ovarian Stimulation: Conclusion

Progestins are a safe and efficient alternative to GnRH analogs for prevention of LH surge. They seem to be cost-effective in cycles where no fresh transfer is planned. The available embryological and neonatal data is reassuring in terms of blastocyst euploidy and neonatal outcomes. Mandatory freeze-all and deferred embryo transfer however increases the cost and also time to live birth in routine patients. Whether or not progestins can totally replace analogs needs larger studies and RCTs.

CONCLUSION

The understanding of new theories of follicular recruitment has led to the development of newer protocols for ovarian stimulation. The available literature is promising and proves their efficacy and safety, especially in certain subset of patients such as cancer patients and women with poor ovarian reserve.

REFERENCES

1. Baerwald AR, Adams GP, Pierson RA. Characteristics of ovarian follicular wave dynamics in women. Biol Reprod. 2003;69:1023-31.
2. Baerwald AR, Adams GP, Pierson RA. A new model for ovarian follicular development during the human menstrual cycle. Fertil Steril. 2003;80:116-22.
3. Baerwald AR, Adams GP, Pierson RA. Ovarian antral folliculogenesis during the human menstrual cycle: a review. Hum Reprod Update. 2012;18:73-91.
4. Hillier SG. Current concepts of the roles of follicle stimulating hormone and luteinizing hormone in folliculogenesis. Hum Reprod. 1994;9:188-91.
5. Yang DZ, Yang W, Li Y, He Z. Progress in understanding human ovarian folliculogenesis and its implications in assisted reproduction. J Assist Reprod Genet. 2013;30:213-9.
6. de Mello Bianchi PH, Serafini P, Monteiro da Rocha A, Assad Hassun P, Alves da Motta EL, Sampaio Baruselli P, et al. Review: follicular waves in the human ovary: a new physiological paradigm for novel ovarian stimulation protocols. Reprod Sci. 2010;17:1067-76.
7. Cakmak H, Rosen MP. Random start ovarian stimulation in patients with cancer. Curr Opin Obstet Gynecol. 2015; 27:215-21.
8. Sonmezer M, Sukur YE, Ates C. Random start ovarian stimulation before gonadotoxic therapies in women with cancer—a systematic review and meta-analysis. Reprod Biomed Online. 2023;47(6):103337.
9. Alexander VM, Martin CE, Schelble AP, Laufer AB, Hardi A, McKenzie LJ, et al. Ovarian stimulation for fertility preservation in women with cancer: a systematic review and meta-analysis comparing random and conventional starts. J Gynecol Obstet Hum Reprod. 2021;50:102080.
10. Kumar P, Rao S, Mundkar A. Random Start Ovarian Stimulation. J Hum Reprod Sci. 2022;15(2):200-3.

11. Qin N, Chen Q, Hong Q, Cai R, Gao H, Wang Y, et al. Flexibility in starting ovarian stimulation at different phases of the menstrual cycle for treatment of infertile women with the use of in vitro fertilization or intracytoplasmic sperm injection. Fertil Steril. 2016;106: 334-41.
12. Guerrero J, Castillo JC, Ten J, Ortiz JA, Lledó B, Orozco D, et al. Random-start ovarian stimulation in an oocyte donation programme: a large, single-centre, experience. Reprod Biomed Online. 2024;48:103572.
13. Anderson RA, Kinniburgh D, Baird DT. Preliminary experience of the use of a gonadotrophin-releasing hormone antagonist in ovulation induction/in-vitro fertilization prior to cancer treatment. Hum Reprod. 1999; 14:2665-8.
14. Gagliato Dde M, Gonzalez-Angulo AM, Lei X, Theriault RL, Giordano SH, Valero V, et al. Clinical impact of delaying initiation of adjuvant chemotherapy in patients with breast cancer. J Clin Oncol. 2014;32:735-44.
15. von Wolff M, Thaler CJ, Frambach T, Zeeb C, Lawrenz B, Popovici RM, et al. Ovarian stimulation to cryopreserve fertilized oocytes in cancer patients can be started in the luteal phase. Fertil Steril. 2009;92(4):1360-5.
16. Kuang Y, Hong Q, Chen Q, Lyu Q, Ai A, Fu Y, et al. Luteal-phase ovarian stimulation is feasible for producing competent oocytes in women undergoing in vitro fertilization/intracytoplasmic sperm injection treatment, with optimal pregnancy outcomes in frozen-thawed embryo transfer cycles. Fertil Steril. 2014;101:105-11.
17. Wang N, Wang Y, Chen Q, Dong J, Tian H, Fu Y, et al. Luteal-phase ovarian stimulation versus conventional ovarian stimulation in patients with normal ovarian reserve treated for IVF: a large retrospective cohort study. Clin Endocrinol. 2016;84:720-8.
18. Li Y, Yang W, Chen X, Li L, Zhang Q, Yang D. Comparison between follicular stimulation and luteal stimulation protocols with clomiphene and HMG in women with poor ovarian response. Gynecol Endocrinol. 2016;32(1): 74-7.
19. Chen H, Wang Y, Lyu Q, Ai A, Fu Y, Tian H, et al. Comparison of live-birth defects after luteal-phase ovarian stimulation vs. conventional ovarian stimulation for in vitro fertilization and vitrified embryo transfer cycles. Fertil Steril. 2015;103(5):1194-1201.e2.
20. Lu BJ, Lin CJ, Lin BZ, Huang L, Chien LT, Chen CH. ART outcomes following ovarian stimulation in the luteal phase: a systematic review and meta-analysis. J Assist Reprod Genet. 2021;38(8):1927-38.
21. Kuang Y, Chen Q, Hong Q, Lyu Q, Ai A, Fu Y, et al. Double stimulations during the follicular and luteal phases of poor responders in IVF/ICSI programmes (Shanghai protocol). Reprod Biomed Online. 2014;29(6):684-91.
22. Moffat R, Pirtea P, Gayet V, Wolf JP, Chapron C, de Ziegler D. Dual ovarian stimulation is a new viable option for enhancing the oocyte yield when the time for assisted reproductive technnology is limited. Reprod Biomed Online. 2014;29(6):659-61.
23. Cardoso MCA, Evangelista A, Sartório C, Vaz G, Werneck CLV, Guimarães FM, et al. Can ovarian double-stimulation in the same menstrual cycle improve IVF outcomes? JBRA Assist Reprod. 2017;21(3):217-21.
24. Liu C, Jiang H, Zhang W, Yin H. Double ovarian stimulation during the follicular and luteal phase in women ≥38 years: a retrospective case-control study. Reprod Biomed Online. 2017;35:678-84.
25. Tsampras N, Gould D, Fitzgerald CT. Double ovarian stimulation (DuoStim) protocol for fertility preservation in female oncology patients. Hum Fertil (Camb). 2017;20(4): 248-53.
26. Polat M, Mumusoglu S, Yarali Ozbek I, Bozdag G, Yarali H. Double or dual stimulation in poor ovarian responders: where do we stand? Ther Adv Reprod Health. 2021;15:26334941211024172.
27. Vaiarelli A, Cimadomo D, Trabucco E, Vallefuoco R, Buffo L, Dusi L, et al. Double Stimulation in the Same Ovarian Cycle (DuoStim) to Maximize the Number of Oocytes Retrieved From Poor Prognosis Patients: A Multicenter Experience and SWOT Analysis. Front Endocrinol (Lausanne). 2018; 9:317.
28. Massin N, Abdennebi I, Porcu-Buisson G, Chevalier N, Descat E, Piétin-Vialle C, et al. The BISTIM study: a randomized controlled trial comparing dual ovarian stimulation (duostim) with two conventional ovarian stimulations in poor ovarian responders undergoing IVF. Hum Reprod. 2023;38(5):927-37.
29. Kuang Y, Chen Q, Fu Y, Wang Y, Hong Q, Lyu Q, et al. Medroxyprogesterone acetate is an effective oral alternative for preventing premature luteinizing hormone surges in women undergoing controlled ovarian hyperstimulation for in vitro fertilization. Fertil Steril. 2015;104(1):62-70.e3.
30. Custodia-Lora N, Callard IP. Progesterone and progesterone receptors in reptiles. Gen Comp Endocrinol. 2002; 127(1):1-7.
31. Evans NP, Richter TA, Skinner DC, Robinson JE. Neuroendocrine mechanisms underlying the effects of progesterone on the oestradiol-induced GnRH/LH surge. Reprod Suppl. 2002;59:57-66.
32. Heikinheimo O, Gordon K, Williams RF, Hodgen GD. Inhibition of ovulation by progestin analogs (agonists vs. antagonists): preliminary evidence for different sites and mechanisms of actions. Contraception. 1996;53: 55-64.
33. Doğan Durdağ G, Çağlar Aytaç P, Alkaş Yağınç D, Yetkinel S, Çok T, Şimşek E. Comparison of fixed and flexible progestin-primed ovarian stimulation protocols to prevent premature luteinization in patients with diminished ovarian reserve. Arch Gynecol Obstet. 2023; 308(2):579-86.

34. Chen Q, Chai W, Wang Y, Cai R, Zhang S, Lu X, et al. Progestin vs. Gonadotropin-Releasing Hormone Antagonist for the Prevention of Premature Luteinizing Hormone Surges in Poor Responders Undergoing in vitro Fertilization Treatment: A Randomized Controlled Trial. Front Endocrinol (Lausanne). 2019;10:796.
35. Ata B, Capuzzo M, Turkgeldi E, Yildiz S, La Marca A. Progestins for pituitary suppression during ovarian stimulation for ART: a comprehensive and systematic review including meta-analyses. Hum Reprod Update. 2021;27:48-66.
36. Huang H, Itaya Y, Samejima K, Ichinose S, Narita T, Matsunaga S, et al. Usefulness of random-start progestin-primed ovarian stimulation for fertility preservation. J Ovarian Res. 2022;15(1):2.
37. Mathieu d'Argent E, Ferrier C, Zacharopoulou C, Ahdad-Yata N, Boudy AS, Cantalloube A, et al. Outcomes of fertility preservation in women with endometriosis: comparison of progestin-primed ovarian stimulation versus antagonist protocols. J Ovarian Res. 2020;13:18.
38. Yang AM, Feng TF, Han Y, Zhao ZM, Wang W, Wang YZ, et al. Progestin-Primed Ovarian Stimulation Protocol for Patients With Endometrioma. Front Endocrinol (Lausanne). 2022;13:798434.
39. Devesa M, Racca A, Clúa E, Casato C, García S, Polyzos NP, et al. Progesterone-primed ovarian stimulation in oocyte donation: a model for elective fertility preservation? Reprod Biomed Online. 2022;44(6):1015-22.
40. Huang P, Tang M, Qin A. Progestin-primed ovarian stimulation is a feasible method for poor ovarian responders undergoing in IVF/ICSI compared to a GnRH antagonist protocol: A retrospective study. J Gynecol Obstet Hum Reprod. 2019;48(2):99-102.
41. Du M, Zhang J, Ren B, Guan Y. Comparison of the neonatal outcomes of progestin-primed ovarian stimulation and flexible GnRH antagonist protocols: a propensity score-matched cohort study. Front Endocrinol (Lausanne). 2023; 14:1156620.
42. La Marca A, Capuzzo M, Sacchi S, Imbrogno MG, Spinella F, Varricchio MT, et al. Comparison of euploidy rates of blastocysts in women treated with progestins or GnRH antagonist to prevent the luteinizing hormone surge during ovarian stimulation. Hum Reprod. 2020; 35(6):1325-31.
43. Yang L, Luo, Lu G, Lin G, Gong F. Euploidy rates among preimplantation genetic testing for aneuploidy cycles with oral dydrogesterone primed ovarian stimulation or GnRH antagonist protocol. Reprod Biomed Online. 2022;45:721-6.
44. Zolfaroli I, Ferriol GA, Mora JH, Cano A. Impact of progestin ovarian stimulation on newborn outcomes: a meta-analysis. J Assist Reprod Genet. 2020;37:1203-12.
45. Evans MB, Parikh T, DeCherney AH, Csokmay JM, Healy MW, Hill MJ. Evaluation of the cost-effectiveness of ovulation suppression with progestins compared with GnRH analogs in assisted reproduction cycles. Reprod Biomed Online. 2019;38(5):691-8.
46. Khurana RK, Rao V, Nayak C, Pranesh GT, Rao KA. Comparing Progesterone Primed Ovarian Stimulation (PPOS) to GnRH Antagonist Protocol in Oocyte Donation Cycles. J Hum Reprod Sci. 2022;15(3):278-83.

Role of Ulipristal and Magnetic Resonance-guided Focused Ultrasound Prior to Fertility Treatment

Dimple Jain

INTRODUCTION

Uterine leiomyomas, or fibroids, are the most common form of benign uterine tumors occurring in 20–40% women of reproductive age.[1] They are hormone sensitive, smooth muscle tumors with a wide heterogeneity in composition, size, and number.[2]

In the majority of cases, fibroids are asymptomatic; the diagnosis is incidental and needs no intervention. However, one-third of cases present with a variety of symptoms depending on their location and size, and require treatment. The most common symptom is abnormal uterine bleeding, usually excessive menstrual bleeding with subsequent anemia, which could be life-threatening. Other symptoms include pelvic pressure, bowel dysfunction, urinary frequency and urgency, urinary retention, low back pain, constipation, dyspareunia, and obstetric complications.[2]

Fibroids are also implicated in causing infertility and miscarriages. Their anatomical location, specifically submucous, and intramural fibroids seem to be the most relevant in affecting fertility. Fibroids can impair fertility through several possible mechanisms including **(Fig. 1)** including alteration of the local anatomy (anatomic distortion of the uterine cavity) with subsequent endometrial function modification; functional changes, such as increased uterine contractility and impairment of the endometrial and myometrial blood supply; and changes to the local hormone milieu which could impair gamete transport and/or reduce blastocyst implantation.[3]

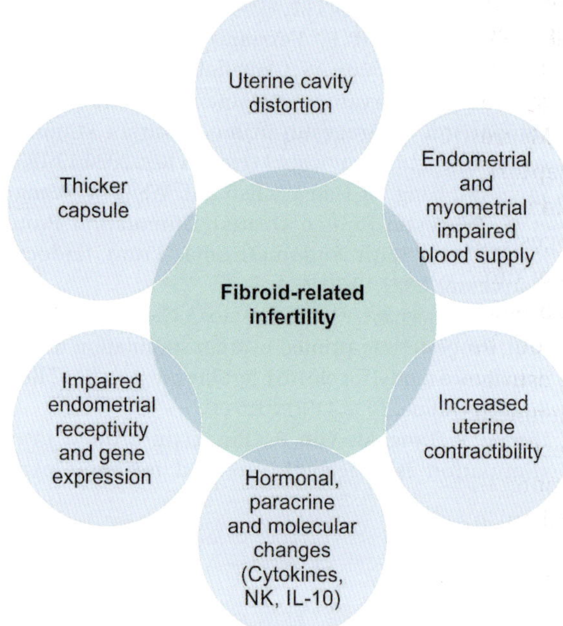

Fig. 1: Uterine fibroids and infertility.

FIBROID TREATMENT MODALITIES

Various modalities are used in the treatment of uterine fibroids. These include surgical (myomectomy, hysterectomy, hysteroscopic resection of fibroids, etc.), and nonsurgical procedures [uterine artery embolization, magnetic resonance imaging (MRI)-guided focused ultrasound, and medical therapy]. The type of treatment is guided by fibroid's characteristics (size, number, and location), patient's age, symptoms, and whether the women desire to preserve fertility or not.

Though surgery remains the mainstay of treatment—it is expensive plus associated with significant surgical morbidity. The need for alternatives to surgical option is eminently real especially for women desiring fertility. Nonsurgical conservative options have gained widespread popularity in the recent years and have been found to be safe and effective in alleviating the symptoms. Medical therapy with progestins, progestin-releasing intrauterine devices, and gonadotropin-releasing hormone agonists (GnRHa) have been used since many years. The newer treatment options including selective progesterone receptor modulators (SPRMs) [ulipristal acetate (UPA)] and magnetic resonance-guided focused ultrasound (MRgFUS) have opened more avenues for controlling the symptoms and reducing the size of fibroids. This chapter summarizes the use of UPA and MRgFUS in the treatment of fibroids and their effect on subsequent fertility in women of reproductive age.

Ulipristal Acetate and Fibroids

Various pharmacological and histological studies have suggested that progesterone and its receptors paly a cardinal role in the growth of fibroids.[4] This fact opened the avenue of using SPRMs for treatment of fibroids. SPRMs are synthetic compounds that bind to progesterone receptors and can exhibit agonistic or antagonistic actions depending on their structure and how it changes progesterone receptor conformation.[5] They are known to act directly on fibroids and exerts proapoptotic and antiproliferative actions thereby decreasing its size. It also acts on the pituitary and inhibits ovulation, suppresses the estrogen levels to midfollicular phase, and induces amenorrhea.[6] Additionally, it is known to have direct effects on the endometrium, which helps in reducing menometrorrhagia. **Flowchart 1** illustrates the different mechanism of action of SPRMs.

Ulipristal Acetate and Uterine Fibroids: Clinical Evidence

Various studies and randomized controlled trials have shown that UPA is effective in reducing the size of fibroids and controlling menorrhagia. It can be used either preoperatively in patients awaiting surgery or it can be used as a long-term management for patients who do not want surgery or have contraindications for surgery.

One of the first trials evaluating the efficacy of UPA in treating uterine fibroids was the PEARL I trial.[7] In this trial, women with symptomatic fibroids were administered UPA for 13 weeks. The trial clearly demonstrated that UPA was effective in controlling the bleeding and caused significant diminution in the size of fibroids. The PEARL II trial compared the efficacy of UPA to GnRH agonists in women with symptomatic fibroids.[8] It was observed that UPA was as effective as GnRH agonists in controlling the menstrual symptoms. The incidence of symptoms of hypoestrogenemia was significantly higher in the analog group. The PEARL III and IV trials proposed the safety and efficacy of long-term intermittent use of UPA in symptomatic women with fibroids who do not wish to undergo surgery.[6,9] It has been observed that menstruation is resumed with 4–5 weeks of discontinuation of UPA, but effects on myoma and uterine mass reduction are sustained for few months. Besides PEARL, many other studies have evaluated the efficacy of UPA therapy for fibroids. Biscione et al. showed that UPA is effective in improving different aspects of daily and sexual life (quality of life) of patients undergoing medical treatment for uterine fibroids.[10]

Fertility Outcomes After Ulipristal Acetate Treatment

Restoring fertility is one of the important goals of UPA treatment in women of reproductive age. Many case reports and retrospective studies have shown that UPA is effective in reducing the size of uterine fibroids and increases the odds of spontaneous conception.

Flowchart 1: Mechanism of action of selective progesterone receptor modulators (SPRMs).

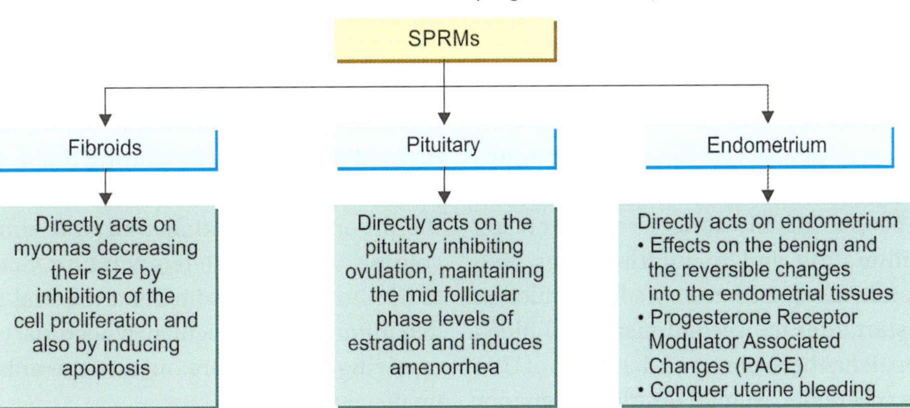

A retrospective analysis by Costa et al. reported a series of 55 pregnancies after UPA treatment in women with symptomatic fibroids.[11] The authors observed that UPA was effective in controlling the symptoms and caused a significant reduction in the size of fibroids. Approximately half of the patients became pregnant without the need for interval surgery. No malformations were reported in the newborns after UPA therapy.

A study by Morgante et al. evaluated the efficacy of UPA treatment in women with submucous fibroids before in vitro fertilization (IVF).[12] Patients with submucous fibroids received 1–3 treatment cycles of UPA depending on their response. The aim was reduction in volume of fibroid and restoration of normal uterine cavity. It was observed that UPA treatment caused significant reduction in fibroid volume (mean reduction 41%) and restores the normal cavity. The pregnancy rates of posttreatment were comparable to the control group with no fibroids. The authors concluded that UPA can restore the normal cavity in women with submucous fibroids and avoids surgery.

Orvieto et al. used UPA treatment in an advanced age women with large intramural fibroid.[13] Embryos were first cryopreserved, following which the patient underwent 12-week course of UPA and subsequent thaw embryo transfer with a successful pregnancy. Kale et al. reported a series of two cases where two women with intramural fibroids and previous IVF failure were administered UPA.[14] Both women showed significant reduction in the size of fibroid and increased distance from endometrial cavity, followed by successful pregnancy post-IVF without the need for surgery.

Ulipristal acetate has not shown to have any adverse effects on the quality of embryos.[15] Neither there have been any reports of subsequent increase in the size of fibroids during pregnancy after UPA treatment. The absence of regrowth during pregnancy, despite high levels of circulating progesterone, may be explained by apoptosis and the prolonged decrease in myoma size observed following UPA therapy.[16]

The PEARL trials demonstrated that effect of UPA on endometrium are reversible and disappear 2 months after discontinuation of treatment.[6-9] Kolanska et al. demonstrated absence of any long-term effects on endometrial proliferation and maturation after UPA therapy.[17] It is generally accepted that assisted reproduction procedures may start after the second menstrual bleed after UPA cessation. It has been observed that effect of UPA lasts for 6 months. Therefore, women desiring pregnancy should undergo assisted reproductive technology (ART) during this time frame.

Ulipristal Acetate: Safety

Though the drug is known to be well tolerated, there had been some concerns about liver toxicity associated with UPA administration. However, a cross-sectional study by Del Forno et al. demonstrated that UPA does not worsen liver function or cause severe organ injury and showed high tolerability and satisfaction profiles.[18] The review conducted by European Medicines Agency (EMA) also confirmed the safety of the drug.[19-21] Currently, the administration of UPA 5 mg a day for up to 3 months is limited to premenopausal women who are not suitable candidates for surgery or uterine fibroid embolization, or who have experienced unsuccessful surgical interventions. Vigorous monitoring of liver functions is recommended in such patients.

Ulipristal Acetate: Conclusion

Ulipristal acetate possesses all favorable characteristics that make it an ideal candidate for fibroid treatment, without the adverse effects commonly associated with reduced estrogen levels and bone density loss. However, larger prospective randomized trials are required to reinforce its efficacy and safety, especially in women desiring pregnancy and planning to undergo ART treatments.

MAGNETIC RESONANCE-GUIDED FOCUSED ULTRASOUND/MAGNETIC RESONANCE-GUIDED HIGH-INTENSITY FOCUSED ULTRASOUND

Magnetic resonance-guided focused ultrasound is a noninvasive thermoablative technique that combines the anatomic detail and thermal monitoring capabilities of MRI with the therapeutic potential of high-intensity focused ultrasound (HI-FU). MRI offers excellent three-dimensional anatomic resolution and real-time thermal monitoring, measuring tissue temperature with an accuracy of ±2°C.[22] HI-FU waves can pass through the anterior abdominal wall and aim at the targeted volume, where tissue temperature increases rapidly up to 60°C or higher, inducing a thermal lesion by protein denaturation and coagulative necrosis, while the skin and overlying tissue layers outside the ablated area remain unaffected.[23,24]

Magnetic resonance-guided focused ultrasound differs from magnetic resonance-guided high-intensity focused ultrasound (MR-HIFU), which is the newer technology. While the former involved heating tumor surface, MR-HIFU involves adequate volumetric heating of the fibroid with real-time feedback which makes it even more precise. Heating every part of the tissue that has been targeted and ablated volumetrically makes it more efficient and quicker.[25] In MR-HIFU, the tumor is divided into small sections which are subsequently subjected to ultrasound beam activity. However, it makes the procedure relatively time-consuming. Highly precise targeting of ultrasound waves on tumor tissue reduces the risk of destroying adjacent tissues.

Magnetic Resonance-guided Focused Ultrasound for Fibroids

Magnetic resonance-guided focused ultrasound has proven to be a successful noninvasive therapy for treating fibroids. The real-time MR imaging and thermal mapping have been key factors for the success of this modality. Multiple studies have demonstrated its rapid therapeutic effects and sustained symptomatic relief without any negative implications on the rate of adverse events. It is especially suitable for women not desiring surgery or for those who have contraindications for surgery.

A retrospective analysis by Jindal et al. evaluating the efficacy of focused ultrasound in 167 women with fibroids and adenomyosis observed significant reduction in fibroid volume around 68 and 75% at 6 and 12 months, respectively; and improvements in symptoms such as menorrhagia, discomfort, pressure symptoms, urine symptoms, and quality of life scores.[26] Six study participants reported successful pregnancies after the procedure. Another retrospective study by Jiang et al. compared the pregnancy outcomes of individual with fibroids following HIFU ablation and laparoscopic myomectomy.[27] The patients in the HIFU group had shorter pregnancy interval and better quality of life.

Though MRgFUS has demonstrated to be effective in treating the fibroids, there had been concerns about future fertility after the treatment. There had been concerns about the effect on ovarian reserve or damage to the endometrium leading to scarring and adhesions. A study Keserci and Duc reported that the level of anti-Müllerian hormone tested 6 months after a HIFU procedure was similar to that of the control group, implying that ovarian vessels had not been destroyed during the procedure.[28] Also, it is suggested that energy of the ultrasound beam is not sufficient to cause permanent damage to the endometrium and pregnancies have been reported after ablation of submucosal fibroids.[29]

A number of successful pregnancies have been reported after MR-HIFU treatment.[30,31] Additionally, it has been observed that unlike myomectomy there are no adhesion formation after HIFU, and there is no risk of uterine wall rupture during pregnancy and labor.[32] Łoziński et al. that showed that MR-HIFU did not increase the rate of spontaneous abortions or pregnancy complications.[25] The same authors also published a case report in which MR-HIFU treatment in a patient with a very early pregnancy was not found to be associated with any complications or adverse effects on pregnancy.[29]

Advantages of Magnetic Resonance-guided Focused Ultrasound

- Outpatient department (OPD) procedure, no hospitalization
- Low complication rate
- Utilizes nonionizing radiation
- Shorter recovery time
- Needs only conscious sedation allowing patients to communicate with the treating physician and halt treatment if needed
- Can be carried out even in anemic patients
- Can be done in patients with contraindications to surgery.

Magnetic Resonance-guided Focused Ultrasound: Safety

Magnetic resonance-guided focused ultrasound has a good safety profile. Careful supervision by the operating physician and detailed preparation of the patient are important in minimizing uncommon severe complications as bowel perforation, skin burns, and deep vein thrombosis. It can be carried out even in anemic patients and those who are at risk for surgical operation. It represents an effective and almost noninvasive approach that may be used as a fertility-preserving technique. **Box 1** enlisted the various possible side-effects or complications associated with the procedure.[33,34]

Also, it is noteworthy that not all fibroids are suitable for HIFU/MRgFUS treatment. A study by Machtinger et al. observed that hyperintense fibroids on T2-weighted

BOX 1: Side effects/complications of magnetic resonance-guided focused ultrasound (MRgFUS).

- Peri-interventional pain (usually low and of short duration) can usually be managed well with analgesia
- Skin burns
- Inflammation of subcutaneous fat tissue and of the abdominal muscles
- Paresthesia of the legs due to irritation of, or damage to, the nerves
- Deep vein thrombosis of the legs (very rare)
- Intestinal lesions or intestinal perforation (extremely rare)
- Discharge of vaginal tissue
- Increased and/or irregular bleeding for around 3 months postprocedure

MRI had lower long-term success rate after ablation.[35] Similarly, septate, subserous, or strongly dorsal fibroids close to sacral nerve have been observed to have poor success rates following MRgFUS.

CONCLUSION

Managing uterine fibroids, especially in the context of fertility treatment, entails a multimodal strategy designed to maximize results while maintaining the ability to procreate. Particularly for women receiving IVF treatments, the use of SPRMs, such as UPA, has demonstrated encouraging benefits in lowering fibroid size and alleviating symptoms. This could improve reproductive outcomes. Furthermore, women desiring fertility preservation may find MRgFUS to be an appealing alternative due to its noninvasive nature, low risk of complications, and quick recovery.

The available literature suggests that MRgFUS and UPA therapy have favorable pregnancy outcomes, giving hope to women who are infertile because of uterine fibroids. However, to completely understand the long-term effects, safety profiles, and ideal patient selection criteria for these therapy modalities, more research, and investigations are necessary. Personalized care that takes into account the unique traits and preferences of each patient is crucial to getting the best results while maintaining fertility.

REFERENCES

1. Donnez J, Jadoul P. What are the implications of myomas on fertility? A need for a debate? Hum Reprod. 2002;17:1424-30.
2. Stewart EA. Uterine Fibroids. Lancet. 2001;357:293-8.
3. Somigliana E, Vercellini P, Daguati R, Pasin R, De Giorgi O, Crosignani PG. Fibroids and female reproduction: a critical analysis of the evidence. Hum Reprod Update. 2007;13(5):465-76.
4. Tamaya T, Fujimoto J, Okada H. Comparison of cellular levels of steroid receptors in uterine leiomyoma and myometrium. Acta Obstet Gynecol Scand. 1985;64(4):307-9.
5. Safrai M, Chill HH, Reuveni Salzman A, Shushan A. Selective Progesterone Receptor Modulators for the Treatment of Uterine Leiomyomas. Obstet Gynecol. 2017;130(2):315-8.
6. Donnez J, Donnez O, Matule D, Ahrendt HJ, Hudecek R, Zatik J, et al. Long-term medical management of uterine fibroids with ulipristal acetate. Fertil Steril. 2016;105(1):165-73.e4.
7. Donnez J, Tomaszewski J, Vázquez F, Bouchard P, Lemieszczuk B, Baró F, et al. Ulipristal acetate versus leuprolide acetate for uterine fibroids. N Engl J Med. 2012;366(5):421-32.
8. Donnez J, Tatarchuk TF, Bouchard P, Puscasiu L, Zakharenko NF, Ivanova T, et al. Ulipristal acetate versus placebo for fibroid treatment before surgery. N Engl J Med. 2012;366(5):409-20.
9. Donnez J, Vázquez F, Tomaszewski J, Nouri K, Bouchard P, Fauser BC, et al. Long-term treatment of uterine fibroids with ulipristal acetate. Fertil Steril. 2014;101(6):1565-73.e1-18.
10. Biscione A, Barra V, Bellone E, Severi FMLS. Ulipristal acetate on quality of life and sexual function of women with uterine fibromatosis. Gynecol Endocrinol. 2020;36:87-92.
11. Costa AR, Carvalho AP, Martins DR, Carvalho MJ, Silva PT, Roque SC, et al. Series of 55 pregnancies following Ulipristal acetate treatment of symptomatic uterine fibroids. J Endometr Pelvic Pain Disord. 2020;12:12(3-4):170-5.
12. Morgante G, Centini G, Troìa L, Orvieto R, De Leo V. Ulipristal acetate before in vitro fertilization: efficacy in infertile women with submucous fibroids. Reprod Biol Endocrinol. 2020;18(1):50.
13. Orvieto R, Zilberberg E, Vanni VS, Botchan A. A novel approach to infertility treatment of advance-age patient with prominent intramural fibroid. Gynecol Endocrinol. 2018;34:551-3.
14. Kale AR. Comparison between Mifepristone and Ulipristal Acetate as an Alternative to Surgical Management of Uterine Fibroids (Leiomyoma) in Symptomatic Patients of Reproductive Age Group in Asian Population. Int J Reprod Contracept Obstet Gynecol. 2018;7:109-13.
15. Wdowiak A. Pre-treatment with Ulipristal acetate before ICSI procedure: a case report. Menopausal Review/Przegląd Menopauzalny. 2013;12(6):496-500.
16. De Gasperis-Brigante C, Singh SS, Vilos G, Kives S, Murji A. Pregnancy outcomes following ulipristal acetate for uterine fibroids: a systematic review. J Obstet Gynaecol Can. 2018;40:1066-76.

17. Kolanska K, Sbeih M, Canlorbe G, Mekinian A, Varinot J, Capmas P, et al. Ulipristal Acetate Modifies miRNA Expression in Both Superficial and Basal Layers of the Human Endometrium. J Clin Med. 2021;10(19):4442.
18. Del Forno S, Degli Esposti E, Salucci P, Leonardi D, Iodice R, Arena A, et al. Liver function, tolerability and satisfaction during treatment with ulipristal acetate in women with fibroids: a single center experience. Gynecol Endocrinol. 2020;36(5):445-7.
19. Branch S. Esmya (ulipristal acetate) for uterine fibroids: monitor liver function in current and recent users; do not initiate treatment in new users or those between treatment courses. Geneva: World Health Organization; 2015.
20. Raine J. Esmya (ulipristal acetate) for symptoms of uterine fibroids: restrictions to use and requirement to check liver function before, during and after treatment. Geneva: World Health Organization; 2015.
21. European Medicines Agency. (2018). Esmya: new measures to minimise risk of rare but serious liver injury.
22. Napoli A, Anzidei M, Ciolina F, Marotta E, Cavallo Marincola B, Brachetti G, et al. MR-guided high-intensity focused ultrasound: current status of an emerging technology. Cardiovasc Intervent Radiol. 2013;36(5):1190-203.
23. Jenne JW, Preusser T, Günther M. High-intensity focused ultrasound: principles, therapy guidance, simulations and applications. Z Med Phys. 2012;22(4):311-22.
24. Xie B, Zhang C, Xiong C, He J, Huang G, Zhang L. High intensity focused ultrasound ablation for submucosal fibroids: A comparison between type I and type II. Int J Hyperthermia. 2015;31(6):593-9.
25. Łoziński T, Filipowska J, Gurynowicz G, Zgliczyńska M, Kluz T, Jędra R, et al. The effect of high-intensity focused ultrasound guided by magnetic resonance therapy on obstetrical outcomes in patients with uterine fibroids—experiences from the main Polish center and a review of current data. Int J Hyperthermia. 2019;36(1):582-90.
26. Jindal S, Jung J, Lee K, Chern B. High-intensity focused ultrasound for the treatment of fibroids: A single-center experience in Singapore. Gynecol Minim Invasive Ther. 2023;12:15-25.
27. Jiang Z, Li Q, Li W, Zhu X, Jiang J, Chen L, et al. A comparative analysis of pregnancy outcomes of patients with uterine fibroids after high intensity focused ultrasound ablation and laparoscopic myomectomy: a retrospective study. Int J Hyperthermia. 2021;38(1):79-84.
28. Keserci B, Duc NM. Magnetic Resonance Imaging Parameters in Predicting the Treatment Outcome of High-intensity Focused Ultrasound Ablation of Uterine Fibroids With an Immediate Nonperfused Volume Ratio of at Least 90. Acad Radiol. 2018;25(10):1257-69.
29. Łoziński T, Filipowska J, Ludwin A, Ciebiera M. The outcome of magnetic resonance-guided high-intensity ultrasound for clinically symptomatic submucosal uterine fibroid performed accidentally in very early pregnancy: a case report. Int J Hyperthermia. 2019;36(1):975-9.
30. Rabinovici J, David M, Fukunishi H, Morita Y, Gostout BS, Stewart EA, et al. Pregnancy outcome after magnetic resonance-guided focused ultrasound surgery (MRgFUS) for conservative treatment of uterine fibroids. Fertil Steril. 2010;93(1):199-209.
31. Zou M, Chen L, Wu C, Hu C, Xiong Y. Pregnancy outcomes in patients with uterine fibroids treated with ultrasound-guided high-intensity focused ultrasound. BJOG. 2017;124 Suppl 3:30-5.
32. Liu X, Xue L, Wang Y, Wang W, Tang J. Vaginal delivery outcomes of pregnancies following ultrasound-guided high-intensity focused ultrasound ablation treatment for uterine fibroids. Int J Hyperthermia. 2018;35(1):510-7.
33. Chen J, Chen W, Zhang L, Li K, Peng S, He M, et al. Safety of ultrasound-guided ultrasound ablation for uterine fibroids and adenomyosis: A review of 9988 cases. Ultrason Sonochem. 2015;27:671-6.
34. Stanford Health Care. Risks of the MRgFUS procedure. 2019. Available from: https://stanfordhealthcare.org/medicaltreatments/m/mr-guided-focused-ultrasound/complications.html
35. Machtinger R, Inbar Y, Cohen-Eylon S, Admon D, Alagem-Mizrachi A, Rabinovici J. MR-guided focus ultrasound (MRgFUS) for symptomatic uterine fibroids: predictors of treatment success. Hum Reprod. 2012;27(12):3425-31.

Chapter

Do all Uterine Septa Need Resection?

Sanket Pisat, Monica Uppal

INTRODUCTION

Embryonic development: The paramesonephric ducts, also called the Müllerian ducts, are critical in the development of the female reproductive system. The paramesonephric ducts give rise to fallopian tubes, uterus, cervix, and the upper two-thirds of vagina. The developing Müllerian ducts fuse laterally that creates a midline septum in the uterine cavity, which undergoes complete bidirectional resorption by week 20 of intrauterine life. Vertical fusion of the fused ducts occurs with the sinovaginal bulb and the lower one-third part of the vagina forms from the canalization of this sinovaginal bulb.[1]

Uterine anomalies: Congenital uterine anomalies (CUA) occur due to disturbances at one or more stages of normal development. The most widely accepted classifications include the American Society for Reproductive Medicine (ASRM), European Society of Human Reproduction and Embryology (ESHRE) and Congenital Uterine Malformation by Experts (CUME).

The CONgenital UTerine Anomalies (CONUTA) classification classifies uterine anomalies as:[2]

- *U0:* Normal uterus
- *U1:* Dysmorphic uterus
- *U2:* Septate uterus
- *U3:* Bicorporeal uterus
- *U4:* Hemiuterus
- *U5:* Aplastic
- *U6:* Unclassified **(Fig. 1)**

Septate uterus: Septate uterus identification is based on 3D ultrasonography (USG) criteria provided by different systems.

ESHRE (CONUTA classification): External contour is normal plus internal indentation below the interostial line exceeds 50% of the myometrial thickness above the interostial line.[3]

ASRM 2021: Internal fundal indentation depth >1 cm with acute angle of indentation (<90°); and subseptate uterus is classified as <1 cm and >90°[3] **(Fig. 2)**.

CUME suggests internal indentation of >1 cm as septate uterus, as it is simplified and most reliable.[4]

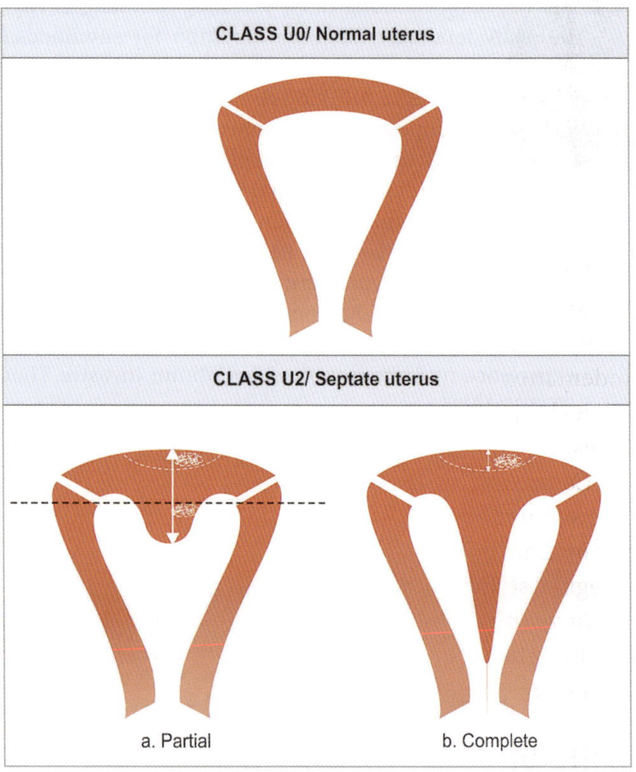

Fig. 1: CONgenital UTerine Anomalies (CONUTA) classification of septate uterus.

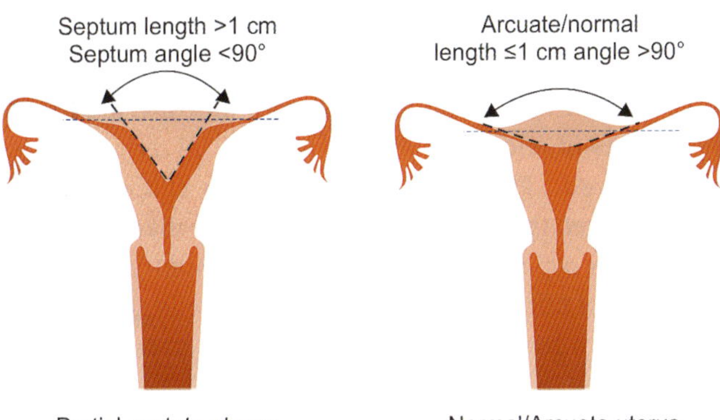

Fig. 2: American Society for Reproductive Medicine (ASRM) classification of septate uterus.

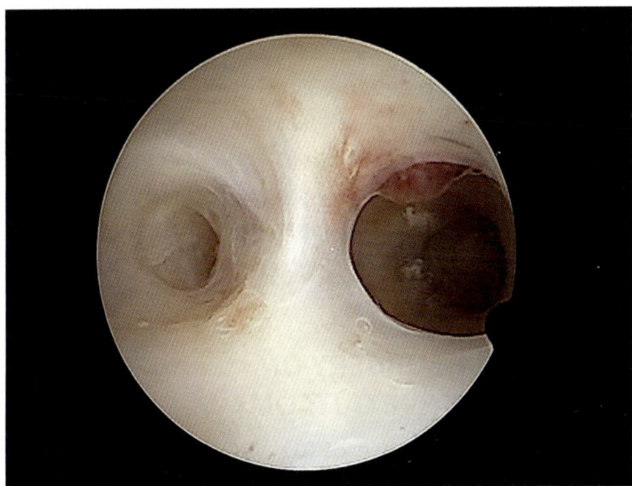

Fig. 3: Complete septate uterus.

If the arrest in resorption occurs early in development, the septum creates a significant division of endometrial cavity versus a halt late in development, where only a mild indentation, like an arcuate uterus may be seen and not clinically significant, and hence septa are of the following types:

Complete septate uterus has a single uterine fundus. The septum extends from the top of the uterine cavity to the internal or external cervical os. This may be seen with a vaginal septum **(Fig. 3)**.

Incomplete/partial septate uterus refers to a single fundus and cervix with septum extending into the cavity but not up to the external os **(Fig. 4)**.

INCIDENCE

Due to the varied defining criteria of uterine anomalies and different modalities of diagnosis, the true incidence of it in the general population remains uncertain. However, a systematic review showed the incidence of uterine anomalies to be 5.5% in the general population, 8% in infertile women, and 13.3% in women with bad obstetric history.[5] Septate uterus accounts for the most common uterine anomaly with a mean incidence of 35% of all uterine anomalies.[6]

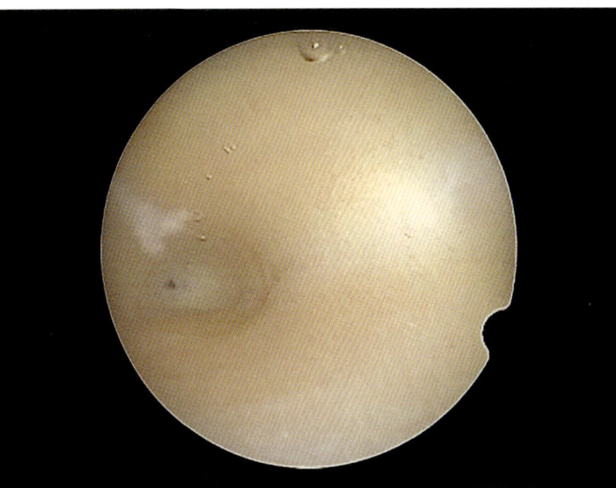

Fig. 4: Partial septate uterus.

DIAGNOSIS

Most cases are diagnosed during the evaluation of subfertility. Various modalities can be used to diagnose the condition.

Hysterosalpingography

Hysterosalpingography is the most commonly used diagnostic modality in the workup of infertility. This shows the internal contour of the endometrial cavity, cervical canal, and fallopian tubes with comment on patency of the tubes. A septate uterus may be seen as a midline indentation of the uterine cavity with the two halves of the cavity not falling very far apart unlike a bircornuate uterus. However, this differentiation needs other diagnostic modalities revealing the external contour of the uterus such as magnetic resonance imaging (MRI) and 3D USG.

Two-dimensional Ultrasonography

Two-dimensional USG is a frequently used diagnostic modality and usually the first technique in the approach to CUA. It shows the presence of two separate endometrial cavities at the fundus and the diagnostic accuracy is about 93.38%.[7]

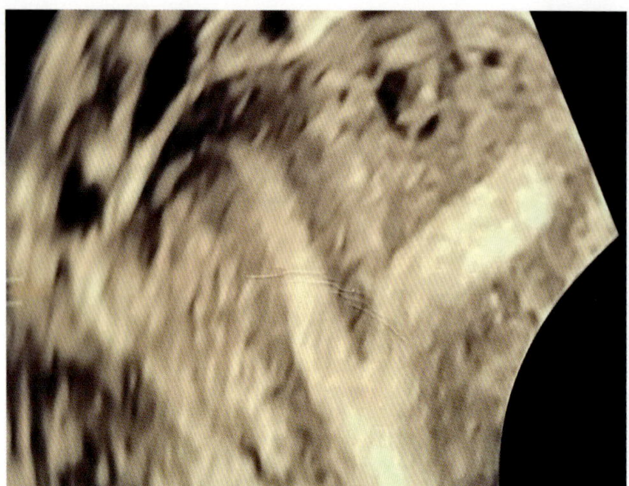

Fig. 5: 3D ultrasonography (USG) of septate uterus with no serosal indentation.

Three-dimensional Ultrasonography

Three-dimensional USG modality enables visualization of the coronal plane, allowing an accurate diagnosis of septate uterus. The uterine fundus appears normal externally, with an internal indentation of endometrium and myometrium. 3D USG has high sensitivity and specificity for diagnosis of septate uterus **(Fig. 5)**.

Magnetic Resonance Imaging

Magnetic resonance imaging provides a better characterization of the uterus but is not frequently employed in the diagnosis of septate uterus. Unlike other major congenital anomalies such as duplication disorders (uterus didelphys), septate uterus is not associated with renal anomalies. Duplication disorders are most often found with skeletal and renal abnormalities and need an MRI for planning further management and surgical assistance.

Hysteroscopy

The direct visualization of endometrial cavity along with preoperative USG or simultaneous laparoscopy forms the gold standard in the diagnosis of CUA.[6] It also offers the advantage to treat the condition in the same procedure after informing the patient.

IMPACT OF SEPTUM ON FERTILITY

The septum varies in its characteristics in terms of width and length. Most often septum is found associated with recurrent pregnancy loss due to an implantation failure. A systematic review on the pathophysiology of septum investigated the histology of septum and revealed that it consists of endometrial and myometrial tissue and is vascularized.[8] This was in contrast to the cohort studies that analyzed the septum hysteroscopically that described septum as a pale, scarcely bleeding structure that was made up of fibrous tissue The glandular cells and stroma in a septum have different morphological characteristics than the rest of the cavity.[9]

- The number of glandular cells and cilia are lower.
- There is incomplete ciliogenesis of the ciliated cells.
- The septum also contains lower levels of the vascular endothelial growth factor (VEGF) receptor that plays an important role in embryo implantation and placentation.
- Two studies revealed the gene expression of HOXA10 genes to be altered in the septate uterus. These genes are important in early implantation of embryos.

Hence septate uterus may result in early pregnancy failure. The septum is a fibromuscular structure and the composition varies with its width and also guides the surgical management.

IMPACT OF SURGERY ON REPRODUCTIVE OUTCOME

With the increasing use of 3D USG, which makes the assessment of uterine morphology more reproducible, the detection of CUA has been increasing. The counseling and management of women diagnosed with uterine septum pose challenges for the following reasons:

- Various definitions and differing criterion of diagnosis
- Several different diagnostic modalities in use with lack of absolute consensus
- Contrasting literature on the benefit of surgery.

While literature on the current practice of management of uterine septum is varying, numerous retrospective and prospective studies have shown a better outcome with operative intervention versus expectant management in women with primary unexplained infertility. Studies found live birth rate (LBR) ranging from 30% to 55%, well above the 17% rate assumed with expectant management in this population.[10] A prospective cohort study involving 127 women having primary infertility with uterine septum had a LBR of 35.3% in the group that underwent septum removal compared with 8% in a matched group of women with expectant management.[11]

A matched controlled study of 2,481 embryo transfers (ET) showed uterine septum to be an independent risk factor for reduced pregnancy rate after IVF.[12] Studies also suggest the role of septum surgery in patients with endometriosis. Even a subtle obstruction of antegrade menstruation predisposes to endometriosis with a very high prevalence rate in current practice.[13] Uterine septum also increases risk of obstetric complications. Meta-analysis of 25 studies found increased risk of preterm delivery, malpresentation, growth restriction, placental abruption, and prenatal mortality in women with uterine septum.[14]

A Cochrane Review in 2017 studied the advantage of hysteroscopic removal of uterine septum in women of reproductive age group and also studied the safety of the procedure. It concluded that even though the surgery is widely performed to improve reproductive outcome in women with infertility, recurrent pregnancy loss and obstetric complications, the literature is inconclusive in the absolute benefit of it.[15]

Multicenter The Randomized Uterine Septum Trial (TRUST) was conducted and randomized women to hysteroscopic management and expectant management. In terms of LBR as outcome, the results were contrary to what was previously believed. This was 35% in the expectant group versus 31% in the surgical group. Other reproductive outcomes such as pregnancy loss and preterm birth were also comparable in the two groups.[16] In the authors' opinion, surgery for septate uterus in correctly selected cases with a prior history of infertility or RPL significantly improves her chances of conception and reduces early pregnancy losses.

SURGERY

Decision of Surgery

Septal resection/septal incision surgery can be rewarding in terms of benefit in improvement of infertility and recurrent pregnancy loss. However, a judicious approach is required for appropriate case selection to ascertain which patients will benefit and those where surgery is unnecessary.

The CONUTA and the ASRM classifications now provide objective assessment criteria for diagnosis of septate uterus. In order to consider surgery, the patient must first fall within the defined criteria mentioned at the beginning of this chapter. Smaller septa may be considered as arcuate uteri, and these patients will not benefit by surgery. In fact, it must be remembered that the normal fundus is arcuate, not flat, and hence any excessive correction entails the risk of perforation or adhesion formation.

Among those patients who do fit into the diagnostic criteria, the authors are of the opinion that an overall clinical picture must be considered before taking a decision to operate, rather than just a preset checklist. In general, patients who are young, newly married, have not had an adequate trial of fertility treatment, and for whom other factors of infertility or recurrent pregnancy loss have not been ruled out are not ideal for septal surgery. On the other hand, patients who are above 30–35 years of age, have been trying for conception for a year or more, for whom other factors have been assessed and ruled out may benefit by septal surgery. Patients with previously failed IVF cycles would also fall into this category.

It must be remembered, and conveyed to the patient, that the mere presence of a septate uterus is not an all-or-none phenomenon to determine its detrimental effect on fertility outcome.

Traditionally, the approach to septal metroplasty was abdominal, which paved the way for modern hysteroscopic procedures. Previously, the surgery for uterine septum was performed only in women with bad obstetric history and via laparotomy and hysterotomy. They included the Jones type, involving transfundal uterine incision, excision of the septum along with a part of the fundal myometrium, and then subsequent repair. The other method was the Bret–Tomkins metroplasty, which involved division of the uterus in the anteroposterior plane and then the division of septum transversely without excision of myometrium. These procedures, even though had good reproductive outcome, exposed the patient to formation of postoperative adhesions, prolonged recovery, and longer wait to conception. It also required a mandatory cesarean section in subsequent pregnancy.

Septal Incision with Hysteroscopic Scissors

Hysteroscopy has been a game changer for patients with septate uterus. Using a hysteroscope and microscissors (3 FR or 5 FR), the septum can be divided under vision in a very short time. This can also be performed as an office procedure, without the need for anesthesia and admission to the hospital.

The incision is carried out from the most dependent part of the septum toward the fundal area. Small cuts are made to divide the septum, until the entire ridge separating the

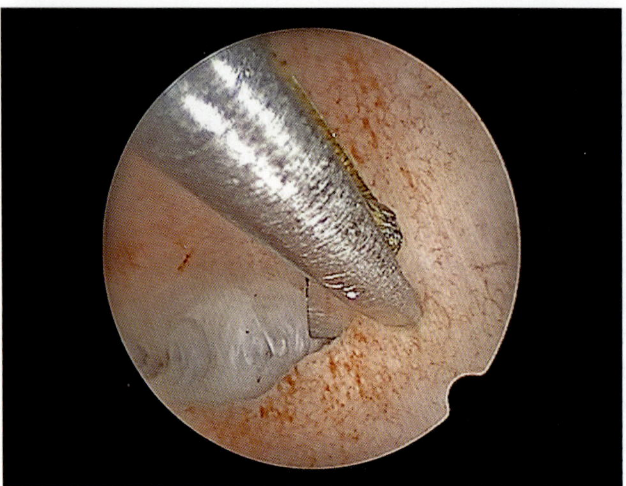

Fig. 6: Septal incision using hysteroscopic scissors.

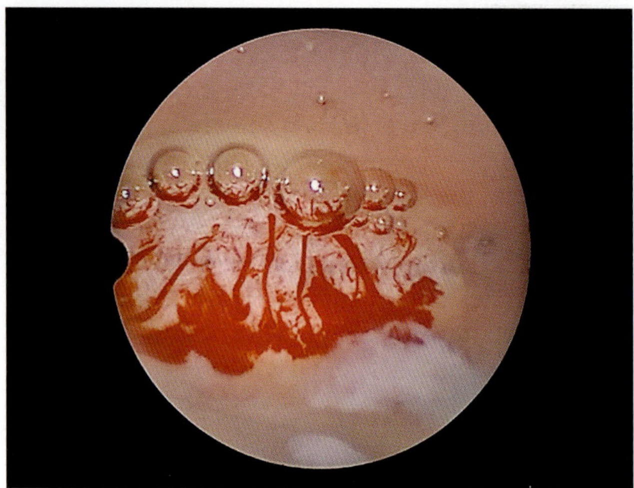

Fig. 8: Vascular septal bed after septal incision.

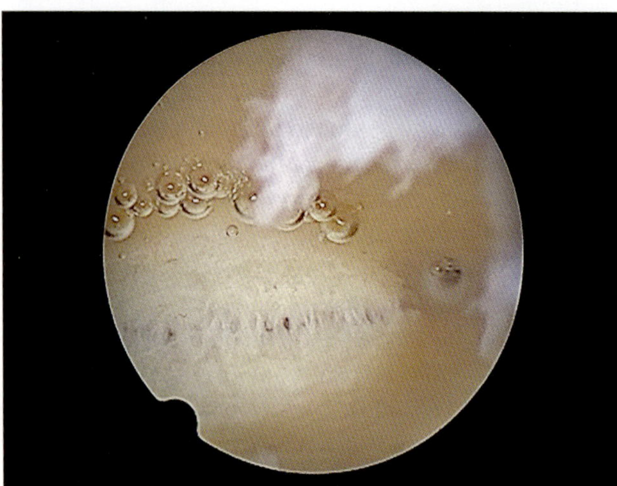

Fig. 7: Complete septal incision.

two ostia is seen to be cut **(Fig. 6)**. The end point of surgery is being able to appreciate both ostia at the same level over the fundus, with a minimal fundal indentation between the two **(Fig. 7)**. It must again be emphasized that a slight indentation between the two ostia is considered normal, not pathological. The other marker is the appearance of fine blood vessels at the base of the septum, indicating that the fibrous zone has been cut, and the well-vascularized muscular zone is now exposed **(Fig. 8)**. Endometrium is now likely to cover this part with a good possibility of implantation of embryo in the future.

Hysteroscopic scissors are usually considered the instrument of choice for this procedure, as there is zero collateral damage to the surrounding endometrium and the possibility of an accidental perforation is less.

SEPTAL INCISION WITH HYSTEROSCOPIC COLLIN'S KNIFE ELECTRODE

Patients with larger septa usually have the lower (inferior) part of the septum as a fibrous band, and the upper (superior) part is vascularized and muscular.

In these septa, there is a possibility of excessive bleeding while performing septal incision with scissors. Some surgeons prefer to operate these cases using a Collin's knife electrode, where current is used to divide the septum and simultaneously ensure hemostasis **(Fig. 9)**. Nowadays, bipolar energy has almost completely replaced the traditional monopolar energy in view of enhanced patient safety and the reduced possibility of fluid overload due to *glycine* overdose.

Septal Incision versus Excision

An ongoing debate exists among surgeons about which procedure is superior: Hysteroscopic septal incision (only dividing the septum in the midline) versus septal resection (en bloc removal of a piece of the septum). Fascilla et al.[9] have reported better outcome with the latter; however, not enough literature exists to change from the traditional incision to the new concept of en bloc excision of septum. Authors in favor of septal incision argue that the septum is, indeed, an embryonic part of the uterus itself and must be left within the uterus rather than subjected to excision.

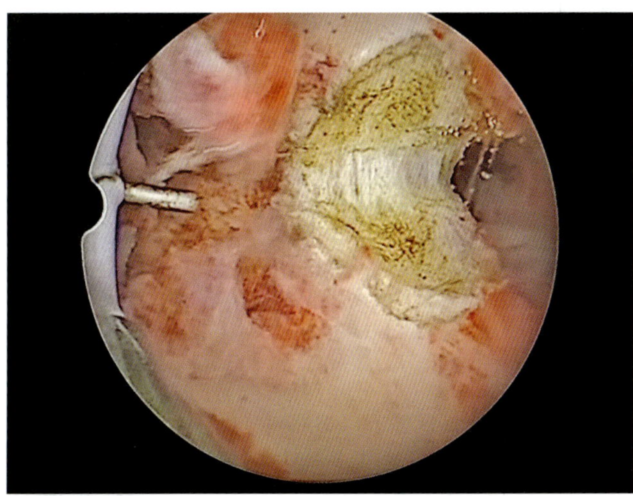

Fig. 9: Incision of large septum using resectoscope.

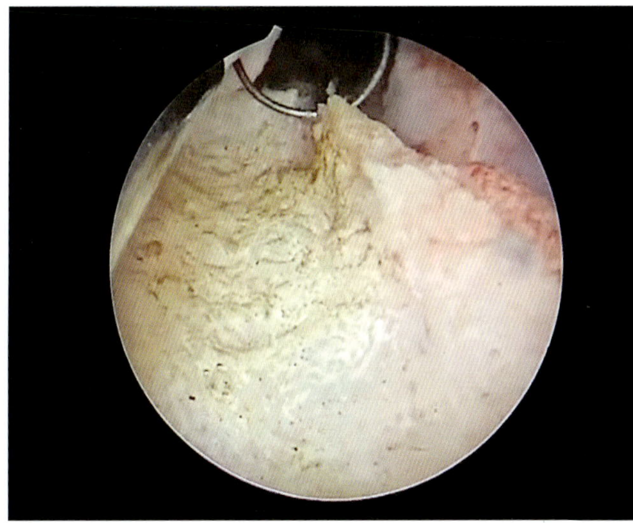

Fig. 10: Resection of residual septal tissue after incision.

In the authors' opinion, most septa will automatically get resorbed into the respective uterine walls immediately after they have been divided. This is so evident intra-operatively that there is hardly any tissue left to perform resection. In these patients, attempting a resection may be both futile and counterproductive.

On the other hand, there are some larger septa in which one finds that after the septum has been divided, there still remain obvious ridges of the septum that are projecting beyond the anterior and posterior endometrial linings **(Fig. 10)**. These ridges may act as fibrous foreign bodies and it is these patients who will probably do better with septal resection than incision.

CONCLUSION

Uterine anomalies, like septate uterus, result from deviations in the process from embryological development from paramesonephric ducts, impacting fertility and obstetric outcomes. The presence and impact of uterine septum on reproductive outcomes remain a complex and multifaceted issue. Varied diagnostic criteria and modalities contribute to challenges in identifying and classifying these anomalies accurately. The incidence of uterine anomalies remains conclusively uncertain, but septate uterus stands out as the most common, affecting approximately 35% of cases. While septate uterus has been implicated in a myriad of reproductive challenges ranging from infertility to recurrent pregnancy loss, the decision to intervene surgically should be judicious and individualized. The efficacy and absolute benefits of surgical intervention continue to be debated, with contrasting studies offering varying results. Furthermore, the evolution from traditional abdominal approaches to modern hysteroscopic procedures has heralded a new era of minimally invasive management, reducing the associated risks and postoperative recovery time. Nevertheless, it remains paramount for clinicians to engage in comprehensive counseling, ensuring patients are informed of the potential benefits, risks, and uncertainties surrounding septum resection. Despite challenges in diagnosis and classification, hysteroscopic removal of the septum emerges as a valuable intervention to enhance fertility outcomes and minimize obstetric complications in women with septate uterus.

REFERENCES

1. Wilson D, Bordoni B. Embryology, mullerian ducts (paramesonephric ducts). In: StatPearls. Treasure Island (FL): StatPearls Publishing; 2024.
2. Grimbizis GF, Gordts S, Di Spiezio Sardo A, Brucker S, De Angelis C, Gergolet M, et al. The ESHRE/ESGE consensus on the classification of female genital tract congenital anomalies. Hum Reprod. 2013;28(8):2032-44.
3. Pfeifer SM, Attaran M, Goldstein J, Lindheim SR, Petrozza JC, Rackow BW, et al. ASRM müllerian anomalies classification 2021. Fertil Steril. 2021;116(5):1238-52.
4. Ludwin A, Martins WP, Nastri CO, Ludwin I, Coelho Neto MA, et al. Congenital Uterine Malformation by Experts (CUME): better criteria for distinguishing between normal/ arcuate and septate uterus? Ultrasound Obstet Gynecol. 2018;51(1):101-9.
5. Chan YY, Jayaprakasan K, Zamora J, Thornton JG, Raine-Fenning N, Coomarasamy A. The prevalence of congenital

uterine anomalies in unselected and high-risk populations: a systematic review. Hum Reprod Update. 2011;17(6): 761-71.

6. Homer HA, Li TC, Cooke ID. The septate uterus: a review of management and reproductive outcome. Fertil Steril. 2000; 73(1):1-4.
7. Alcázar JL, Carriles I, Cajas MB, Costa S, Fabra S, Cabrero M, et al. Diagnostic Performance of Two-Dimensional Ultrasound, Two-Dimensional Sonohysterography and Three-Dimensional Ultrasound in the Diagnosis of Septate Uterus—A Systematic Review and Meta-Analysis. Diagnostics (Basel). 2023;13(4):807.
8. Rikken JF, Leeuwis-Fedorovich NE, Letteboer S, Emanuel MH, Limpens J, van der Veen F, et al. The pathophysiology of the septate uterus: a systematic review. BJOG. 2019;126(10): 1192-9.
9. Fascilla FD, Resta L, Cannone R, De Palma D, Ceci OR, Loizzi V, et al. Resectoscopic metroplasty with uterine septum excision: a histologic analysis of the uterine septum. J Minim Invasive Gynecol. 2020;27(6):1287-94.
10. Wang R, Danhof NA, Tjon-Kon-Fat RI, Eijkemans MJ, Bossuyt PM, Mochtar MH, et al. Interventions for unexplained infertility: a systematic review and network meta-analysis. Cochrane Database Syst Rev. 2019;9(9):CD012692.
11. Tonguc EA, Var T, Batioglu S. Hysteroscopic metroplasty in patients with a uterine septum and otherwise unexplained infertility. Int J Gynaecol Obstet. 2011;113(2):128-30.
12. Tomaževič T, Ban-Frangež H, Virant-Klun I, Verdenik I, Požlep B, Vrtačnik-Bokal E. Septate, subseptate and arcuate uterus decrease pregnancy and live birth rates in IVF/ICSI. Reprod Biomed Online. 2010;21(5):700-5.
13. Piriyev E, Römer T. Coincidence of uterine malformations and endometriosis: a clinically relevant problem? Arch Gynecol Obstet. 2020;302:1237-41.
14. Venetis CA, Papadopoulos SP, Campo R, Gordts S, Tarlatzis BC, Grimbizis GF. Clinical implications of congenital uterine anomalies: a meta-analysis of comparative studies. Reprod Biomed Online. 2014;29(6):665-83.
15. Rikken JF, Kowalik CR, Emanuel MH, Mol BW, Van der Veen F, van Wely M, et al. Septum resection for women of reproductive age with a septate uterus. Cochrane Database Syst Rev. 2017;1(1):CD008576.
16. Rikken JF, Kowalik CR, Emanuel MH, Bongers MY, Spinder T, Jansen FW, et al. Septum resection versus expectant management in women with a septate uterus: an international multicentre open-label randomized controlled trial. Hum Reprod. 2021;36(5):1260-7.

SECTION

Dilemmas and Debates in Assisted Reproduction

Should Fresh Embryo Transfer be Eliminated Completely: Pros and Cons of Freeze-all

Pinky R Shah, Charumati V Pekhale

INTRODUCTION

In vitro fertilization (IVF) is being practised for >40 years now. Controlled ovarian stimulation (COS) to recruit multiple follicles is the crux of IVF cycle to improve the IVF outcome.[1] Conventional IVF practice with fresh embryo transfer (ET) was followed for many years. However, possible role of supraphysiological sex steroids in IVF treatment in reduction of endometrial receptivity and IVF success rates have been studied and reported.[2] The advent of vitrification, a nonequilibrium method of cryopreservation, which avoids ice crystal formation, allowed the embryologists to freeze-all embryos at various stages. The high post-thaw survival rates and higher pregnancy rates observed in frozen embryo transfer (FET) cycles due to its more physiological environment for embryos led to emergence of freeze-all policy at many IVF centers worldwide.[3] With freeze-all policy, entire cohort of embryos can be frozen and transferred at a later date when the endometrial environment is optimal.[4] It is postulated that the IVF success depends on embryo quality, embryo-endometrium talk, and endometrial receptivity[5] and freeze-all policy assures improved, physiological-endometrial environment for high implantation and pregnancy rates. Whether freeze-all policy can be adopted universally for all patients needs further research. This chapter will discuss about pros and cons of freeze-all policy and should fresh ET be eliminated completely, or it can be reserved for selected cases without having compromised pregnancy results.

PROS OF FREEZE-ALL POLICY AND FROZEN EMBRYO TRANSFER

Prevention of Ovarian Hyperstimulation Syndrome

Ovarian hyperstimulation syndrome (OHSS) is a severe iatrogenic complication that can occur during ovarian stimulation in 1–14% of IVF-ART (assisted reproductive techniques) cycles[6] and poses a significant risk to the patient. To mitigate the risk of OHSS, one approach is to electively cryopreserve all embryos and transfer them in nonstimulated cycles. This strategy avoids the increase in endogenous human chorionic gonadotropin (hCG) levels associated with fresh transfer cycles, effectively preventing the development of OHSS. Preventing OHSS is crucial and constitutes a key aspect of its management. In recent years along with many strategies to reduce OHSS risk, the most effective is avoiding hCG trigger and giving gonadotropin-releasing hormone (GnRH) agonist trigger for final oocyte maturation combining it with freeze-all policy has significantly minimized the risk of OHSS.[7,8]

Improved Endometrial Receptivity with Freeze-all Policy

Evidence suggests that the elevated levels of estradiol (E2) and progesterone during COS can cause biochemical and morphological changes that may impair endometrial receptivity. Consequently, these changes can lead to a lack of synchrony between the embryo and the endometrium, resulting in reduced implantation rates during IVF and intracytoplasmic sperm injection (ICSI) treatments.[2,9,10] Higher levels of E2 due to multifolliculogenesis have been associated with alterations in endometrial maturation and implantation, with negative impact on gene expression and endometrial angiogenesis.[11] During the final follicular phase, subtle increases in progesterone levels are associated with advancements in the ultrastructural morphology and echogenicity of the endometrium.[12,13] These increased progesterone levels appear to have a negative impact on embryo implantation.[14,15] In comparison, frozen-thawed cycles, which involve the precise control of endometrial development and priming, show better endometrial receptivity than COS cycles with gonadotropins.[16] This observation suggests that adopting a freeze-all policy may favor patients by enhancing endometrial receptivity.

Controlled Ovarian Stimulation and Uterine Contractility

It is well-established that uterine contractions (UC) occurring during ET can have a negative impact on the outcomes of IVF treatments.[16] Moreover, supraphysiologic levels of hormones observed during COS can further increase the occurrence of UC.[17] Studies have indicated that uterine contractility is significantly higher in stimulated cycles compared to natural cycles.[18] It is plausible to suggest that during FET, when hormonal levels are lower, UC may be reduced compared to fresh embryo transfer (ET). This could be attributed to the fact that high levels of circulating E2 in IVF patients have been associated with increased UC.[19] Notably, the impact of UC appears to be more pronounced during cleavage-stage ET, as contractility gradually decreases and reaches a nearly quiescent state by the time of blastocyst transfer.[20]

Increased Time for Preimplantation Genetic Testing

Advancements in IVF techniques like preimplantation genetic testing (PGT) for aneuploidy (PGT-A) have significantly improved the overall pregnancy rates by enabling the selective transfer of euploid blastocysts.[21] To facilitate this process, the freeze-all strategy has been employed, which involves cryopreserving all embryos after biopsy and conducting PGT on the entire cohort of embryos. This strategy allows sufficient time for the PGT-A results to reach the clinician, and subsequently, the transfer of a euploid embryo can be scheduled in a subsequent cycle.

Uterine Pathology

There are various uterine pathologies that can be diagnosed during ovarian stimulation, which have been associated with decreased fertility rates.

Polyps

Studies suggest that polyps can have a negative impact on fertility by affecting endometrial receptivity.[22] In case the polyp is detected during ovarian stimulation, the embryos can be cryopreserved. Such cases can undergo polyp removal followed by frozen–thaw ET at a later date.

Adenomyosis

Adenomyosis may have a negative influence on the outcomes of assisted reproductive technology.[23] The most commonly used approach for managing adenomyosis in this context is the administration of depot GnRH agonist (GnRHa) for a duration of 3–6 months, either alone or in combination with cytoreductive surgery. It has been suggested that using vitrified embryos and transferring them after treatment with a GnRHa may increase pregnancy rates.[24]

Hydrosalpinx

Patients with hydrosalpinx experience impaired pregnancy outcomes when undergoing IVF treatment. In such cases, freezing the embryos and undergoing salpingectomy before ET has been shown to improve the chances of achieving a successful birth after IVF treatment.[25]

Nonconventional Start of Ovarian Stimulation

New strategies for ovarian stimulation, including random-start protocols, dual stimulation has emerged in the field of ART. Random-start ovarian stimulation is currently being used in cancer patients to minimize delays between ovarian stimulation and cancer therapies, with no significant differences in the number of retrieved oocytes as compared to the conventional stimulation.[26] Dual stimulation involves continuing ovarian stimulation after the first oocyte retrieval, allowing for two stimulations to be performed within the same cycle.[27,28] Dual stimulation can be beneficial in cases of poor ovarian reserve. In cases of "nonconventional start" stimulation, where there is asynchrony between endometrial receptivity and embryo development, all oocytes/embryos need to be cryopreserved and transferred at a later time. This approach has become possible due to advancements in embryo and oocyte vitrification techniques, enabling total disarticulation of the ovarian stimulation and the ET.

Increased Flexibility in Cycle Timing

One of the advantages of FET is the ability to store embryos for an extended period, which provides increased flexibility in determining the timing of the ET. This flexibility allows optimal scheduling based on the preferences and personal circumstances of the patient, as well as the availability of the fertility clinic. Also, in FET cycles, IVF practitioners have flexibility in oocyte retrieval and need less stringent monitoring of IVF cycle.

Obstetric Complications

It is postulated that frozen-thaw transfer cycles being nonstimulated cycles are more conducive to early embryogenesis and placentation in comparison to fresh ET cycles and thus associated with lesser risk of some antepartum complications.

Systematic review of 11 observational studies compared obstetric and perinatal outcomes in singleton pregnancies in fresh verses FET. The review found much lower relative risk of antepartum hemorrhage, small for gestation age, low birth weight, and perinatal mortality in FET cycles. Thus, FETs were associated with better obstetric and perinatal outcome.[29]

CONS OF FREEZE-ALL POLICY AND FROZEN EMBRYO TRANSFER

Increased Costs

One drawback of FET is the additional costs (approximately 30% higher) associated with the freezing, storage, and thawing processes. Cryopreservation requires specialized equipment, skilled personnel, and the maintenance of liquid nitrogen (LN2) storage tanks. Patients may also require additional medications and monitoring during the frozen cycle, which can contribute to the overall expenses of IVF treatment.

Psychological Impact

The emotional and psychological aspects of fertility treatment are significant considerations. The waiting period between embryo freezing and transfer in FET cycles can be emotionally challenging for individuals and couples. The uncertainty and anticipation during this waiting period may lead to increased levels of anxiety, depression, and stress. The prolonged treatment timeline associated with FET can also impact patients' overall well-being and quality of life.

Prolonged Treatment Timelines

One of the drawbacks of FET is the extended treatment timeline compared to fresh transfers. Following the freezing of embryos, patients need to undergo an additional cycle for endometrial preparation before the actual ET can take place.

Uncertainty Regarding Embryo Viability

There are certain uncertainties regarding embryo viability associated with the cryopreservation procedure itself. Cryodamage, toxicity of cryoprotectants, potential equipment failure or LN2 supply failure, packaging breach, and contamination in storage are some of the negative effects that can occur during the cryopreservation process.[30] Various factors such as embryo quality at freezing, post-thaw conditions, and the procedure of cryopreservation itself can affect the result of cryopreservation. These variables can impact the survival rates of the embryos affecting the implantation rates.[31,32] The time to pregnancy also poses increase in the risk of epigenetic changes in the embryo.

Large for Gestational Age and High Birth Weight

Certain studies and meta-analyses have indicated that there is a higher incidence of large for gestational age (LGA) and high birth weight in babies born after FET.[33-35] These studies do not support implantation of universal freeze-all policy.

SHOULD FRESH EMBRYO TRANSFER BE ELIMINATED COMPLETELY? FREEZE-ALL FOR ALL?

Freeze-all policy has shown to have many advantages such as reduction in OHSS rate, better endometrial receptivity, and better implantation and pregnancy rates due to filtering out borderline embryos with lower implantation potential post freezing-thawing physical effects.[36] Blockeel et al., looked upon the SWOT (strengths, weaknesses, opportunities, and threats) analysis of a freeze-all strategy. They concluded that more well-designed clinical trials are needed before shifting to freeze-all for all from current IVF practice.[37] Roque et al. suggested in view of freeze-all not being suited for all patients, more detailed evaluation of pros and cons is needed of cost, risks, and potential benefits.[38,39] Studies have been carried out in normal- or high-responder patients,[40] while extrapolation of same outcome cannot be done for poor responders' patients.

E-Freeze, a multicentric randomized trial in the United Kingdom (UK) conducted over 18 clinics from

2016 to 2019 on 619 couples, compared elective freezing of embryos verses fresh ET in IVF. There was no evidence of a statistically significant difference in outcomes in the elective freeze group compared to the fresh ET group: Healthy baby rate, OHSS, live birth rate, and miscarriage rates. They found poor adherence of patients in elective freeze-all group and also elective freeze was not likely to be cost-effective in the UK NHS (National Health Service). The E-Freeze trial concluded that elective freeze-all should only be adopted if there is a definite clinical indication and not for everyone considering cost, efficacy, and safety into account.[41]

The Cochrane Review in 2021 concluded that freeze-all policy is associated with lower risk of OHSS (for an OHSS rate of 3% following the conventional strategy, the rate following the "freeze-all" strategy would be 1%) but was associated with higher risk of hypertensive disorders of pregnancy and LGA baby. Time to pregnancy is likely to be shorter in fresh ET cycles. There was moderate quality of evidence in terms of cumulative live births rates and ongoing pregnancy rates, one strategy being superior to another.[42]

Concerns regarding the children born after FET: The available research on the long-term effects of children born after FET is still relatively limited, and further studies are necessary to comprehensively assess various health aspects and outcomes. Genomic integrity of embryos can be influenced by cryopreservation technique due to increased reactive oxygen species, exposure to low temperature and cryoprotectants, intracellular crystallization and the incorporation of the calcium-zinc DNA-protamine complex. Thus, studies on long-term outcome of children born with frozen-thaw ET are needed.[43] While there is a considerable body of research on the safety and health of children conceived through fresh ET, the specific effects of FET on long-term health parameters require more investigation.

CONCLUSION

Elective freeze-all poses many advantages. In view of lack of evidence of its role for all patients, it should be reserved for patients with risk of OHSS, high serum progesterone on day of trigger, suspected uterine pathology in IVF stimulated cycles, those undergoing PGT, and in patients with random-start protocols. Elective freeze-all is associated with increase in cost, waiting time, and potential increase in epigenetic risks, and increase in hypertensive disorders and LGA babies. Thus, with available evidence, elective freeze-all policy for all is not justified. More multicentric trials are needed before introducing elective freeze-all policy for all.

REFERENCES

1. Siristatidis C, Sergentanis TN, Kanavidis P, Trivella M, Sotiraki M, Mavromatis I, et al. Controlled ovarian hyperstimulation for IVF: impact on ovarian, endometrial and cervical cancer—a systematic review and meta-analysis. Hum Reprod Update. 2013;19:105-23.
2. Devroey P, Bourgain C, Macklon NS, Fauser BC. Reproductive biology and IVF: ovarian stimulation and endometrial receptivity. Trends Endocrinol Metab. 2004; 15:84-90.
3. Serdarogullari M, Coban O, Boynukalin FK, Bilgin EM, Findikli N, Bahceci M. Successful application of a single warming protocol for embryos cryopreserved by either slow freezing or vitrification techniques. Syst Biol Reprod Med. 2019;65:12-19.
4. Saupstad M, Freiesleben NLC, Skouby SO, Andersen LF, Knudsen UB, Petersen KB, et al. Preparation of the endometrium and timing of blastocyst transfer in modified natural cycle frozen-thawed embryo transfers (mNC-FET): a study protocol for a randomised controlled multicentre trial. BMJ Open. 2019;9:e031811.
5. Roque M, Lattes K, Serra S, Solà I, Geber S, Carreras R, et al. Fresh embryo transfer versus frozen embryo transfer in in vitro fertilization cycles: a systematic review and meta-analysis. Fertil Steril. 2013;99:156-62.
6. de Mouzon J, Goossens V, Bhattacharya S, Castilla JA, Ferraretti AP, Korsak V, et al.; European IVF-Monitoring (EIM); Consortium for the European Society on Human Reproduction and Embryology (ESHRE). Assisted reproductive technology in Europe, 2007: results generated from European registers by ESHRE. Hum Reprod. 2012; 27:954-66.
7. Devroey P, Polyzos NP, Blockeel C. An OHSS-Free Clinic by segmentation of IVF treatment. Hum Reprod. 2011; 26:2593-7.
8. Kol S, Humaidan P. GnRH agonist triggering: recent developments. Reprod Biomed Online. 2013;26:226-30.
9. Bourgain C, Devroey P. The endometrium in stimulated cycles for IVF. Hum Reprod Update. 2003;9:515-22.
10. Kolibianakis E, Bourgain C, Albano C, Osmanagaoglu K, Smitz J, Van Steirteghem A, et al. Effect of ovarian stimulation with recombinant follicle-stimulating hormone, gonadotropin releasing hormone antagonists, and human chorionic gonadotropin on endometrial maturation on the day of oocyte pick-up. Fertil Steril. 2002;78:1025-9.
11. Groothuis PG, Dassen HH, Romano A, Punyadeera C. Estrogen and the endometrium: lessons learned from gene expression profiling in rodents and human. Hum Reprod Update. 2007;13:405-17.

12. Nikas G, Develioglu OH, Toner JP, Jones HW Jr. Endometrial pinopodes indicate a shift in the window of receptivity in IVF cycles. Hum Reprod. 1999;14:787-92.
13. Venetis CA, Kolibianakis EM, Papanikolaou E, Bontis J, Devroey P, Tarlatzis BC. Is progesterone elevation on the day of human chorionic gonadotrophin administration associated with the probability of pregnancy in in vitro fertilization? A systematic review and meta-analysis. Hum Reprod Update. 2007;13:343-55.
14. Kiliçdag EB, Haydardedeoglu B, Cok T, Hacivelioglu SO, Bagis T. Premature progesterone elevation impairs implantation and live birth rates in GnRH-agonist IVF/ICSI cycles. Arch Gynecol Obstet. 2010;281:747-52.
15. Huang R, Fang C, Xu S, Yi Y, Liang X. Premature progesterone rise negatively correlated with birth rate in IVF cycles with GnRH agonist: an analysis of 2,566 cycles. Fertil Steril. 2012;98:664-70.e2.
16. Richter KS, Shipley SK, McVearry I, Tucker MJ, Widra EA. Cryopreserved embryo transfers suggest that endometrial receptivity may contribute to reduced success rates of later developing embryos. Fertil Steril. 2006;86:862-6.
17. Fanchin R, Righini C, Olivennes F, Taylor S, de Ziegler D, Frydman R. Uterine contractions at the time of embryo transfer alter pregnancy rates after in-vitro fertilization. Hum Reprod. 1998;13:1968-74.
18. Fanchin R, Ayoubi JM, Olivennes F, Righini C, de Ziegler D, Frydman R. Hormonal influence on the uterine contractility during ovarian stimulation. Hum Reprod. 2000;15 (Suppl 1):90-100.
19. Zhu L, Li Y, Xu A. Influence of controlled ovarian hyperstimulation on uterine peristalsis in infertile women. Hum Reprod. 2012;27:2684-9.
20. Moraloglu O, Tonguc E, Var T, Zeyrek T, Batioglu S. Treatment with oxytocin antagonists before embryo transfer may increase implantation rates after IVF. Reprod Biomed Online. 2010;21:338-43.
21. Lee E, Illingworth P, Wilton L, Chambers GM. The clinical effectiveness of preimplantation genetic diagnosis for aneuploidy in all 24 chromosomes (PGD-A): systematic review. Hum Reprod. 2015;30:473-83.
22. Galliano D, Bellver J, Díaz-García C, Simón C, Pellicer A. ART and uterine pathology: how relevant is the maternal side for implantation? Hum Reprod Update. 2015;21: 13-38.
23. Vercellini P, Consonni D, Dridi D, Bracco B, Frattaruolo MP, Somigliana E. Uterine adenomyosis and in vitro fertilization outcome: a systematic review and meta-analysis. Hum Reprod. 2014;29:964-77.
24. Park CW, Choi MH, Yang KM, Song IO. Pregnancy rate in women with adenomyosis undergoing fresh or frozen embryo transfer cycles following gonadotropin-releasing hormone agonist treatment. Clin Exp Reprod Med. 2016; 43:169-73.
25. Strandell A, Lindhard A, Waldenström U, Thorburn J. Hydrosalpinx and IVF outcome: cumulative results after salpingectomy in a randomized controlled trial. Hum Reprod. 2001;16:2403-10.
26. Ubaldi FM, Capalbo A, Vaiarelli A, Cimadomo D, Colamaria S, Alviggi C, et al. Follicular versus luteal phase ovarian stimulation during the same menstrual cycle (DuoStim) in a reduced ovarian reserve population results in a similar euploid blastocyst formation rate: new insight in ovarian reserve exploitation. Fertil Steril. 2016;105:1488-95.e1.
27. Cakmak H, Katz A, Cedars MI, Rosen MP. Effective method for emergency fertility preservation: random-start controlled ovarian stimulation. Fertil Steril. 2013;100: 1673-80.
28. Cardoso MCA, Evangelista A, Sartório C, Vaz G, Werneck CLV, Guimarães FM, et al. Can ovarian double-stimulation in the same menstrual cycle improve IVF outcomes? JBRA Assist Reprod. 2017;21:217-21.
29. Maheshwari A, Pandey S, Shetty A, Hamilton M, Bhattacharya S. Obstetric and perinatal outcomes in singleton pregnancies resulting from the transfer of frozen thawed versus fresh embryos generated through in vitro fertilization treatment: A systematic review and meta-analysis. Fertil Steril. 2012;98(2):368-77.e1-9.
30. Bhattacharya S. Maternal and perinatal outcomes after fresh versus frozen embryo transfer-what is the risk-benefit ratio? Fertil Steril. 2016;106(2):241-3.
31. Wong KM, Mastenbroek S, Repping S. Cryopreservation of human embryos and its contribution to in vitro fertilization success rates. Fertil Steril. 2014;102(1):19-26.
32. Yin H, Jiang H, He R, Wang C, Zhu J, Li Y. The effects of blastocyst morphological score and blastocoele re-expansion speed after warming on pregnancy outcomes. Clin Exp Reprod Med. 2016;43(1):31-7.
33. Pinborg A, Henningsen AA, Loft A, Malchau SS, Forman J, Andersen AN. Large baby syndrome in singletons born after frozen embryo transfer (FET): is it due to maternal factors or the cryotechnique? Hum Reprod. 2014;29:618-27.
34. Sazonova A, Källen K, Thurin-Kjellberg A, Wennerholm UB, Bergh C. Obstetric outcome in singletons after in vitro fertilization with cryopreserved/thawed embryos. Hum Reprod. 2012;27:1343-50.
35. Maheshwari A, Raja EA, Bhattacharya S. Obstetric and perinatal outcomes after either fresh or thawed frozen embryo transfer: an analysis of 112,432 singleton pregnancies recorded in the Human Fertilisation and Embryology Authority anonymized dataset. Fertil Steril. 2016;106:1703-8.
36. Shih W, Rushford DD, Bourne H, Garrett C, McBain JC, Healy DL, et al. Factors affecting low birthweight after assisted reproduction technology: Difference between transfer of fresh and cryopreserved embryos suggests an adverse effect of oocyte collection. Hum Reprod. 2008; 23(7):1644-53.

37. Blockeel C, Drakopoulos P, Santos-Ribeiro S, Polyzos NP, Tournaye H. A fresh look at the freeze-all protocol: A SWOT analysis. Hum Reprod. 2016;31(3):491-7.
38. Roque M, Valle M, Kostolias A, Sampaio M, Geber S. Freeze-all cycle in reproductive medicine: Current perspectives. JBRA Assist Reprod. 2017;21(1):49-53.
39. Roque M, Valle M, Guimarães F, Sampaio M, Geber S. Freeze-all policy: Fresh vs. frozen-thawed embryo transfer. Fertil Steril. 2015;103(5):1190-3.
40. Chen ZJ, Shi Y, Sun Y, Zhang B, Liang X, Cao Y, et al. Fresh versus frozen embryos for infertility in the polycystic ovary syndrome. N Engl J Med. 2016;375(6):523-33.
41. Maheshwari A, Bell JL, Bhide P, Brison D, Child T, Chong HY, et al. Elective freezing of embryos versus fresh embryo transfer in IVF: a multicentre randomized controlled trial in the UK (E-Freeze). Hum Reprod. 2022;37(3):476-87.
42. Zaat T, Zagers M, Mol F, Goddijn M, van Wely M, Mastenbroek S. Fresh versus frozen embryo transfers in assisted reproduction. Cochrane Database Syst Rev. 2021;2:CD011184.
43. Kopeika J, Thornhill A, Khalaf Y. The effect of cryopreservation on the genome of gametes and embryos: Principles of cryobiology and critical appraisal of the evidence. Hum Reprod Update. 2015;21(2):209-27.

Chapter

Varicocele: To Ligate or not to Ligate?

Vikash Kumar

INTRODUCTION

Varicocele is defined as an abnormal dilatation and tortuosity of veins in the pampiniform plexus. Among the correctable causes of male infertility, it is the most common pathology.[1] Usual incidence of varicoceles is around 15–20% of all males. It is more common in infertile males, found in about 40% of infertile males. Varicocele is prevalent in 80% of secondary infertility patients.[2,3] Association of varicocele and male infertility is still debatable, but there are ample studies now to correlate it. A study conducted by the World Health Organization (WHO) reported the prevalence of varicocele in infertility patients with normal and abnormal semen parameters as 11.7% and 25.4%, respectively.[4]

Varicocele repair is widely used in the management of male-factor infertility, however, the effectiveness of varicocelectomy has been a matter of debate, and there is still no consensus. In fact, it has been seen as the most common correctable cause in male-factor infertility. Controversy over the role of varicocele surgery in the management of infertility is primarily due to two reasons: Mainly, lack of defined etiological mechanisms of varicocele affecting spermatogenesis and absence of well-designed trial showing benefit of surgery. With the latest development of surgical techniques in correction of varicocele (especially microscopic varicocelectomy) and better understanding of the pathophysiology affecting sperm functions and parameters, its role has been evaluated in various studies.

There is expanding evidence that varicocele is detrimental to male fertility. Varicocele is known to cause impaired semen parameters and it is more common in infertile males where semen parameters improve after varicocelectomy. Due to advances in assisted reproductive technique, the role of varicocelectomy is reduced significantly. The major advantage of varicocelectomy is that it offers onetime cure for patients seeking to further multiple pregnancies. Also, the risks of treatment are small.

PATHOPHYSIOLOGY OF VARICOCELE AND ITS EFFECTS

Testicular dysfunction due to varicocele is mainly attributed to venous reflux and testicular temperature elevation. In the recent past, research into pathophysiology of varicoceles has focused on the following factors namely oxidative stress-related damage [reactive oxygen species (ROS) level], tissue hypoxia, and hormonal imbalances. Oxidative stress may lead to damage to sperm membrane and DNA.[5-7]

Reactive Oxygen Species

The ROS amount was found higher in the semen samples of men with varicoceles, irrespective of their fertility status by Weese et al.[5] Mostafa et al. observed that surgical treatment of varicocele improves ROS.[6]

Tissue Hypoxia

In patients with varicocele, there is significantly higher level of hypoxia-inducible factor-1 (HIF-1), one of the principal regulators to hypoxia as found by Lee et al.[7]

Hormonal Imbalances

Varicoceles may alter hormonal milieu that can have damaging effects on spermatogenesis. The level of testosterone is lower in affected individuals established in various studies. Reduction in testosterone production is due to adverse effect on the Leydig cells in the testes. Varicocelectomy leads to improvement in the serum testosterone level, with the mean increase between 100 and 140 ng/mL following varicocelectomy, and it shows positive impact in >80% of patients. Hypogonadal (testosterone <300 ng/mL) men were benefited the most in form of increase in testosterone level after varicocelectomy.

Hence persons with high-grade varicoceles might eventually have testicular failure, leading to lower hormonal production, oligospermia, and testicular atrophy. Sperm nuclear DNA integrity is also affected and reduced due to varicocele, which has been linked to reduced sperm motility, counts, viability, and abnormal morphology.[8,9]

WHICH SEMEN PARAMETERS ARE AFFECTED USUALLY?

Clinically detected varicocele was found to be a significant risk factor for decreased sperm count, motility, and morphology in adult infertile men.[10] All improve after surgery as per latest literature. Isolated sperm defect is not due to varicocele.

EVALUATION

Clinical examination is still the most important evaluation tool, and it can be confirmed with color Doppler. On contrary, Doppler-proven clinically insignificant varicoceles do not require treatment. Dubin and Amelar[11] devised a useful clinical grading system for palpable varicoceles. Grade 1 varicoceles are defined as those palpable only during a Valsalva maneuver. Grade 2 varicoceles are palpable even without the Valsalva maneuver. Grade 3 varicoceles are visible on visual inspection only.

SURGERY FOR VARICOCELE

Several treatments are available for varicocele. Two basic approaches to the management of varicocele have been percutaneous embolization and surgery. Surgical ligation is showing better results and in that also microscopic varicocelectomy is treatment of choice among surgical options.

Current evidence indicates that microsurgical varicocelectomy is the most effective technique with higher success rate and lowest complication rate among the varicocelectomy techniques. There is still debate in the literature regarding the outcomes of various techniques: A meta-analysis by Cayan et al. suggested that surgical intervention is better than embolization regarding spontaneous pregnancy rates (41.97% for microsurgical vs. 33.2% for embolization, p value = 0.001) and recurrence rates (1.07% for microsurgery vs. 12.70% from embolization, p value = 0.001).[12]

Different options for the management of couples with male-factor infertility associated with a varicocele are varicocele repair, intrauterine insemination (IUI), and in vitro fertilization/intracytoplasmic sperm injection (IVF/ICSI). Various important factors are taken into consideration to decide the method of management. Among the various treatment modalities available, varicocele repair has the advantage of reversing the pathological condition leading to permanent cure for infertility, as opposed to other modality (IUI/IVF) required for each attempt to achieve pregnancy. Other factors to be considered in the management of infertility include the age of female partner and unknown long-term health effects of IVF and ICSI on the offspring resulting from these techniques. Varicocelectomy is a more cost-effective treatment modality compared to IVF/ICSI.[13] Ultimately not treating a varicocele may result in progressive decline in semen parameters, hence further aggravating the infertility issue in a couple.[14]

RECOMMENDATIONS AND GUIDELINES

Although controversy exists, most experts in male reproductive medicine agree that correction of clinically significant varicocele in infertile men can enhance male fertility status leading to improved testicular function, testosterone production, enhanced semen profile, sperm chromatin integrity, and pregnancy rates through natural intercourse or reproductive outcome through assisted reproductive technique. Several well-designed meta-analysis in the recent past have shown positive outcome on semen parameters and pregnancy after varicocelectomy.

Among different studies, one study worth discussion is by Cayan et al. It was a prospective study on 540 infertile males with clinically palpable varicocele. All patients underwent microsurgical varicocelectomy and were followed up for more than 1 and 2 years on the two outcomes, postoperative semen quality and conception, respectively. 50% increase in total motile sperm count was considered as positive response and was observed in 271 patients (50%). Spontaneous pregnancy rate was 36.6% and was achieved with mean time to conception of 7 months (range 1–19). Among the males requiring IVF and ICSI, 31% required only IUI or had spontaneous pregnancy. Among IUI candidates 42% gained the potential for spontaneous pregnancy.[15] Hence after analyzing this study, it was stated that varicocelectomy has significant potential to reduce indication of assisted reproductive technology and also to downstage or shift the level of assisted reproductive technology needed in cases of male-factor infertility.

The American Urological Association (AUA) and American Society of Reproductive Medicine (ASRM) guideline recommend varicocele surgery for infertile man with clinically palpable varicocele and at least one or two abnormal semen parameters with the female partner having either normal or potential treatable fertility[16] as per guidelines for the best practice policy committee in 2001. European Urological Association (EAU) guidelines in 2014 indicated that varicocele repair should be considered in cases of clinical varicocele, oligospermia, infertility duration >2 years, and otherwise unexplained infertility in a couple.[17]

Some studies and meta-analyses had shown limited benefits on fertility in patients treated for varicocele,[18,19] but recent scientific evidence had shown that varicocele treatment improves semen parameters and pregnancy rates, when an appropriate selection of patients is made.[20,21] In the study published on global survey involving 574 experts from 59 countries showed wide difference in opinion regarding varicocele management and nonuniform adherence to guidelines.[20] Latest AUA and EAU guidelines recommend treating varicocele in selected set of patients with specific indications.[16,22]

SPECIAL SITUATIONS OF VARICOCELE WITH INFERTILITY

Bilateral Varicocele and Infertility

For this condition of bilateral varicocele, both sides should be repaired simultaneously. Even in situation with clinically significant left varicocele but only a subclinical right varicocele, it has been observed that repairing both sides may ultimately be beneficial in achieving a pregnancy.

Role of Varicocelectomy in Azoospermia

Should azoospermia patients with varicocele be operated? In patients of nonobstructive azoospermia (NOA), varicocele surgery will show benefit if testis size is normal and it is a clinically grade 3 varicocele. Medical history, genetic testing, and hormonal examinations are needed to differentiate between obstructive azoospermia (OA) and NOA. As per latest meta-analysis, an increase in sperm retrieval rate was observed in men with NOA who underwent varicocelectomy versus who did not undergo surgery [odds ratio (OR): 2.65; 95% confidence interval (CI) 1.69–4.14; 5 < 0.0001].[23] 19 NOA patients who underwent testicular biopsy and varicocelectomy were assessed in a study.[24] 15 were unilateral and 4 bilateral. Semen analysis was done after 3 months. Hypospermatogenesis in 3 patients, maturation arrest in 6, and germ cell aplasia in 10 were observed. After mean follow-up of 7.4 months, motile sperms were identified in 7 (36.4%) of NOA patients. Out of 7, 2 had hypospermatogenesis, 4 had maturation arrest, and 1 had Sertoli cell-only syndrome. One patient had natural pregnancy (5.3%) with hypospertmatogenesis.[24]

Subclinical Varicocele and Infertility

Varicocele surgery for subclinical varicoceles is not recommended as per current guidelines, and varicocele surgery for grade 1 varicoceles has to be selected after proper discussion in view of the lower likelihood of significant benefit.[20]

IMPORTANT PRACTICE GUIDELINES

- Do not rush into varicocele surgery.
- Diagnose the varicocele but offer the choice of medical therapy especially in young couples with short trying time.
- Consider varicocele ligation if adequate trial therapy does not lead to pregnancy.
- Do not operate a varicocele if count is excellent and motility alone is very poor.
- Do not operate if count and motility is good and only isolated teratozoospermia.

CONCLUSION

Varicoceles are relatively common in the adult male population in general and the infertile male population in particular. Infertile male with palpable varicocele and at least one abnormal semen parameter seeking to establish fertility should undergo surgical varicocelectomy. Among the various modes of therapy, microsurgical ligation is the gold standard and should be the procedure of choice. Varicoceles among the different causes of male infertility are correctable pathology and give an opportunity to easily improve sperm count and function, which should not be overlooked if present.

REFERENCES

1. Su JS, Farber NJ, Vij SC. Pathophysiology and treatment options of varicocele: an overview. Andrologia. 2021;53: e13576.
2. Alsaikhan B, Alrabeeah K, Delouya G, Zini A. Epidemiology of varicocele. Asian J Androl. 2016;18:179-81.
3. Jarow JP, Coburn M, Sigman M. Incidence of varicoceles in men with primary and secondary infertility. Urology. 1996; 47:73-6.
4. The influence of varicocele on parameters of fertility in a large group of men presenting to infertility clinics. World Health Organization. Fertil Steril. 1992;57:1289-93.
5. Weese DL, Peaster ML, Himsl KK, Leach GE, Lad PM, Zimmern PE. Stimulated reactive oxygen species generation in the spermatozoa of infertile men. J Urol. 1993; 149:64-7.
6. Mostafa T, Anis TH, El-Nashar A, Imam H, Othman IA. Varicocelectomy reduces reactive oxygen species levels and increases antioxidant activity of seminal plasma from infertile men with varicocele. Int J Androl. 2001;24:261-5.
7. Lee JD, Jeng SY, Lee TH. Increased expression of hypoxia-inducible-factor-1α in the internal spermatic vein of patients with varicocele. J Urol. 2006;175:1045-8.
8. Franco G, Misuraca L, Ciletti M, Leonardo C, De Nunzio C, Palminteri E, et al. Surgery of male infertility: an update. Urologia. 2014;81:154-64.
9. Agarwal A, Cannarella R, Saleh R, Boitrelle F, Gül M, Toprak T, et al. Impact of Varicocele Repair on Semen Parameters in Infertile Men: A Systematic Review and Meta-Analysis. World J Mens Health. 2023;41:289-310.
10. Agarwal A, Sharma R, Harlev A, Esteves SC. Effect of varicocele on semen characteristics according to the new 2010 World Health Organization criteria: a systematic review and meta-analysis. Asian J Androl. 2016;18(2):163-70.
11. Dubin L, Amelar RD. Varicocele size and results of varicocelectomy in selected subfertile men with varicocele. Fertil Steril. 1970;21:606-9.
12. Cayan S, Shavakhabov S, Kadioğlu A. Treatment of Palpable Varicocele in Infertile Men: A Meta-Analysis to Define the Best Technique. J Androl. 2009;30:33-40.
13. Sclegal PN. Is assisted reproduction the optimal treatment for varicocele-associated infertility? A cost-effective analysis. Urology. 1997;49:83-90.
14. Chehval MJ, Purcell MH. Deterioration of semen parameters over time in men with untreated varicocele: evidence of progressive testicular damage. Fertil Steril. 1992;57:174-7.
15. Cayan S, Erdemir F, Ozbey I, Turek PJ, Kadioğlu A, Tellaloğlu S. Can varicocelectomy significantly change the way couples use assisted reproductive technologies? J Urol. 2002;167(4):1749-52.
16. Practice Committee of the American Society for Reproductive Medicine. Report on Varicocele and Infertility. Fertil Steril. 2008;90:S247-9.
17. Jungwirth A, Diemer T, Dohle GR, Giwercman A, Kopa Z, Tournaye H, et al. Guidelines on male infertility: European Association of Urology guidelines. Arnhem: European Association of Urology; 2015.
18. Evers JLH, Collins JA. Assessment of Efficacy of Varicocele Repair for Male Subfertility: A Systematic Review. Lancet. 2003;361:1849-52.
19. Abdel-Meguid TA, Al-Sayyad A, Tayib A, Farsi HM. Does Varicocele Repair Improve Male Infertility? An Evidence-Based Perspective from a Randomized, Controlled Trial. Eur Urol. 2011;59:455-61.
20. Shah R, Agarwal A, Kavoussi P, Rambhatla A, Saleh R, Cannarella R, et al. Consensus and Diversity in the Management of Varicocele for Male Infertility: Results of a Global Practice Survey and Comparison with Guidelines and Recommendations. World J Mens Health. 2023; 41(1):164-97.
21. Çayan S, Şahin S, Akbay E. Paternity Rates and Time to Conception in Adolescents with Varicocele Undergoing Microsurgical Varicocele Repair vs Observation Only: A Single Institution Experience with 408 Patients. J Urol. 2017;198:195-201.
22. Minhas S, Bettocchi C, Boeri L, Capogrosso P, Carvalho J, Cilesiz NC, et al; EAU Working Group on Male Sexual and Reproductive Health. European Association of Urology Guidelines on Male Sexual and Reproductive Health: 2021 Update on Male Infertility. Eur Urol. 2021;80:603-20.
23. Berookhim BM, Schlegel PN. Azoospermia due to spermatogenic failure. Urol Clin North Am. 2014;41:97-113.
24. Lee JS, Park HJ, Seo JT. What is the indication of varicocelectomy in men with nonobstructive azoospermia? Urology. 2007;69:352-5.

How Many Embryos to Transfer: Is There a Consensus?

Anand Nanavati, Kriti Sharma

INTRODUCTION

In vitro fertilization (IVF) has proven to be a boon for many infertile couples in the past few decades. On one hand where it has given hopes to many, it has also introduced many risks. One of the major complications in IVF since its inception has been multiple gestation and its associated perinatal and maternal complications. Controlled ovarian stimulation is the integral part of all IVF programs, which often results in multiple good-grade embryos available for transfer. It is a common practice in almost all clinics to transfer more than one embryo in a cycle to enhance the success rates. However, this practice of transferring more than one embryo also results in higher incidences of iatrogenic twins and high-order multiple gestations, which cause significant maternal and perinatal morbidity. While strict transfer policies have eliminated the risk of high-order multiples, the incidence of twin pregnancy is still unchanged. Selective fetal reduction is often being used to reduce these multiple gestations, but the procedure is invasive and is associated with its own cons. Ideally, the aim of any assisted reproductive treatment is to achieve a healthy single baby. The morbidity and risks associated with multiple pregnancies have led clinicians to limit the number of embryos transferred and many countries now resort to single-embryo transfer (SET). However, the perceived disadvantage of reduced pregnancy rate with SET still discourages adoption of this policy universally.

CONSEQUENCES OF MULTIPLE PREGNANCIES

Multiple pregnancies have been the major side effect of assisted reproductive treatments. These have significant impact on the maternal and fetal health and also tremendous psychosocial effect and financial burden on the family. It has been observed that compared to a singleton, a twin is about five times more likely to die in the first year of life and has 10 times higher risk of having a lifelong handicap (cerebral palsy, mental retardation). **Box 1** summarizes the various consequences of multiple pregnancies.

BOX 1: Impact of multiple pregnancies.

Maternal health	***Infant***	***Psychosocial***
• Spontaneous abortions • GDM • PIH • Preterm labor • APH, PPH • Cesarean section • Increased maternal morbidity and mortality	• Preterm birth • LBW/SGA • IUGR • *Complications related to preterm birth*: RDS, Interventricular hemorrhage, sepsis, jaundice, ROP • Perinatal mortality • NICU care	• Financial burden • Obstetric cost and cost of NICU • Cost of taking care of multiple children • Postpartum depression • Relationship stress

(APH: antepartum hemorrhage; GDM: gestational diabetes mellitus; NICU: neonatal intensive care unit; IUGR: intrauterine growth restriction; LBW: low birth weight; PIH: pregnancy-induced hypertension; PPH: postpartum hemorrhage; RDS: respiratory distress syndrome; ROP: retinopathy of prematurity; SGA: small for gestational age)

FACTORS TO DECIDE THE NUMBER OF EMBRYOS TO BE TRANSFERRED

To avoid the maternal, fetal, and neonatal morbidity associated with multiple pregnancies, it is advisable to limit the number of embryos transferred so as to reduce the incidence of multiple pregnancies but at the same time maintaining the acceptable success rates of IVF treatment.

Multiple factors should be considered while deciding the number of embryos to be transferred in a particular patient. These factors can be divided into two categories—namely, patient-related factors and embryo-related factors.

Patient-related Factors

Age

Age is the important determinant of IVF success as the chances of having euploid embryos decrease with advancing age. The general trend is to transfer more numbers of embryos in women with advanced age to achieve better success rates. However, it is difficult to unravel the specific impact of age on live birth rates (LBRs) with respect to number of embryos transferred, as most studies comparing the outcome of SET versus double-embryo transfer (DET) have included young patients with good prognosis.

It has been observed that if elective single-embryo transfer (eSET) and DET are compared after a single cycle, DET is associated with higher LBR. However, if sequential SET are compared to DET, results favor SET. In a meta-analysis conducted by Ma et al.,[1] which included 85 studies [14 randomized controlled trials (RCTs) and 71 observational studies], it was observed that LBR was higher after a DET in patients aged <35 years and 35–40 years. However, in patients aged ≥40 years, such differences were not observed. Similarly, multiple pregnancy rates (MPRs) were lower in women aged <35 years receiving SET or those aged 35–40 years, whereas the difference was not significant in women ≥40 years old. The risk of obstetric and neonatal complications was lower with SET compared to DET.

The Cochrane Systematic Review included 17 RCTs and data on 2,505 patients.[2] However, majority of the women included in the studies were under 36 years old with expected good prognosis. No significant differences in cumulative LBR (CLBR) were observed after two consecutive SETs versus one DET, whereas MPR after repeated SET was significantly lower, compared to that of DET.

The latest American Society for Reproductive Medicine (ASRM) guideline (ASRM 2021) recommends SET for patients younger than 35 years of age regardless of the stage of the embryo. The guideline strongly recommends eSET also for patients aged 35–37 years. For older patients, one or more embryos can be transferred depending on the embryo stage at the time of transfer.[3]

Advanced maternal age is associated with increased obstetric risks including preterm birth, low birth weight, hypertensive disorders, stillbirth, and cesarean delivery. As these risks are even more aggravated in multiple pregnancies, avoidance of multiple pregnancies is more important in this group of patients. These specific health risks should be evaluated and considered at the time of planning assisted reproductive technology (ART) treatment.

Previous Failed Cycles

Previously failed treatment is one of the factors that provokes the clinician to transfer more embryos in one attempt to enhance the success rates in subsequent cycles. It has been observed that chances of LBR in each cycle decrease with the increasing number of ART attempts. McLernon et al., in a large population-based observational cohort study, observed that LBR gradually decreased from 28.5% in the first cycle to 16.8% in the fifth cycle of ART.[4] In another study conducted by Thurin et al., it was observed that the odds of ongoing implantation decrease with each unsuccessful ART attempt.[5] However, when other prognostic factors like age and number of available embryos are kept in mind, the number of failed treatment attempts is observed to be a weak prognostic factor.[6]

Currently, there are no prospective studies analyzing the impact of the number of previous unsuccessful ART treatments on LBR with respect to number of embryos transferred. There is no strong evidence which support that previous failed cycle is an indication for transferring multiple embryos. No difference in clinical pregnancy rate was observed between SET and DET in patients with previous failed attempts.[7] However, one may consider transferring multiple embryos (maximum three cleavage-stage embryos or two blastocysts), as time taken to clinical pregnancy is shorter due to less number of attempts. But careful counseling and the risks associated with multiple pregnancies must be explained to the couple.

Duration of Infertility

Duration of infertility is an important factor and one of the main criteria for the decision to initiate ART. However, it does not seem to affect the reproductive outcomes when analyzing the results with respect to the number of embryos transferred.

Previous Pregnancy/Live Birth

A live birth from previous ART or spontaneous pregnancy may increase the chance of having a positive pregnancy in the subsequent ART cycle, but the evidence toward this is low.[8] In a clinical setting, a couple having a living child usually may opt for another single pregnancy due to social, financial, psychological, and personal reasons. Hence a thorough discussion regarding SET versus DET must be done, risk of multiple pregnancies with multiple-embryo transfer must be considered.

Donor Oocyte/Donor Embryo

In a clinical setting, one may consider SET in patients opting for donor oocyte/embryo. The donors selected usually are from a younger age-group, i.e., 23–35 years. Hence the chances of obtaining euploid embryos are higher.[9] Also, considering the risk of hypertensive disorders and preterm deliveries being higher among women opting donor oocytes over self-oocytes, one should counsel the patients carefully and consider minimizing the multiple pregnancy risks.

Surrogate Mother/Gestational Carrier

Considering the increased risk of hypertensive disorders and preterm deliveries associated with donor embryo in surrogate mothers, it is advisable to opt for a SET. A SET may prevent multiple pregnancies and complications related to that for the surrogate and indirectly may be beneficial financially and legally for both parties.[10,11]

Poor-reserve Patients

In patients with poor ovarian reserve, multiple cycles of egg retrieval may be required to obtain the correct number of embryos in order to achieve a live birth. The number of embryos needed to achieve a live birth also depends on patient's age. The clinician may consider DET (blastocyst) or up to three cleavage-stage embryo transfer in the above group of patients in order to minimize the number of attempts needed for a clinical pregnancy. Thorough counseling of the patient must be done taking into account her age, quality of embryos, and risks of multiple pregnancies.

In some cases, women do not opt for pooling of embryos. They prefer transferring a single embryo rather than multiple embryos at a time due to the fear of losing the limited number of embryos in a single attempt. This may be taken into account if the clinician cannot definitively rule out other factors such as uterine, endometrial, or immunological factors. A SET may be considered in this scenario after thorough counseling with the couple.

Embryo-related Factors

The number of embryos to be transferred may be decided by the quality of the embryos and also the stage at which the embryos are transferred.

Various noninvasive and invasive assessment techniques are used to find the embryo with the highest reproductive potential. Morphological scoring at different stages of preimplantation development is the most practiced approach to evaluate the embryo's developmental quality. The implantation rates are higher among higher-grade embryos. Hence the clinician may decide on the number of embryos to be transferred depending on the grading of the embryos. Most clinicians consider SET for good-quality embryos and multiple embryos to be transferred for lower-grade embryos. Grading is usually done by a qualified embryologist using a standard grading system, which makes it simpler to identify good-quality embryos.

A cleavage-stage embryo is categorized as good quality on day-2 by having four equally sized mononucleated blastomeres in a three-dimensional tetrahedral arrangement, with <10% fragmentation. Similarly, a good-quality day 3 embryo should have eight equally sized mononucleated blastomeres with <10% fragmentation.[12]

The grading system for blastocysts is adapted from the original Gardner scale. In this system, the embryo score results from the degree of expansion (scores 1–6) as well as the inner cell mass (ICM) (grades A, B, and C) and trophectoderm (TE) (grades A, B, and C).[13]

American Society for Reproductive Medicine recommends SET for patients younger than 35 years of age regardless of the stage of the embryo. It also recommends eSET for patients aged 35–37 years. For older patients, one or more embryos can be transferred depending on the embryo stage, at the time of transfer. **Table 1** summarizes the latest ASRM recommendation of number of embryos to be transferred based on age of the patient, stage of the embryo, and euploidy status.[3]

A meta-analysis on perinatal outcomes for patients who had a blastocyst transfer versus cleavage-stage transfer revealed that the risk of preterm delivery was higher in patients undergoing blastocyst transfer

TABLE 1: Number of embryos to transfer based on age, stage of embryo, and euploidy status.[3]

Recommendations for the limit to the number of embryos to transfer				
	Age			
Prognosis	***<35***	***35–37***	***38–40***	***41–42***
Cleavage-stage embryos				
Euploid*	1	1	1	1
Other favorable†	1	1	≤3	≤4
Embryos not euploid* or favorable†	≤2	≤3	≤4	≤5
Blastocysts				
Euploid*	1	1	1	1
Other favorable†	1	1	≤2	≤3
Embryos not euploid* or favorable†	≤2	≤2	≤3	≤3

*Demonstrated euploid embryos, best prognosis.

†Other favorable = Any ONE of these criteria; fresh cycle: Expectation of one or more high-quality embryos available for cryopreservation or previous live birth after a prior transfer with sibling embryo(s); FET cycle: Availability of vitrified day 5 or day 6 blastocysts, euploid embryos, first FET cycle, or previous live birth after an IVF cycle.

(FET: frozen embryo transfer; IVF: in vitro fertilization)

compared to cleavage-stage transfer. However, the meta-analysis concluded that the risk of fetal growth restriction and small for gestational age was lesser among those with a blastocyst transfer.[14]

Therefore, one may consider transferring a single blastocyst in order to reduce the multiple pregnancy risk, which in turn increases preterm delivery.

ADVANCED TECHNOLOGIES FOR BETTER EMBRYO SELECTION

Traditionally embryos have been selected based on morphology, but morphological selection is not always predictive of implantation potential. Preimplantation genetic testing (PGT), time-lapse imaging, artificial intelligence (AI), and metabolomics are additional tools, which may can help in better selection of an euploid embryo with highest implantation potential.

Role of Preimplantation Genetic Testing in Embryo Selection

Conventionally embryos have been selected based on morphological grading systems. However, it has been observed that morphological selection of embryos is not 100% accurate and approximately 20% of day 5 embryos transferred based on morphological selection alone may be aneuploid.[15] Aneuploidy is the major cause of implantation failure and miscarriages in ART cycles.[16] Preimplantation genetic testing for aneuploidies (PGT-A) along with comprehensive chromosome screening (CCS) allows to select euploid embryos and thus can be a useful tool in embryo selection for eSET. TE biopsy at blastocyst stage is currently the preferred method for screening.

A prospective randomized study by Scott et al. observed that 96% of aneuploid embryos fail to implant compared to 41% of euploid embryos.[17] In a randomized trial conducted by Forman et al., which included 175 women <43 years of age, it was observed that transfer of one euploid embryo results in similar pregnancy rates compared to transfer of two unscreened embryos (69% after euploid eSET compared to 72% after untested DET, p value = 0.6).[18] The incidence of twin pregnancies, preterm deliveries, and neonatal intensive care unit (NICU) admissions was significantly lesser in the euploid eSET group. Schoolcraft et al. observed that use of CCS can improve eSET success rates in women with advanced maternal age (>35 years). In another study conducted by Gonzalez et al., it was observed that euploid blastocysts implant irrespective of their morphology after next-generation sequencing (NGS)-(PGT-A) testing in women with advanced age.[19]

One may consider SET, if PGT has been done on the embryos and after ruling out uterine and endometrial factors.

However, in spite of various studies proving the benefit of PGS in embryo selection, the technology has not gained widespread use. The additional costs of the procedure, the need for cryopreservation of all embryos, and the fact that euploidy does not guarantee pregnancy and successful live birth are the factors limiting its use.

A newer technology called noninvasive chromosome screening (NICS) uses spent culture media to isolate cell-free embryonic DNA, which is then tested for aneuploidies. The advantage of this technique over conventional PGT is that it is totally noninvasive and does not disturb the growth of the embryo.

Time-lapse Monitoring for Embryo Selection

Traditionally, embryos have been assessed by direct observation under the inverted microscope. Though this method is simple, it is subject to interobserver variability and it provides information of the embryo only at the time of assessment. Time-lapse technology is a new milestone in the field of assisted reproduction as it allows for continuous noninvasive observation of embryos. It allows monitoring the embryos without disturbing the culture conditions. The continuous monitoring and the large number of pictures available provide thorough information about the embryo development. It also enables observation of specific developmental events such as multinucleation, direct division (division from one to three cells), and cell fusion. Observing these events is crucial, as they are associated with a low implantation potential.[20] The embryos can thus be selected based on morphological, dynamic, and morphokinetic criteria using some predictive programs and algorithms.[21]

An association between embryo aneuploidy and time-lapse markers has also been assessed in various studies. It has been observed that euploid embryos follow tight kinetic parameters whereas aneuploid embryos have an unpredictable development outside the optimal range and show a higher degree of fragmentation.

A number of studies have compared outcomes after embryo selection by morphokinetic versus morphological assessment. Though some researchers found increased success and LBRs using time lapse, many others did not find any improved outcomes using this technology.[22,23] Retrospective study by Fishel et al., which compared a single blastocyst transfer using time-lapse versus double-blastocyst transfer using conventional methods, showed that in patients <38 years of age, the LBRs were lower in the single time-lapse-based embryo transfer as compared to the other group. A similar difference was observed in those >38 years of age. MPRs were increased by 30–40% after a DET compared to SET regardless of age, incubator type, and embryo stage.[24] In conclusion, time-lapse technology does not aid in deciding about the number of embryos to be transferred.

Though the concept of time-lapse monitoring sounds promising, more prospective studies are needed to prove its efficacy and safety before this can be applied in routine clinical use.[25]

Artificial Intelligence for Embryo Selection

Both direct visualization and time-lapse methods of embryo selection grade embryos based on their ability to reach particular stages of development in timely manner. However, these morphological grading systems remain limited in their ability to predict live birth. AI using routinely generated images or time-lapse videos can help to grade embryos more accurately and objectively and can thus help in better embryo selection for eSET. AI can also have a role in analyzing data from noninvasive metabolomics and secretory profiles from embryo culture media. Though, many studies have shown that AI can help in improving the accuracy of manual grading and predicting development to blastocyst, its usefulness in increasing the LBR is yet to be demonstrated.[26,27]

Metabolomics for Embryo Selection

Metabolomics in ART refers to metabolite product found in specific biological material or media. They are a group of small nonproteinaceous compounds including metabolic intermediates, adenosine triphosphate, hormones, or metabolites. They are more informative than genomics, transcriptomics, or proteomics, as they represent the final product of cell regulatory system and so are closer to the functional phenotype. Metabolomics profiling of embryo is done using spent culture media. Though the technique has helped in better understanding of nutritional environment of oocytes and embryos, it is yet to be proved beneficial for improving ongoing pregnancy and LBR.[28]

CONCLUSION

The ultimate goal of infertility treatment is a single healthy baby. Multiple pregnancies is one of the major complications of IVF, and there is a global recognition of the need to reduce the incidence of same. The decision for the number of embryos to be transferred should be a shared one with the couple and one should take into account not only medical factors discussed above but also social, financial, and psychological factors into account. For poor-prognosis patients with repeated implantation failures or insufficient funds for several transfer cycles, the decision for transferring multiple embryos in order to achieve clinical pregnancy in a short period of time may be considered.

RECOMMENDATIONS ON THE NUMBER OF EMBRYO TRANSFER: AMERICAN SOCIETY REPRODUCTIVE MEDICINE[3]

Box 2 gives the recommendations on the number of embryo transfer by ASRM.

BOX 2: Recommendations on the number of embryo transfer by American Society Reproductive Medicine (ASRM).

A. *Patients with a favorable prognosis:*
- Transfer of a euploid embryo should be limited to one, regardless of patient age
- Patients <35 years of age should be strongly encouraged to receive a single-embryo transfer, regardless of the embryo stage
- For patients between 35 and 37 years of age, strong consideration should be made for a single-embryo transfer
- For patients between 38 and 40 years of age, no more than three untested cleavage-stage embryos or two blastocysts should be transferred
- Patients 41–42 years of age should plan to receive no more than four untested cleavage-stage embryos or three blastocysts

B. *Other scenarios:*
- In each of the preceding age groups, patients who do not meet the criteria for a favorable prognosis may have an additional embryo transferred according to their individual circumstances. The patient must be counseled regarding the additional risk of twin or higher-order multiple pregnancy
- If otherwise favorable patients fail to conceive after multiple cycles with high-quality embryo(s) transferred, the physicians and patients may consider proceeding with an additional embryo to be transferred
- Patients with a coexisting medical condition for which a multiple pregnancy may increase the risk of significant morbidity should not have more than one embryo transferred
- In the rare cases in which the number of embryos or blastocysts transferred exceeds the recommended limits, both the counseling and the justification must be documented in the patient's permanent medical record
- In women ≥43 years of age, there are insufficient data to recommend a limit on the number of embryos to transfer when the patient uses her own oocytes. Caution should be exercised as the risk associated with multiple pregnancies increases dramatically with advancing maternal age

C. In donor–oocyte cycles, the age of the donor should be used to determine the appropriate number of embryos to transfer. For example, when the donor is <38 years of age and other favorable criteria exist, single-embryo transfer should be planned

D. Single-embryo transfer should be strongly recommended in all gestational carrier (GC) cycles, given the health risks associated with multiple gestations for the GC. At a minimum, it is recommended to follow age-related limits on the number of embryos to transfer in GC cycles, on the basis of the age of the woman who produced the oocytes (either the intended parent or oocyte donor)

E. In frozen embryo transfer (FET) cycles, favorable characteristics should be on the basis of the age of the woman when the embryos were cryopreserved and include the presence of high-quality vitrified embryos, euploid embryos, first FET cycle, or previous live birth after a prior transfer with sibling embryo(s)

REFERENCES

1. Ma S, Peng Y, Hu L, Wang X, Xiong Y, Tang Y, Tan J, Gong F. Comparisons of benefits and risks of single embryo transfer versus double embryo transfer: a systematic review and meta-analysis. Reprod Biol Endocrinol. 2022;20:20.
2. Kamath MS, Mascarenhas M, Kirubakaran R, Bhattacharya S. Number of embryos for transfer following in vitro fertilisation or intra-cytoplasmic sperm injection. Cochrane Database Syst Rev. 2020;8:CD003416.
3. Practice Committee of the American Society for Reproductive Medicine and the Practice Committee for the Society for Assisted Reproductive Technologies. Guidance on the limits to the number of embryos to transfer: a committee opinion. Fertil Steril. 2021;116:651-654.
4. McLernon DJ, Steyerberg EW, Te Velde ER, Lee AJ, Bhattacharya S. Predicting the chances of a live birth after one or more complete cycles of in vitro fertilisation: population based study of linked cycle data from 113 873 women. BMJ. 2016;355:i5735.
5. Thurin A, Hardarson T, Hausken J, Jablonowska B, Lundin K, Pinborg A, et al. Predictors of ongoing implantation in IVF in a good prognosis group of patients. Hum Reprod. 2005;20:1876-80.
6. Roberts S, McGowan L, Hirst W, Brison D, Vail A, Lieberman B. Towards single embryo transfer? Modelling clinical outcomes of potential treatment choices using multiple data sources: predictive models and patient perspectives. Health Technol Assess. 2010;14:1-237.
7. Monteleone PA, Mirisola RJ, Gonçalves SP, Baracat EC, Serafini PC. Outcomes of elective cryopreserved single or double embryo transfers following failure to conceive after fresh single embryo transfer. Reprod Biomed Online. 2016;33:161-7.
8. Luke B, Brown MB, Wantman E, Stern JE, Baker VL, Widra E, et al. Application of a validated prediction model for in vitro fertilization: comparison of live birth rates and multiple birth rates with 1 embryo transferred over 2 cycles vs 2 embryos in 1 cycle. Am J Obstet Gynecol. 2015;212:676.e1-7.
9. Fishel S, Campbell A, Montgomery S, Smith R, Nice L, Duffy S, et al. Live births after embryo selection using morphokinetics versus conventional morphology: a retrospective analysis. Reprod Biomed Online. 2017;35(4):407-16.
10. Swanson K, Debbink M, Letourneau JM, Kuppermann M, Einerson BD. Association of multifetal gestation with obstetric and neonatal outcomes in gestational carrier pregnancies. J Assist Reprod Genet. 2021;38:661-7.

11. Shenfield F, Pennings G, Cohen J, Devroey P, De Wert G, Tarlatzis B; ESHRE Task Force on Ethics and Law. ESHRE Task Force on Ethics and Law 10: surrogacy. Hum Reprod. 2005;20(10):2705-7.
12. ALPHA Scientists in Reproductive Medicine; ESHRE Special Interest Group of Embryology. The Istanbul consensus workshop on embryo assessment: proceedings of an expert meeting. Reprod Biomed Online. 2011;22:632-46.
13. Gardner DK, Schoolcraft WB, Wagley L, Schlenker T, Stevens J, Hesla J. A prospective randomized trial of blastocyst culture and transfer in in-vitro fertilization. Hum Reprod. 1998;13:3434-40.
14. Maheshwari A, Kalampokas T, Davidson J, Bhattacharya S. Obstetric and perinatal outcomes in singleton pregnancies resulting from the transfer of blastocyst-stage versus cleavage-stage embryos generated through in vitro fertilization treatment: a systematic review and meta-analysis. Fertil Steril. 2013;100(6):1615-21.
15. Forman EJ, Upham KM, Cheng M, Zhao T, Hong KH, Treff NR, et al. Comprehensive chromosome screening alters traditional morphology-based embryo selection: a prospective study of 100 consecutive cycles of planned fresh euploid blastocyst transfer. Fertil Steril. 2013;100:718-24.
16. Schoolcraft WB, Katz-Jaffe MG. Comprehensive chromosome screening of trophoectoderm with vitrification facilitates elective single-embryo transfer for infertile women with advanced maternal age. Fertil Steril. 2013;100:615-9.
17. Scott RT Jr, Ferry K, Su J, Tao X, Scott K, Treff NR. Comprehensive chromosome screening is highly predictive of the reproductive potential of human embryos: a prospective blinded nonselection study. Fertil Steril. 2012;97:870-5.
18. Forman EJ, Hong KH, Franasiak JM, Scott RT Jr. Obstetrical and neonatal outcomes from the BEST Trial: single embryo transfer with aneuploidy screening improves outcomes after in vitro fertilization without compromising delivery rates. Am J Obstet Gynecol. 2014;10:157.
19. Viñals Gonzalez X, Odia R, Naja R, Serhal P, Saab W, Seshadri S, et al. Euploid blastocysts implant irrespective of their morphology after NGS-(PGT-A) testing in advanced maternal age patients. J Assist Reprod Genet. 2019;36:1623-9.
20. Barrie A, Homburg R, McDowell G, Brown J, Kingsland C, Troup S. Preliminary investigation of the prevalence and implantation potential of abnormal embryonic phenotypes assessed using time-lapse imaging. Reprod Biomed Online. 2017;34:455-62.
21. Kirkegaard K, Ahlström A, Ingerslev HJ, Hardarson T. Choosing the best embryo by time lapse versus standard morphology. Fertil Steril. 2015;103:323-32.
22. Adamson GD, Abusief ME, Palao L, Witmer J, Palao LM, Gvakharia M. Improved implantation rates of day 3 embryo transfers with the use of an automated time-lapse-enabled test to aid in embryo selection. Fertil Steril. 2016;105:369-75.
23. Goodman LR, Goldberg J, Falcone T, Austin C, Desai N. Does the addition of time-lapse morphokinetics in the selection of embryos for transfer improve pregnancy rates? A randomized controlled trial. Fertil Steril. 2016;105:275-85.
24. Fishel S, Campbell A, Montgomery S, Smith R, Nice L, Duffy S, et al. Live births after embryo selection using morphokinetics versus conventional morphology: a retrospective analysis. Reprod Biomed Online. 2017;35(4):407-16.
25. Armstrong, S, Bhide, P, Jordan V, Pacey A, Marjoribanks J, Farquhar C. Time-lapse systems for embryo incubation and assessment in assisted reproduction. Cochrane Database Syst Rev. 2019;5:CD011320.
26. Ver Mileya M, Hall JMM, Diakiw SM, Johnston A, Nguyen T, Perugini D, et al. Development of an artificial intelligence-based assessment model for prediction of embryo viability using static images captured by optical light microscopy during IVF. Hum Reprod. 2020;35:770-84.
27. Chavez Badiola A, Flores-Saifee Farias A, Mendizabal-Ruiz G, Garcia-Sanchez R, Drakeley AJ, Garcia-Sandoval JP. Predicting pregnancy test results after embryo transfer by image feature extraction and analysis using machine learning. Scientific reports 2020; 10:4394.
28. Siristatidis CS, Sertedaki E, Vaidakis D. Metabolomics for improving pregnancy outcomes in women undergoing assisted reproductive technologies. Cochrane Database Syst Rev. 2017;5:CD011872.

Intracytoplasmic Sperm Injection: Should it be Routinely done for all?

Pooja Patil, Manisha Takhtani Kundnani

INTRODUCTION

The invention of intracytoplasmic sperm injection (ICSI) has been one of the major breakthroughs in the field of assisted reproduction and it has totally revolutionized the treatment of male factor infertility. The technique was first described by Palmero GD and the first human pregnancy and live birth using this technique was achieved in 1992.[1] Ever since then, ICSI has become the mainstay of treating couples with male factor infertility. However, the last three decades have seen tremendous increase in the use of this technology even in couples with nonmale factor. A study by Boulet et al. observed that the use of ICSI increased fourfold between 1996 and 2012 in nonmale factor infertility.[2] In a report by Adamson et al., it was observed that in some countries ICSI is done in 100% of in vitro fertilization (IVF) cycles irrespective of the cause of infertility.[3] Whether the use of ICSI is justified in couples with a normal male factor and whether it actually translates to increased live birth rates is a matter of debate and there is a clear lack of well-designed randomized controlled trials (RCTs) analyzing the possible benefits of ICSI in these couples.[4]

INTRACYTOPLASMIC SPERM INJECTION FOR NONMALE FACTOR INFERTILITY

Though the initial and original indication for ICSI was to overcome moderate-to-severe male factor infertility, its use has expanded in the last few years to many nonmale factor indications. The proposed indications include unexplained infertility, couples with previous total fertilization failure (TFF) with conventional IVF, couples with advanced age, poor responders with low oocyte yield, preimplantation genetic testing (PGT), fertilization after in vitro maturation (IVM), and fertilization of cryopreserved oocytes. Some practitioners use ICSI for all IVF cases irrespective of the cause of infertility. The rationale for use of ICSI in these indications except PGT is to avoid fertilization failures and get more number of embryos. However, the evidence demonstrating the effectiveness of ICSI in these cases compared to conventional IVF is scarce when the ultimate outcome—the live birth rate—is considered.

Intracytoplasmic Sperm Injection Versus IVF in Couples with Unexplained Infertility

The rationale for use of ICSI in couples with unexplained infertility is that ICSI may help overcome potential fertilization barriers that may be the cause of infertility in these women. Two independent studies by Hershlag et al. and Jaroudi et al. observed better fertilization rates and lesser incidences of fertilization failure with ICSI than conventional insemination on sibling oocytes in women with otherwise unexplained infertility.[5,6] However, the effect on implantation, clinical pregnancy, and live birth rate could not be ascertained. A RCT conducted by Aboulghar et al. comparing ICSI with conventional insemination in unexplained infertility did not reveal any difference in pregnancy rates between the two groups.[7] A meta-analysis by Johnson et al. analyzed 11 RCTs comparing ICSI to conventional insemination in women with unexplained infertility.[8] Fertilization rates per retrieved oocyte was observed. In five of these studies, sibling oocytes were assigned to ICSI or conventional insemination before assessment of maturity. A 30% higher fertilization rates was observed with ICSI fertilized oocytes. The incidence of fertilization failure was eight times higher in the conventional insemination group. However, no clear advantage for ICSI in terms of reproductive outcomes was observed.

Overall, the evidence regarding the superiority of ICSI over conventional IVF in unexplained infertility is limited. Though ICSI is associated with increased fertilization rates and decreased fertilization failure, the current evidence does not show any significant increase in live birth rates with the use of ICSI. Also, it was observed that 30 unwanted cases of ICSI are required to decrease one case of unexpected failed fertilization.[9]

Intracytoplasmic Sperm Injection Versus IVF in Women with Advanced Age

The proportion of women >35 years of age undergoing IVF is constantly on the rise. It has been theorized that oocytes from women with advanced age may have defects of zona or cytoplasm that may hamper the fertilization with conventional IVF. However, a retrospective study by Tannus et al. observed similar fertilization rates, clinical pregnancy, and live birth rates in women with advanced age when ICSI was compared to conventional insemination.[10]

No studies evaluate the efficacy of ICSI over conventional IVF in poor quality oocytes in improving live birth rates.

Intracytoplasmic Sperm Injection Versus IVF in Couples with Previous Total Fertilization Failure

Total fertilization failure is a frustrating situation for both the clinician and the patient. It leads to cycle termination and adds to significant financial and psychological burden on the couple. The underlying issue with TFF could be oocyte activation defect, nonviable, or abnormal sperms. In some cases, TFF occurs due to poor oocyte quality or defects in the cytoplasm or genetic factors. Various retrospective studies have shown that the subsequent fertilization rates with conventional inseminations in such cases range between 30 and 97%.[11-13] And thus ICSI is often advocated in these cases in order to reduce the risk of subsequent failed fertilization. However, it is advisable that couples with TFF should undergo further investigations such as deoxyribonucleic acid (DNA) fragmentation index and other clinical and genetic factors which can affect oocyte quality, rather than believing that ICSI is the only way out.

Westerlaken et al. allocated sister oocytes to either conventional insemination or ICSI after previous TFF with conventional insemination. The subsequent fertilization rates after conventional insemination was 11% and after ICSI was 48%.[14] ICSI can therefore increase the fertilization rates when TFF or lower than expected fertilization has happened with previous conventional insemination.

Intracytoplasmic Sperm Injection Versus IVF in Women Undergoing PGT

For PGT, ICSI is usually the recommended technique of insemination. The rationale behind use of ICSI before PGT is to ensure monospermic fertilization and also avoid contamination from extraneous sperm attached to zona pellucida, especially when polymerase chain reaction (PCR) is used.[15,16] It also avoids contamination from maternal granulosa cells, especially when PGT is performed for single gene defects. However with newer techniques like next-generation sequencing, this risk of contamination is less of concern. It has recently been observed that sperm DNA fails to amplify under PGT processing conditions and therefore the risk of sperm contamination with IVF is negligible.[17,18]

Various studies have shown that the number of embryos available for biopsy, aneuploidy, and mosaicism rates and the number of complete and incomplete diagnosis after PGT are similar after conventional insemination, ICSI, or split insemination.[17,19-21] This was true for both PGT for aneuploidies and PGT for monogenic diseases. Thus, ICSI is just adopted on the basis of fear of contamination rather than strong scientific evidence.

Intracytoplasmic Sperm Injection Versus IVF in Poor Responders/ Less Number of Oocytes Retrieved

Poor responders are patients with a few or low number of eggs retrieved which may present a real dilemma regarding the technique of insemination. These poor responders have reduced pregnancy rates compared with normal responders. ICSI is commonly recommended in cases with poor response and low oocyte yield in order to improve fertilization rates and have more number of embryos. Some studies have shown higher fertilization rates after ICSI than after a conventional IVF. However, many other studies have observed similar outcomes with ICSI and conventional insemination in terms of fertilization rate, fertilization failure, embryo quality, number of embryos, clinical pregnancy, and miscarriage rates in women with poor oocyte yield[22,23] (<6 oocytes retrieved).

The Society for Assisted Reproductive Technology Clinic Outcome Reporting System (SART CORS) registry (2004–11) concluded that ICSI does not improve odds of live birth in women with elevated FSH.[24] On the contrary, in women with diminished ovarian reserve, ICSI was associated with decreased live birth rate when compared to conventional insemination (20.4% in ICSI vs. 21.9% in conventional insemination).

Intracytoplasmic Sperm Injection after IVM

In vitro maturation of immature oocytes can lead to hardening of zona pellucida and therefore ICSI has been suggested as preferred method of fertilization after IVM.[25,26] Though ICSI is associated with better fertilization rates for IVM oocytes, the developmental competence of the resulting embryos may be impaired as was suggested in a study by Söderström-Anttila et al.[27] The implantation rates and the clinical pregnancy rates were higher in IVM oocytes inseminated conventionally. Larger trials comparing effect of IVF or ICSI on IVM oocytes are needed for conclusive interpretation.

Intracytoplasmic Sperm Injection for Frozen Oocytes

Oocyte freezing requires removal of surrounding cumulus cells before freezing. This can lead to alterations in zona which can hamper the fertilization with conventional insemination. So ICSI has been the preferred method of fertilization of frozen oocytes. The data comparing conventional insemination to ICSI for frozen oocytes is scarce.[28]

Intracytoplasmic Sperm Injection for All

Many clinics follow a policy of ICSI for all assisted reproductive technology (ART) cycles irrespective of the etiology of infertility. The reasons behind using ICSI indiscriminately include avoidance of total fertilization failure, potential increase in the number of available embryos, and subsequent increase in the cumulative pregnancy and LBR per treatment cycle. However, most of the available literature does not prove any advantage of ICSI over conventional IVF in terms of treatment outcomes such as cumulative live birth rate (CLBR) for nonmale factor infertility couples.

A retrospective study compiling data from 155 ART clinics in Latin America including 39,564 ICSI cycles and 10,249 IVF cycles showed that fertilization and pregnancy rates were similar with ICSI and conventional IVF.[29] Similar findings were observed in a retrospective study which analyzed data from >500 clinics in United States.[30] Additionally, the use of ICSI did not reduce the risk of TFF even in elderly women (>40 years) and in those with low oocyte yield. A meta-analysis of all the available data till 2020 comparing IVF and ICSI in nonmale factor infertility did not reveal any significant differences with respect to the fertilization rate, implantation rate, clinical pregnancy rate, and LBR. On the contrary, conventional insemination was observed to be superior to ICSI in older women.[31]

INTRACYTOPLASMIC SPERM INJECTION FOR NONMALE FACTOR INFERTILITY: SWOT ANALYSIS

Bosch et al. designed a SWOT (Strengths, Weaknesses, Opportunities, and Threats) analysis to evaluate the available published evidence on possible use of ICSI for nonmale factor infertility.[32] The results of the analysis are summarized in **Figure 1**.

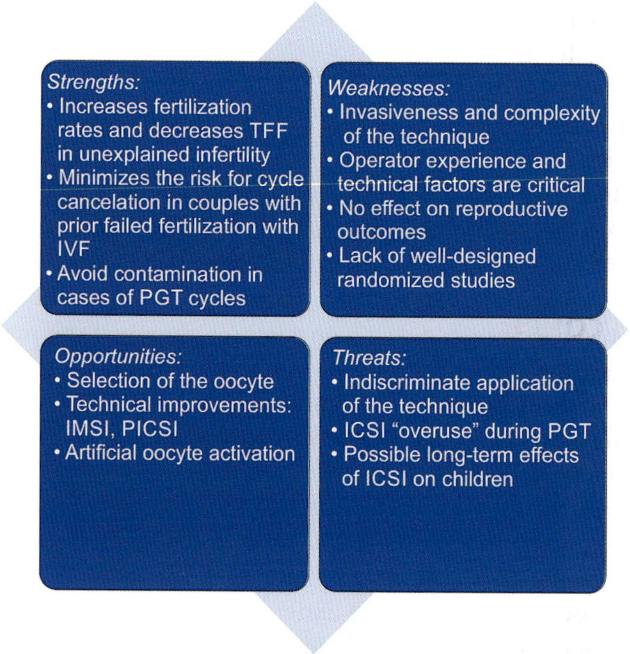

Fig. 1: A SWOT analysis of ICSI versus IVF for nonmale factor infertility in assisted reproduction. (ICSI: intracytoplasmic sperm injection; IMSI: intracytoplasmic morphologically selected sperm injection; IVF: in vitro fertilization; PGT: preimplantation genetic testing; PICSI: physiological intracytoplasmic sperm injection; SWOT: strengths, weaknesses, opportunities, and threats; TFF: total fertilization failure)

TABLE 1: Conventional insemination versus ICSI in nonmale factor infertility: summary of main findings.

Indication	*Evidence*
Unexplained infertility	• Though ICSI is associated with better fertilization rates, no significant effect on pregnancy rates and live birth rates is observed • Approximately 30 unwanted cases of ICSI are required to prevent one case of total fertilization failure
Advanced maternal age	Most available data fail to demonstrate an advantage of ICSI over conventional IVF in terms of fertilization rate, embryo development rate, pregnancy, and live birth rates
Decreased ovarian reserve/poor responders	Comparable fertilization rate, fertilization failure, implantation rate, clinical pregnancy rate, and live birth rate are observed after conventional insemination and ICSI
Previous total fertilization failure	ICSI has better fertilization rates in cases with past history of TFF
Preimplantation genetic testing	No significant differences in contamination rates of the washing medium samples after conventional insemination or ICSI are reported
Frozen oocytes	ICSI is used as a routine and data comparing conventional insemination and ICSI in frozen oocytes is scarce
IVM oocytes	Not enough data available comparing conventional insemination and ICSI for IVM

(ICSI: intracytoplasmic sperm injection; IVM: in vitro maturation; TFF: total fertilization failure)

INTRACYTOPLASMIC SPERM INJECTION FOR NONMALE FACTOR INFERTILITY: OTHER CONCERNS

Intracytoplasmic sperm injection is an invasive technique which requires additional expertise, resources, effort, and time. It thus adds to the overall cost of the procedure. Also, there are concerns regarding its safety including subjective sperm selection, injury during sperm injection, and injection of foreign material into the ooplasm. Additionally, there have been concerns about the potential effects on congenital abnormalities and developmental issues as well as epigenetic changes in children conceived by ICSI.

CONCLUSION

Intracytoplasmic sperm injection is widely used technique to overcome male factor infertility; however, evidence proving its superiority in nonmale factor is scarce or lacking. It is often performed for reasons of caution and consistency. Determining concrete parameters that indicate which patients may benefit from ICSI outside male factor is challenging and controversial. Most available literature shows similar or comparable outcomes to conventional insemination. The procedure involves higher costs, invasiveness, and technical difficulties and thus should be reserved for couples with severe male factor infertility and should not be used routinely for all ART cases.

Table 1 summarizes the main observations comparing conventional insemination and ICSI in nonmale factor infertility.

REFERENCES

1. Palmero GD, Joris H, Devroey P, Van steirteghem AC. Pregnancies after intracytoplasmic injection of single spermatozoon into an oocyte. Lancet. 1992;340(8810):17-8.
2. Boulet SL, Mehta A, Kissin DM, Warner L, Kawwass JF, Jamieson DJ. Trends in use of and reproductive outcomes associated with intracytoplasmic sperm injection. JAMA. 2015;313(3):255-63.
3. Adamson GD, de Mouzon J, Chambers GM, Zegers-Hochschild F, Mansour R, Ishihara O, et al. International Committee for Monitoring Assisted Reproductive Technology: world report on assisted reproductive technology, 2011. Fertil Steril. 2018;110(6):1067-80.
4. van Rumste MM, Evers JL, Farquhar CM. ICSI versus conventional techniques for oocyte insemination during IVF in patients with non-male factor subfertility: a Cochrane review. Hum Reprod. 2004;19(2):223-7.
5. Hershlag A, Paine T, Kvapil G, Feng H, Napolitano B. In vitro fertilization intracytoplasmic sperm injection split: an insemination method to prevent fertilization failure. Fertil Steril. 2002;77:229-32.
6. Jaroudi K, Al-Hassan S, Al-Sufayan H, Al-Mayman H, Qeba M, Coskun S. Intracytoplasmic sperm injection and conventional in vitro fertilization are complementary techniques in management of unexplained infertility. J Assist Reprod Genet. 2003;20:377-81.
7. Aboulghar MA, Mansour RT, Serour GI, Sattar MA, Amin YM. Intracytoplasmic sperm injection and conventional in vitro fertilization for sibling oocytes in cases of unexplained infertility and borderline semen. J Assist Reprod Genet. 1996;13:38-42.
8. Johnson LN, Sasson IE, Sammel MD, Dokras A. Does intracytoplasmic sperm injection improve the fertilization

rate and decrease the total fertilization failure rate in couples with well-defined unexplained infertility? A systematic review and meta-analysis. Fertil Steril. 2013;100:704-11.
9. Bhattacharya S, Hamilton MP, Shaaban M, Khalaf Y, Seddler M, Ghobara T, et al. Conventional in-vitro fertilisation versus intracytoplasmic sperm injection for the treatment of non-male-factor infertility: a randomised controlled trial. Lancet. 2001;357(9274):2075-9.
10. Tannus S, Son WY, Gilman A, Younes G, Shavit T, Dahan MH. The role of intracytoplasmic sperm injection in non-male factor infertility in advanced maternal age. Hum Reprod. 2017;32:119-24.
11. Roest J, Van Heusden AM, Zeilmaker GH, Verhoeff A. Treatment policy after poor fertilization in the first IVF cycle. J Assist Reprod Genet. 1998;15:18-21.
12. Lipitz S, Rabinovici J, Goldenberg M, Bider D, Dor J, Mashiach S. Complete failure of fertilization in couples with mechanical infertility: implications for subsequent in vitro fertilization cycles. Fertil Steril. 1994;61:863-6.
13. Kinzer DR, Barret B, Powers RD. Prognosis for clinical pregnancy and delivery after total fertilization failure during conventional in vitro fertilization of intracytoplasmic sperm injection. Fertil Steril. 2008;90:284-8.
14. Westerlaken Van der, Helmerhorst F, Dieben S, Naaktgeboren N. Intracytoplasmic sperm injection as treatment for unexplained total fertilization failure or low fertilization after conventional in vitro fertilization. Fertil Steril. 2005;83:612-7.
15. Harton GL, Magli MC, Lundin K, Montag M, Lemmen J, Harper JC, et al. ESHRE PGD Consortium/Embryology Special Interest Group—best practice guidelines for polar body and embryo biopsy for preimplantation genetic diagnosis/screening (PGD/PGS). Hum Reprod. 2011; 26(1): 41-6.
16. Practice Committees of the American Society for Reproductive Medicine and the Society for Assisted Reproductive Technology. Intracytoplasmic sperm injection (ICSI) for non-male factor indications: a committee opinion. Fertil Steril. 2020;114:239-45.
17. De Munck N, El Khatib I, Abdala A, El-Damen A, Bayram A, Arnanz A, et al. Intracytoplasmic sperm injection is not superior to conventional IVF in couples with non-male factor infertility and preimplantation genetic testing for aneuploidies (PGT-A). Hum Reprod. 2020;35(2):317-27.
18. Lynch C, Cater E, Charitou M, Forbes H, Griffin D, Gordon T. Intracytoplasmic sperm injection is not necessary as a preventive measure against paternal cell contamination in preimplantation genetic testing. Reprod Biomed Online. 2019;39:e24-5.
19. Palmerola KL, Vitez SF, Amrane S, Fischer CP, Forman EJ. Minimizing mosaicism: assessing the impact of fertilization method on rate of mosaicism after next-generation sequencing (NGS) preimplantation genetic testing for aneuploidy (PGT-A). J Assist Reprod Genet. 2019;36:153-7.
20. Deng J, Kuyoro O, Zhao Q, Behr B, Lathi RB. Comparison of aneuploidy rates between conventional in vitro fertilization and intracytoplasmic sperm injection in in vitro fertilization-intracytoplasmic sperm injection split insemination cycles. F S Rep. 2020;1:277-81.
21. Feldman B, Aizer A, Brengauz M, Dotan K, Levron J, Schiff E, et al. Pre-implantation genetic diagnosis-should we use ICSI for all? J Assist Reprod Genet. 2017;34(9): 1179-83.
22. Moreno C, Ruiz A, Simon C, Pellicer A, Remohi J. Intracytoplasmic sperm injection as a routine indication in low responder patients. Hum Reprod. 1998;13:2126-9.
23. Luna M, Bigelow C, Duke M, Ruman J, Sandler B, Grunfeld L, et al. Should ICSI be recommended routinely in patients with four or fewer oocytes retrieved? J Assist Reprod Genet. 2011;28:911-5.
24. Butts SF, Owen C, Mainigi M, Senapati S, Seifer DB, Dokras A. Assisted hatching and intracytoplasmic sperm injection are not associated with improved outcomes in assisted reproduction cycles for diminished ovarian reserve: an analysis of cycles in the United States from 2004 to 2011. Fertil Steril. 2014;102:1041-7.
25. Hwang JL, Lin YH, Tsai YL. In vitro maturation and fertilization of immature oocytes: a comparative study of fertilization techniques. J Assist Reprod Genet. 2000; 17:39-43.
26. Nagy ZP, Cecile J, Liu J, Loccufier A, Devroey P, Van Steirteghem A. Pregnancy and birth after intracytoplasmic sperm injection of in vitro matured germinal-vesicle stage oocytes: case report. Fertil Steril. 1996;65:1047-50.
27. Söderström-Anttila V, Makinen S, Tuuri T, Suikkari AM. Favourable pregnancy results with insemination of in vitro matured oocytes from unstimulated patients. Hum Reprod. 2005;20:1534-40.
28. Gook DA, Edgar DH. Human oocyte cryopreservation. Hum Reprod Update. 2007;13:591-605.
29. Schwarze JE, Jeria R, Crosby J, Villa S, Ortega C, Pommer R. Is there a reason to perform ICSI in the absence of male factor? Lessons from the Latin American Registry of ART. Hum Reprod Open. 2017;2017:hox013.
30. Zagadailov P, Hsu A, Seifer DB, Stern JE. Differences in utilization of intracytoplasmic sperm injection (ICSI) within human services (HHS) regions and metropolitan megaregions in the U.S. Reprod Biol Endocrinol. 2017; 15:45.
31. Geng T, Cheng L, Ge C, Zhang Y. The effect of ICSI in infertility couples with non-male factor: a systematic review and meta-analysis. J Assist Reprod Genet. 2020;37: 2929-45.
32. Bosch E, Espinós JJ, Fabregues F, Fontes J, García-Velasco J, Llácer J, et al. ALWAYS ICSI? A SWOT analysis. J Assist Reprod Genet. 2020;37(9):2081-92.

Chapter

Hysteroscopy Before IVF: Should it be done for all?

Shefali Bansal Madhav

INTRODUCTION

For successful implantation of embryo and healthy placentation, evaluating the uterine factor, uterine cavity, and endometrium are important. Structural abnormalities of the uterine cavity can negatively affect implantation or may cause spontaneous abortion. Abnormalities or intrauterine lesions have been found more commonly in women undergoing infertility treatment or with history of spontaneous abortions as compared to the general fertile population. These abnormalities may be responsible for infertility or even miscarriages. Proper diagnosis and treatment of various structural abnormalities is crucial in any patient undergoing infertility management. Therefore, it is very important to assess the uterine cavity before any assisted reproductive technology (ART) procedure.[1]

Intrauterine abnormalities may be diagnosed using various techniques. Hysterosalpingography (HSG), transvaginal sonography (TVS)/sonohysterography (SHG), and hysteroscopy are different modalities used for the same. HSG has high sensitivity (98%), but low specificity (34.9%).[2] TVS has more specificity (96.3%) and sensitivity (98%) than HSG.[3] Three-dimensional ultrasound has high sensitivity for submucosal myomas and Müllerian anomalies, but reduced sensitivity and specificity for polyps (61.1% and 91.5%, respectively) relative to hysteroscopy.[4] Hysteroscopy is considered as gold standard for diagnosing intrauterine abnormalities, such as polyp, septum, adhesions, and Müllerian abnormalities. The other main advantage of hysteroscopy is that the abnormalities can be corrected in the same setting. Office or miniature hysteroscope can also be used in office setting even without anesthesia.[5]

However, whether hysteroscopy should be used as a routine procedure in the infertility workup is still unclear and there is no consensus on its efficacy and effectiveness in improving the prognosis of unselected infertile couples. The NICE (National Institute for Health and Care Excellence) guidelines have advised caution against offering hysteroscopy as a primary investigation in all infertility patients (NICE, 2013).[6]

Certain questions still need to be answered. Whether all infertility patients may be appropriate candidates for hysteroscopy? At which stage of the infertility workup [e.g., at initial assessment, when an intrauterine abnormality is suspected by noninvasive methods, prior to timed intercourse/intrauterine insemination (IUI), prior to first in vitro fertilization/intracytoplasmic sperm injection (IVF/ICSI), or after one or more failed IVF/ICSI, etc.] hysteroscopy should be done?

HYSTEROSCOPY IN INFERTILITY WITHOUT ANY SUSPECTED UTERINE ABNORMALITY

Various studies have shown an increased pregnancy rate following routine hysteroscopy in women undergoing fertility treatment. There may be different reasons for this finding:

- There may be undiagnosed or hidden abnormalities which were not picked up on HSG, ultrasonography (USG), or saline infusion sonography (SIS). The incidence of such abnormalities varies between 9.7 and 43.3% in various studies.[7-9] Two-dimensional USG (2D USG) may not differentiate between hyperplastic endometrium, submucous fibroid, or a large polyp. Also, Müllerian abnormalities may be missed on 2D USG. Also, USG might miss submucosal fibroids in cases of multiple fibroids.[10] The see and treat approach of hysteroscopy may increase the chances of positive outcome in such patients.

- Secondly, use of saline during hysteroscopy may flush the harmful antiadhesive glycoprotein molecules on the endometrium surface, such as cyclooxygenase-2 (COX-2), mucin-1 (MUC-1), and integrin $\alpha v\beta 3$.[11]
- Thirdly, cervical dilation and passage of hysteroscope through the cervical canal can lyse any cervical adhesions. This may also overcome any cervical stenosis and will help with easy embryo transfer during the subsequent cycles.[12]
- Fourthly, mechanical injury or endometrium scratching effect of the hysteroscopy procedure may increase endometrium receptivity in subsequent cycles by modulation of expression of gene and coding factors, such as lycodile in a laminate $\alpha 4$, integrin $\alpha 6$, and metallic metalloproteinases.[13,14]

However, El-Toukhy et al. in a multicentric randomized controlled (RCT) trial did not observe any significant improvement in IVF outcomes in patients who underwent pre-IVF hysteroscopy as compared to controls. This multicenter RCT of pre-IVF hysteroscopy was conducted in women with two but <4 IVF failures (Trophy trial, 2014).[15]

The inSIGHT trial which was a multicenter, randomized controlled trial included women with a normal transvaginal ultrasound of the uterine cavity and no previous hysteroscopy. 750 women were randomly assigned to either hysteroscopy with treatment of detected intracavitary abnormalities before starting IVF (hysteroscopy group) or immediate start of the IVF treatment (immediate IVF group). They found a comparable live birth rate between the 2 groups (53% vs. 51%). Hence, the authors concluded that routine hysteroscopy does not improve live birth rates in infertile women with a normal transvaginal ultrasound of the uterine cavity scheduled for a first IVF treatment and women with a normal transvaginal ultrasound should not be offered routine hysteroscopy.[16]

Contrary to this, a systematic review and meta-analysis by Hou et al. observed improved live birth and clinical pregnancy rates following outpatient hysteroscopy in infertile women undergoing ART with normal TVS or HSG. The most commonly missed lesions were endometrial polyps, submucosal fibroids, and endometritis. They suggested that since hysteroscopy is more accurate and well-tolerated procedure, it can be included in evaluation of uterine cavity.[17]

OPERATIVE HYSTEROSCOPY IN INFERTILE WOMEN WITH UTERINE ABNORMALITIES

Various studies have shown that clinical pregnancy rate increases in infertile women diagnosed with intracavitary abnormalities (i.e., endometrial polyps, intrauterine adhesions, uterine septa, and submucous fibroids) detected at USG, HSG, or SIS, who underwent operative hysteroscopy compared with those who underwent diagnostic hysteroscopy only. The specific mechanisms of action through which each one of these intrauterine abnormalities disturbs this essential reproductive process are, as yet, poorly understood.

- *Endometrial polyps and submucous myoma:* Recent papers have shown that apart from mechanical factors both endometrial polyps and submucosal myomas may adversely affect reproduction through a global decrease in endometrial *HOX* gene expression.[18] The American Society for Reproductive Medicine (ASRM) has given grade B evidence that it may be reasonable to offer myomectomy for submucous fibroids for improving clinical pregnancy rates.[19] Evidence shows that removal of ultrasound diagnosed endometrium polyps in otherwise unexplained infertility women prior to IUI can result in better pregnancy rates.[20]
- *Uterine malformations such as septate uterus and uterine synechiae* were found in >3% of a study population with a negative TVS. USG may have low sensitivity to diagnose these anomalies. However, these anomalies may be associated with increased chances of miscarriage.[21] Hysteroscopy alone may not be able to differentiate between septate and bicornuate uterus. Addition of laparoscopy is useful to differentiate between these two Müllerian abnormalities.

  Current ASRM guideline has given grade C evidence about positive impact of septum resection in women undergoing fertility treatment. However, Cochrane review states that high quality evidence is lacking regarding the resection of septum in unselected patients for infertility management.[22]
- Intrauterine adhesions (Asherman syndrome) can cause defective placentation, threatened miscarriage, and preterm labor. Hysteroscopic adhesiolysis with postoperative estrogen followed by progesterone therapy has been shown to improve endometrium pregnancy rate and reduce pregnancy losses.[23]

- *Endometritis* can cause asynchronous endometrium, delayed maturation with defective implantation, recurrent pregnancy losses, and recurrent implantation failure.[24,25] Hysteroscopic signs of endometritis are found in 4% of the patients. While diagnosis is made by histology, endometritis can be suspected by TVS based on endometrial thickening, presence of free fluid in the pelvis and painful uterine mobilization during imaging, or at hysteroscopy by the presence of edema and focal or diffuse hyperemia.[26]
- *Intrauterine synechiae,* frequently referred to as Asherman syndrome, can be a source of abnormal placentation, recurrent miscarriage, and preterm labor. Hysteroscopic adhesiolysis followed by postoperative estrogen followed by progesterone, balloon therapy, and second-look hysteroscopy with adhesiolysis have all been used for treatment of recurrent synechiae after initial adhesiolysis.[27,28]
- *Cesarean isthmoceles:* Cesarean isthmocele can cause abnormal postmenstrual bleeding which can have negative effect on cervical mucus sperm and implantation.

  Hysteroscopic excision of isthmocele can improve the pregnancy rate and reduce miscarriage rate in these patients.[28]
- *Adenomyosis* may be associated with abnormal hysteroscopic findings, such as hypervascularized endometrium, irregular endometrium, cystic hemorrhagic lesions, and pitting endometrium on hysteroscopy. These findings in combination with sonographic or magnetic resonance imaging (MRI) findings along with patient history may be important to assess the endometrium receptivity and implantation potential.[29]

CONCLUSION

Hysteroscopy is considered as gold standard for intracavitary evaluation but whether it improves reproductive outcomes relative to ultrasound or SIS in unselected patients is still unclear. Two recent trials, inSIGHT[16] and TROPHY,[15] did not show any benefit from using routine hysteroscopy. However, these studies had several limitations that may affect their generalizability. Also, subfertility's heterogeneous causes like ovarian reserve and male factor inherently make it difficult for any single test to demonstrate relevance. Timely evaluation and effective therapy are still central to optimizing the conditions for successful implantation and pregnancy.

REFERENCES

1. Taylor E, Gomel V. The uterus and fertility. Fertil Steril. 2008;89:1-16.
2. Preutthipan S, Linasmita V. A prospective comparative study between hysterosalpingography and hysteroscopy in the detection of intrauterine pathology in patients with infertility. J Obstet Gynaecol Res. 2003;29:33-7.
3. Shalev J, Meizner I, Bar-Hava I, Dicker D, Mashiach R, Ben-Rafael Z. Predictive value of transvaginalsonography performed before routine diagnostic hysteroscopy for evaluation of infertility. Fertil Steril. 2000;73:412-7.
4. Apirakviriya C, Rungruxsirivorn T, Phupong V, Wisawasukmongchol W. Diagnostic accuracy of 3D-transvaginal ultrasound in detecting uterine cavity abnormalities in infertile patients as compared with hysteroscopy. Euro J Obstet Gynecol Repro Biol. 2016; 200:24-8.
5. Bettocchi S, Ceci O, Di Venere R, Masciopinto V, Nappi L, Pansini V, et al. Operative office hysteroscopy without anesthesia: analysis of 4863 cases performed with mechanical instruments. J Am Assoc Gynecol Laparosc. 2004;11:59-61.
6. National Collaborating Centre for Women's and Children's Health (UK). Fertility: Assessment and Treatment for People with Fertility Problems. London: Royal College of Obstetricians and Gynaecologists; 2013.
7. Roma Dalfo´ A, Ubeda B, Ubeda A, Monzon M, Rotger R, Ramos R, et al. Diagnostic value of hysterosalpingography in the detection of intrauterine abnormalities: a comparison with hysteroscopy. Am J Roentgenol. 2004;183:1405-9.
8. El-Nashar IH, Nasr A. The role of hysteroscopy before intracytoplasmic sperm injection (ICSI): a randomized controlled trial. Fertil Steril. 2011;96(3):S266.
9. Elsetohy KA, Askalany AH, Hassan M, Dawood Z. Routine office hysteroscopy prior to ICSI vs. ICSI alone in patients with normal transvaginal ultrasound: a randomized controlled trial. Arch Gynecol Obstet. 2015;291:193-9.
10. Shawki HE, Elmorsy M, Eissa MK. Routine office hysteroscopy prior to ICSI and its impact on assisted reproduction program outcome: a randomized controlled trial. Middle East Fertil Soc J. 2012;17:14-21.
11. Takahashi K, Mukaida T, Tomiyama C, Oka C. High pregnancy rate after hysteroscopy with irrigation in uterine cavity prior to blastocyst transfer in patients who have failed to conceive after blastocyst transfer. Fertil Steril. 2000;74(3):S206.
12. El-Toukhy T, Sunkara S, Khalaf Y. Local endometrial injury and IVF outcome: a systematic review and meta-analysis. Reprod Bio Med Online. 2012;25:345-54.
13. Mirkin S, Arslan M, Churikov D, Corica A, Diaz J, Williams S, et al. In search of candidate genes critically expressed in the human endometrium during the window of implantation. Hum Reprod. 2005;20:2104-17.

14. Almog B, Shalom-Paz E, Dufort T, Tolandi T. Promoting implantation by local injury to the endometrium. Fertil Steril. 2010;94:2026-9.
15. El-Toukhy T, Campo R, Sunkara SK, Khalaf Y, Coomarasamy A. A multi-centre randomised controlled study of pre-IVF outpatient hysteroscopy in women with recurrent IVF implantation failure: trial of Outpatient Hysteroscopy—[TROPHY] in IVF. Reprod Health. 2009;6:20.
16. Smit J, Kasius J, Eijkemans M, Koks C, van Golde R, Nap A, et al. Hysteroscopy before in-vitro fertilisation (inSIGHT): a multicentre, randomized controlled trial. Lancet. 2016;387:2622-9.
17. Hou JH, Lu BJ, Huang YL, Chen CH, Chen CH. Outpatient hysteroscopy impact on subsequent assisted reproductive technology: a systematic review and meta-analysis in patients with normal transvaginal sonography or hysterosalpingography images. Reprod Biol Endocrinol. 2024;22(1):18.
18. Rackow BW, Taylor HS. Submucosal uterine leiomyomas have a global effect on molecular determinants of endometrial receptivity. Fertil Steril. 2010;93:2027-34.
19. Practice Committee of the American Society for Reproductive Medicine. Removal of myomas in asymptomatic patients to improve fertility and/or reduce miscarriage rate: a guideline. Fertil Steril. 2017;108:416-25.
20. Bosteels J, Kasius J, Weyers S, Broekmans FJ, Mol BW, D'Hooghe TM. Hysteroscopy for treating subfertility associated with suspected major uterine cavity abnormalities. Cochrane Database Syst Rev. 2013;1:CD009461.
21. Cholkeri-Singh A, Sasaki KJ. Hysteroscopy for infertile women: a review. J Minim Invasive Gynecol. 2015;22:353-62.
22. Practice Committee of the American Society for Reproductive Medicine. Uterine septum: a guideline. Fertil Steril. 2016;106:530-40.
23. Goldenberg M, Sivan E, Sharabi Z, Mashiach S, Lipitz S, Seidman DS. Reproductive outcome following hysteroscopic management of intrauterine septum and adhesions. Hum Reprod. 1995;10:2663-5.
24. McQueen D, Bernardi L, Stephenson M. Chronic endometritis in women with recurrent early pregnancy loss and/or fetal demise. Fertil Steril. 2014;101:1026-30.
25. Johnston-MacAnanny E, Hartnett J, Engmann L, Nulsen J, Sanders M, Benadiva C. Chronic endometritis is a frequent finding in women with recurrent implantation failure after in vitro fertilization. Fertil Steril. 2010;93:437-41.
26. Di Spiezio Sardo A, Di Carlo C, Minozzi S, Spinelli M, Pistotti V, Alviggi C, et al. Efficacy of hysteroscopy in improving reproductive outcomes of infertile couples: a systematic review and meta-analysis. Hum Reprod Update. 2016;22:479-96.
27. Robinson J, Colimon L, Isaacson K. Postoperative adhesiolysis therapy for intrauterine adhesions (Asherman's syndrome). Fertil Steril. 2008;90:409-14.
28. Gubbini G, Centini G, Nascetti D, Marra E, Moncini I, Bruni L, et al. Surgical hysteroscopic treatment of cesarean-induced isthmocele in restoring fertility: prospective study. J Minim Invasive Gynecol. 2011;18: 234-7.
29. Dakhly D, Ghada A, Moety A, Saber W, Gad Allah S, Hashem A, et al. Accuracy of hysteroscopic endomyometrial biopsy in diagnosis of adenomyosis. J Min Invasive Gynecol. 2016;23:364-71.

Noncavity-distorting Intramural Fibroids: To Remove or Not?

Mukesh Gupta

INTRODUCTION

Uterine leiomyomas (also referred to as fibroids or myomas) are the most common pelvic neoplasm in females.[1] They are noncancerous monoclonal tumors arising from the smooth muscle cells and fibroblasts of the myometrium. They arise in reproductive age females and, when symptomatic, typically present with symptoms of abnormal uterine bleeding, infertility, and/or pelvic pain/pressure. Fibroids are seen in about 30% of infertile women and they may be the sole cause of infertility in approximately 2–3%.[2] The available evidence supports removal of submucous (SM) and possibly cavity-distorting intramural (IM) fibroids to improve fertility outcomes.[3] However, the controversy revolves around removal of noncavity-distorting (NCD) IM fibroids in otherwise asymptomatic infertile patients. The chapter aims to review the effect of NCD IM fibroids on fertility and assisted reproductive technology (ART) outcomes.

CLASSIFICATION OF FIBROIDS

Depending on their location in the uterus, fibroids are classified as cervical, submucosal (SM), subserosal (SS), and intramural (IM) fibroids.

The International Federation of Gynecology and Obstetrics (FIGO) classifies fibroids into several types.[4] According to this classification, type 0, 1, and 2 are SM fibroids. Type 3 is an IM fibroid and it is distinguished from type 2 by doing a hysteroscope with the lowest possible intrauterine pressure necessary to allow visualization. There should not be any bulge into the endometrial cavity. Type 4 is the classical IM fibroid. Type 5 even though >50% is IM is often classified as SS. Types 6 and 7 are SS fibroids. **Figure 1** depicts different types of fibroids according to FIGO classification.

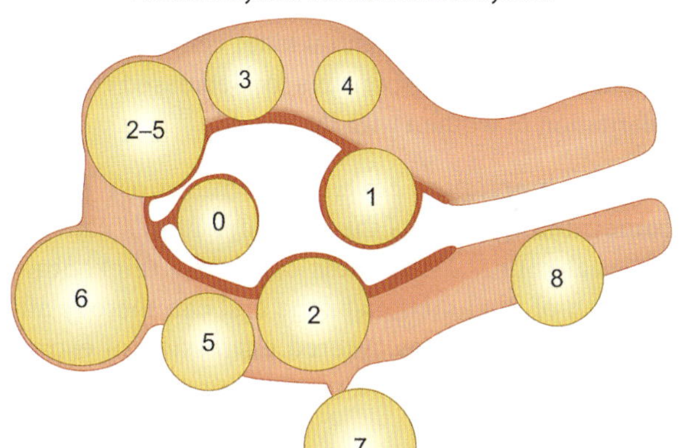

Submucous (SM)	0	Pedunculated intracavitary	
	1	<50% intramural	
	2	≥50% intramural	
	3	Contacts endometrium; 100% intramural	
Other (O)	4	Intramural	
	5	Subserous ≥50% intramural	
	6	Subserous <50% intramural	
	7	Subserous pedunculated	
	8	Other (specify, e.g., cervical and parasitic)	
Hybrid (contact both the endometrium and the serosal layer)		Two numbers are listed and separated by a hyphen. By convention, the first refers to the relationship with the endometrium while the second refers to the relationship to the serosa. One example is below	
		2–5	Submucous and subserous, each with less than half the diameter in the endometrial and peritoneal cavities, respectively

Fig. 1: The International Federation of Gynecology and Obstetrics (FIGO) classification of fibroids.

NONCAVITY-DISTORTING INTRAMURAL FIBROIDS: HOW IT AFFECTS FERTILITY?

Multiple theories have been proposed as to how NCD IM fibroids may affect fertility. It has been suggested that IM fibroids cause inflammation and endometrial vascular disorders which makes intrauterine environment nonconducive for embryo implantation.[5,6] **Figure 2** depicts the possible causes of subfertility with IM fibroids.

Effect on implantation: Intramural fibroids have been found to be associated with reduction of HOXA10 and glycodelin. Both these factors are involved in the implantation process. HOXA10 is responsible for cellular differentiation[7,8] while glycodelin[9-12] promotes angiogenesis and suppresses natural killer cells. A decrease in these factors may be responsible for decreased chances of implantation in women with IM fibroids.[13,14]

Effect on junctional zone: The innermost layer of myometrium that abuts the endometrium is called the junctional zone.[15] IM fibroids can cause thickening or disruption of the junctional zone and can thereby affect reproductive outcomes. Altered expression of estrogen and progesterone receptors may be responsible for increase thickness of junctional zone.[16,17] Additionally, a decrease in the number of natural killer cells and increase in the number of macrophage is observed in the endometrium next to the IM fibroid.[18]

Altered myometrial peristalsis: Disruption of junctional zone in women with IM and SM fibroids can cause increase in myometrial peristalsis during the midluteal phase.[13] The increase in peristalsis is observed in type 3 and type 4a fibroids compared to type 4b. Different modalities can be used to measure uterine peristalsis (UP) namely intrauterine pressure measurement, transvaginal ultrasound, and cine magnetic resonance imaging (cMRI).[19] In a study done by Yoshino et al., it was observed that women with increased uterine peristaltic frequency (≥2 movements within 3 minutes) were unlikely to get pregnant compared to those with less peristaltic frequency.[20]

Fibroid pseudocapsule: The pseudocapsule around the fibroid is shown to have upregulation of neurotransmitters, cytokines, and growth factors which can further increase the UP.[21] This can also result in pregnancy complications like premature uterine contraction causing preterm labor in women with large IM fibroid.[22]

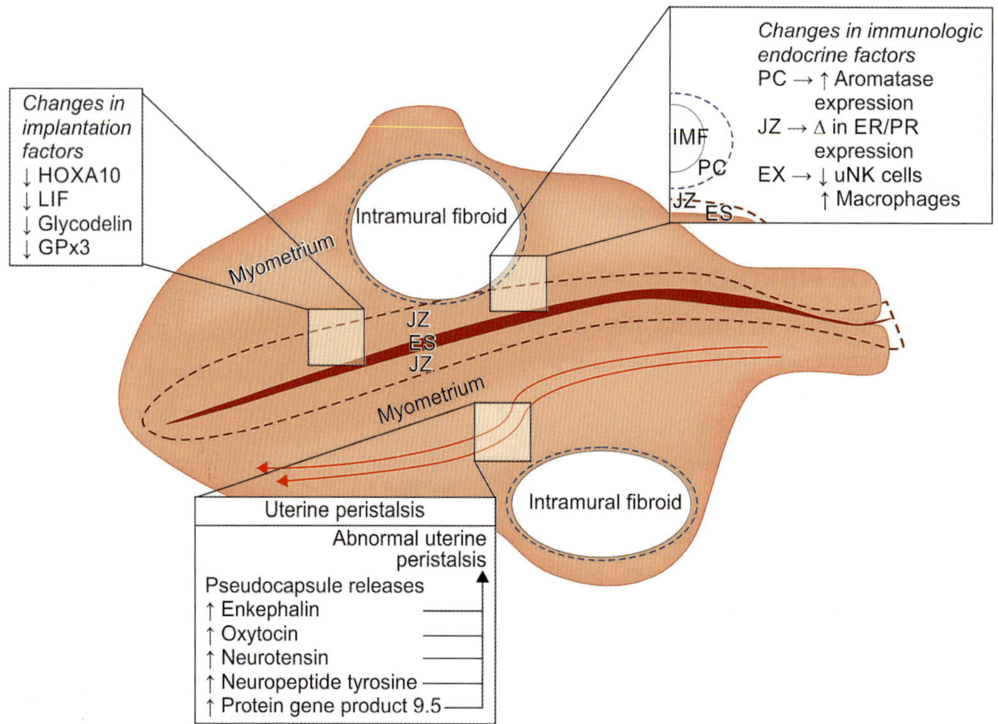

Fig. 2: Possible causes of subfertility with intramural fibroids (IMFs).(JZ: junctional zone; PC: pseudocapsule)
Source: Reprinted from Pier BD, Bates GW. Potential causes of subfertility in patients with intramural fibroids. Fertil Res Pract. 2015;1:12.

NONCAVITY-DISTORTING INTRAMURAL FIBROIDS AND INFERTILITY

There is enough evidence to prove that SM fibroids (type 1 and 2) have deleterious effect on fertility, and surgical resection of these can improve reproductive outcomes. Similarly, SS fibroids (type 5, 6, and 7) usually do not cause any harmful effects on fertility potential. However, the effects of type 3 and 4 (NCD IM fibroids) is unclear and controversial.

While some researchers have observed detrimental effects of NCD IM fibroids on pregnancy outcomes, many others have not found any difference in fertility outcomes in women with or without NCD IM fibroids. Yan et al.[23] and Khalaf et al.[24] observed significant reduction in clinical pregnancy rates (cPRs) and live birth rates (LBRs) in women with NCD IM fibroids undergoing assisted reproductive treatment. Besides the poor PR, a significant reduction in implantation rate (IR) and a higher miscarriage rates (MRs) was observed in these women. Surrey et al. observed a significantly reduced IR in women with fibroids who were <40 years of age. However, no difference in IR was observed in women >40 years of age.[25]

In contrast to these studies, many other researchers did not observe any significant difference in fertility outcomes in women with or without fibroids. Different studies by Klatsky et al.,[26] Yarali et al.,[27] Oliveira et al.,[28] and Bozdag et al.[29] reported comparable implantation and cPRs between women with or without IM fibroids. Aboulghar et al. observed that PR were lower in women with fibroids <5 mm away from endometrial lining but no significant difference was observed with fibroids >5 mm away from endometrium.[30]

Meta-analysis by Sunkara et al. and Wang et al. reported significant reduction in cPR and LBR in women with IM fibroids.[31,32] However Sunkara et al. found no reduction in IR or increase in MRs. Wang et al. on the other hand demonstrated a decrease in IR and increase in MR with IM fibroids.

Size, Location, and Number of Intramural Fibroid and Fertility

Several studies have evaluated the effect of size of fibroid on the reproductive outcomes. Yan et al. observed a significant reduction in IR, cPR, and LBR in women with fibroid diameter >2 cm.[23] Christopoulos et al. and Vimercati et al. reported that NCD fibroids of >3 cm and 4 cm respectively can have adverse impact on the pregnancy outcomes.[33,34] Another study by Oliveira et al. supported the same findings.[28]

However, no correlation was found between the number and location of IM fibroids and the reproductive outcomes after IVF/ICSI treatment.

IS REMOVAL OF INTRAMURAL FIBROIDS BENEFICIAL?

Myomectomy is major surgery with significant surgical morbidities. The risks and benefits of the surgery must be kept in mind before planning the procedure. While few authors have found significant improvement in fertility outcomes after myoma removal for NCD IM fibroids, many others do not recommend to do the procedure routinely.

Bulletti et al. reported higher PR and LBR postlaparoscopic myomectomy among patients with IM fibroids >5 cm, compared to the nonsurgical group (LBR 42% vs. 12%).[35] Campo et al. also reported significantly better reproductive outcomes after surgery.[36] Yoshino et al. identified women IM fibroids with increased UP by doing cMRI. They reported significant reduction in UP and better pregnancy outcomes after myomectomy.[20] Kolankaya et al. stated that most surgeons recommend surgery for big fibroids (>7 cm) or in women with multiple failed IVF cycles.[37]

Aboulghar et al. however did not observe any improvement in the cPR after surgery for IM fibroids.[30] Carranza-Mamane B et al. also advised against surgery for NCD IM fibroids regardless of the size of the fibroid.[38] A systematic review by Pritts et al. concluded that removal of NCD IM fibroids does not increase the cPR and LBR significantly.[39] Cochrane database systematic review also did not report any improvement in fertility outcomes after the surgery regardless of the location of the fibroid.[40] Many other authors recommend surgery for cases like multiple implantation failure, recurrent miscarriages, or fibroid-related obstetric complications.

A recent systematic review and meta-analysis by Rikhraj et al. reported that patients with NCD IM fibroids had 44% lower odds of live birth and 32% lower odds of clinical pregnancy.[41] However, whether removal of these fibroids improves IVF outcomes or not needs to be evaluated in further well-designed prospective studies.

RECOMMENDATIONS AND CONCLUSION

In contrast to submucosal fibroids, there are no clear recommendations concerning NCD IM fibroids. There is no consensus as to whether IM fibroids should be removed in women with infertility. Many clinicians would recommend removal of IM fibroids if they are ≥5 cm in diameter. Although IM fibroids are reported to be associated with poorer pregnancy outcomes, women who underwent myomectomy for IM fibroids experienced no benefit with regard to pregnancy outcomes compared to controls. Regrettably, studies addressing this specific question and included in the Cochrane analysis are scarce and do not provide precise recommendations. The procedure should be discussed individually with each patient, and other alternatives to myomectomy including gonadotropin-releasing hormone (GnRH) agonist, ulipristal acetate, magnetic resonance-guided focused ultrasound (MRgFUS), and uterine artery embolization should be considered and discussed as per the case.

REFERENCES

1. Baird DD, Dunson DB, Hill MC, Cousins D, Schectman JM. High cumulative incidence of uterine leiomyoma in black and white women: ultrasound evidence. Am J Obstet Gynecol. 2003;188(1):100-7.
2. Buttram VC Jr, Reiter RC. Uterine leiomyomata: etiology, symptomatology, and management. Fertil Steril. 1981; 36(4):433-45.
3. Lasmar RB, Barrozo PR, Dias R, Oliveira MA. Submucous myomas: a new presurgical classification to evaluate the viability of hysteroscopic surgical treatment—preliminary report. J Minim Invasive Gynecol. 2005;12(4):308-11.
4. Munro MG, Critchley HO, Fraser IS. The two FIGO systems for normal and abnormal uterine bleeding symptoms and classification of causes of abnormal uterine bleeding in the reproductive years: 2018 revisions. Int J Gynaecol Obstet. 2018;143:393-408.
5. Pier BD, Bates GW. Potential causes of subfertility in patients with intramural fibroids. Fertil Res Pract. 2015;1:12.
6. Cakmak H, Taylor HS. Implantation failure: molecular mechanisms and clinical treatment. Hum Reprod Update. 2011;17:242-53.
7. Matsuzaki S, Canis M, Darcha C, Pouly JL, Mage G. HOXA-10 expression in the mid-secretory endometrium of infertile patients with either endometriosis, uterine fibromas or unexplained infertility. Hum Reprod. 2009;24(12):3180-7.
8. Alizadeh Z, Faramarzi S, Saidijam M, Alizamir T, Esna-Ashari F, Shabab N, et al. Effect of intramural myomectomy on endometrial HOXA10 and HOXA11 mRNA expression at the time of implantation window. Iran J Reprod Med. 2013;11(12):983-8.
9. Seppälä M, Koistinen H, Koistinen R, Chiu PC, Yeung WS. Glycosylation related actions of glycodelin: gamete, cumulus cell, immune cell and clinical associations. Hum Reprod Update. 2007;13(3):275-87.
10. Ben-Nagi J, Miell J, Mavrelos D, Naftalin J, Lee C, Jurkovic D. Endometrial implantation factors in women with submucous uterine fibroids. Reprod Biomed Online. 2010; 21(5):610-5.
11. Richlin SS, Ramachandran S, Shanti A, Murphy AA, Parthasarathy S. Glycodelin levels in uterine flushings and in plasma of patients with leiomyomas and polyps: implications for implantation. Hum Reprod. 2002;17(10): 2742-7.
12. Farimani Sanoee M, Alizamir T, Faramarzi S, Saidijam M, Yadegarazari R, Shabab N, et al. Effect of myomectomy on endometrial glutathione peroxidase 3 (GPx3) and glycodelin mRNA expression at the time of the implantation window. Iran Biomed J. 2014;18(2):60-6.
13. Brosens I, Derwig I, Brosens J, Fusi L, Benagiano G, Pijnenborg R. The enigmatic uterine junctional zone: the missing link between reproductive disorders and major obstetrical disorders? Hum Reprod. 2010;25(3):569-74.
14. Ciavattini A, Di Giuseppe J, Stortoni P, Montik N, Giannubilo SR, Litta P, et al. Uterine fibroids: pathogenesis and interactions with endometrium and endomyometrial junction. Obstet Gynecol Int. 2013;2013:173184.
15. Hricak H, Alpers C, Crooks LE, Sheldon PE. Magnetic resonance imaging of the female pelvis: initial experience. AJR Am J Roentgenol. 1983;141(6):1119-28.
16. Ishikawa H, Reierstad S, Demura M, Rademaker AW, Kasai T, Inoue M, et al. High aromatase expression in uterine leiomyoma tissues of African-American women. J Clin Endocrinol Metab. 2009;94(5):1752-6.
17. Jakimiuk AJ, Bogusiewicz M, Tarkowski R, Dziduch P, Adamiak A, Wróbel A, et al. Estrogen receptor alpha and beta expression in uterine leiomyomas from premenopausal women. Fertil Steril. 2004;82(Suppl 3):1244-9.
18. Kitaya K, Yasuo T. Leukocyte density and composition in human cycling endometrium with uterine fibroids. Hum Immunol. 2010;71:158-63.
19. Kuijsters NPM, Methorst WG, Kortenhorst MSQ, Rabotti C, Mischi M, Schoot BC. Uterine peristalsis and fertility: current knowledge and future perspectives: a review and meta-analysis. Reprod Biomed Online. 2017;35(1):50-71.
20. Yoshino O, Hayashi T, Osuga Y, Orisaka M, Asada H, Okuda S, et al. Decreased pregnancy rate is linked to abnormal uterine peristalsis caused by intramural fibroids. Hum Reprod. 2010;25(10):2475-9.
21. Malvasi A, Cavallotti C, Nicolardi G, Pellegrino M, Dell'Edera D, Vergara D, et al. NT, NPY and PGP 9.5 presence in myomettrium and in fibroid pseudocapsule and their possible impact on muscular physiology. Gynecol Endocrinol. 2013;29(2):177-81.
22. Shavell VI, Thakur M, Sawant A, Kruger ML, Jones TB, Singh M, et al. Adverse obstetric outcomes associated with

sonographically identified large uterine fibroids. Fertil Steril. 2012;97(1):107-10.

23. Yan L, Yu Q, Zhang YN, Guo Z, Li Z, Niu J, et al. Effect of type 3 intramural fibroids on in vitro fertilization-intracytoplasmic sperm injection outcomes: a retrospective cohort study. Fertil Steril. 2018;109(5):817-822.e2.
24. Khalaf Y, Ross C, El-Toukhy T, Hart R, Seed P, Braude P. The effect of small intramural uterine fibroids on the cumulative outcome of assisted conception. Hum Reprod. 2006;21(10):2640-4.
25. Surrey ES, Lietz AK, Schoolcraft WB. Impact of intramural leiomyomata in patients with a normal endometrial cavity on in vitro fertilization-embryo transfer cycle outcome. Fertil Steril. 2001;75:405-10.
26. Klatsky PC, Lane DE, Ryan IP, Fujimoto VY. The effect of fibroids without cavity involvement on ART outcomes independent of ovarian age. Hum Reprod. 2007;22(2):521-6.
27. Yarali H, Bukulmez O. The effect of intramural and subserosal uterine fibroids on implantation rate and clinical pregnancy rate in patients having ICSI. Arch Gynecol Obstet. 2002;266:30-3.
28. Oliveira FG, Abdelmassih VG, Diamond MP, Dozortsev D, Melo NR, Abdelmassih R. Impact of subserosal and intramural uterine fibroids that do not distort the endometrial cavity on the outcome of in vitro fertilization-intracytoplasmic sperm injection. Fertil Steril. 2004;81(3): 582-7.
29. Bozdag G, Esinler I, Boynukalin K, Aksu T, Gunalp S, Gurgan T. Single intramural leiomyoma with normal hysteroscopic findings does not affect ICSI-embryo transfer outcome. Reprod Biomed Online. 2009;19(2):276-80.
30. Aboulghar MM, Al-Inany HG, Aboulghar MA, Serour GI, Mansour RT. The effect of IM fibroids on the outcome of IVF. Middle East Fertil Soc J. 2004;9:263-7.
31. Sunkara SK, Khairy M, El-Toukhy T, Khalaf Y, Coomarasamy A. The effect of intramural fibroids without uterine cavity involvement on the outcome of IVF treatment: a systematic review and meta-analysis. Hum Reprod. 2010;25(2):418-29.
32. Wang X, Chen L, Wang H, Li Q, Liu X, Qi H. The Impact of Noncavity-Distorting Intramural Fibroids on the Efficacy of In Vitro Fertilization-Embryo Transfer: An Updated Meta-Analysis. Biomed Res Int. 2018;2018:8924703.
33. Christopoulos G, Vlismas A, Salim R, Islam R, Trew G, Lavery S. Fibroids that do not distort the uterine cavity and IVF success rates: an observational study using extensive matching criteria. BJOG. 2017;124(4):615-21.
34. Vimercati A, Scioscia M, Lorusso F, Laera AF, Lamanna G, Coluccia A, et al. Do uterine fibroids affect IVF outcomes? Reprod Biomed Online. 2007;15(6):686-91.
35. Bulletti C, De Ziegler D, Polli V, Flamigni C. The role of leiomyomas in infertility. J Am Assoc Gynecol Laparosc. 1999;6(4):441-5.
36. Campo S, Campo V, Gambadauro P. Reproductive outcome before and after laparoscopic or abdominal myomectomy for subserous or intramural myomas. Eur J Obstet Gynecol Reprod Biol. 2003;110:215-9.
37. Kolankaya A, Arici A. Myomas and assisted reproductive technologies: when and how to act? Obstet Gynecol Clin North Am. 2006;33:145-52.
38. Carranza-Mamane B, Havelock J, Hemmings R; Reproductive endocrinology and infertility committee; special contributor. The management of uterine fibroids in women with otherwise unexplained infertility. J Obstet Gynaecol Can. 2015;37(3):277-85.
39. Pritts EA, Parker WH, Olive DL. Fibroids and infertility: an updated systemic review of evidence. Fertil Steril. 2009; 91:1215-23.
40. Metwally M, Cheong YC, Horne AW. Surgical treatment of fibroids for subfertility. Cochrane Database Syst Rev. 2012;11:CD003857.
41. Rikhraj K, Tan J, Taskin O, Albert AY, Yong P, Bedaiwy MA. The Impact of Noncavity-Distorting Intramural Fibroids on Live Birth Rate in In Vitro Fertilization Cycles: A Systematic Review and Meta-Analysis. J Womens Health (Larchmt). 2020;29(2):210-9.

Chapter

Endometrioma and Infertility: To Excise or Not?

Charumati V Pekhale, Pinky R Shah

INTRODUCTION

Endometriosis is presence of endometrial tissue at ectopic sites other than uterus. Its chronic inflammatory disease and common gynecological condition of unknown origin commonly present with pelvic pain, dysmenorrhea, and subfertility. It affects about 10% childbearing age group patients presenting in gynecology outpatient department, not only causes symptoms and subfertility but also affects quality of life.[1] Endometriosis causes subfertility by attributing to pelvic adhesions, tubal blockages, and altered anatomy. Ovarian endometriomas (OMAs: cyst formed within the ovary with ectopic endometrial tissue) are seen in around 17–44% of patients diagnosed with endometriosis. It is frequently found in the severe form of the disease.[2,3] The monthly fecundity rate in women with endometriosis has been documented to range from 2 to 10%, a figure lower than the 15–20% reported for healthy women. Additionally, there is an inverse relationship between the severity of the disease and fecundity, where the greater the severity, the lower the fecundity.[4] Without intervention, approximately 50% of women with mild endometriosis can conceive. However, for those with moderate endometriosis, only 25% can conceive, and only a few with severe disease can conceive.[5] Consequently, the probability of pregnancy is closely linked to the severity of endometriosis. Existence of endometrioma in patients with subfertility makes its challenging and delicate situation where decision of surgery to address the cyst serves as clinical dilemma which needs a delicate balance between benefits and adverse impact of surgery on ovarian reserve. This chapter will address potential benefits, risks involved with surgery, and evidence-based discussion of endometrioma cyst excision, to do or not to do prior in vitro fertilization (IVF) treatment!

ENDOMETRIOMA AND SUBFERTILITY

Endometriosis leads to immunological, biochemical, endocrine, and genetic derangements and also is associated with poor oocyte/embryo quality and endometrium.[6-8] Studies have concluded that roughly 25–50% of infertile women have endometriosis, and about 30–50% of women with endometriosis are infertile.[9,10] OMAs accounting for 35% of benign ovarian cysts present with chronic pelvic pain and dyspareunia.[11] Options available for endometrioma include conservative management, medical, and surgical management. Various surgical routes are laparotomy, laparoscopy, and robotic surgery. Laparoscopy is most preferred method due to early recovery, short stay, and being acceptable method of excision and resection of cyst and being able to obtain a histological diagnosis.[12] There are different school of thoughts when it comes to addressing endometrioma cyst in patients with subfertility. Some prefer conservative management and not doing surgery and other prefer surgical option believing that surgery at early stage of cyst will be beneficial.[13]

ENDOMETRIOMA AND POSSIBLE MECHANISM ASSOCIATED WITH INFERTILITY

Chronic Inflammation

Endometriosis is a chronic inflammatory condition which is linked to dysregulation of immune system, and is associated with increase in T cells, immune cell numbers, mast cells, natural killer cells, along with elevated growth factors, chemokines, and cytokines in peritoneal fluid.[14-16] Endometrioma is associated with defective folliculogenesis, poor oocyte quality, and impaired ovarian function affected by heightened state of inflammation.[17]

Oocyte and Embryo Quality

Endometriomas and associated pelvic endometriosis may adversely affect oocyte and embryo quality. Due to altered follicular environment, associated with raised interleukin-6 (IL-6), progesterone, reduced vascular endothelial growth factor (VEGF) there is impairment in oocyte quality, leading to reduced embryo quality and its development potential.[18] Embryo development is slower in women with endometriosis in comparison with tubal disease. Women who had moderate-to-severe endometriosis showed similar pregnancy rates with donor egg programmed when compared with other donor egg recipients.[8,19]

Effect on Ovarian Reserve

Ovarian endometrioma is associated with reduction in ovarian reserve by various ways:

- Due to inflammatory reaction and chronic inflammatory condition, it leads to tissue oxidative stress, fibrosis, and thus finally leading to follicle depletion.[20]
- Primordial follicles are found to reduce on histology of the ovarian tissue which thus impacts the response to gonadotropin injections in IVF treatment.[21]
- Negative effect on ovarian reserve is due to chronic mechanical stretching of the ovarian cortex and free iron radicals which could be toxic post its diffusion through endometrioma.[22]

Effect on Endometrial Receptivity

Endometrioma is associated alerted receptivity due to associated progesterone resistance, reduction in cell apoptosis, increased cell proliferation, thus leading to dysregulation of biomarkers which are associated with endometrial receptivity.[23]

BENEFITS OF SURGERY FOR ENDOMETRIOMA BEFORE IN VITRO FERTILIZATION

- *Improved access to dominant follicles during ovum pick-up:* It helps more in huge endometrioma beyond 4–5 cm in size and also in patients where ovary is fixed, and surgery can facilitate access to the follicles. More number of follicles can be aspirated and thus a greater number of embryos can be formed and available for embryo transfer and further increasing pool of frozen embryos.
- *Decrease in the risk of pelvic abscess:* Endometriotic cyst fluid can serve as an excellent culture for organisms and increase the spread of organisms leading to pelvic abscess. Study suggested that risk of pelvic abscess for patients undergoing ovum pick-up with endometrioma is below 1.7 %. Risk of accidental puncturing the endometriotic cyst at the time of ovum pick-up was reported up to 2.8% but no case of pelvic infection was reported.[24] With proper surgical expertise and antibiotic cover, risk can be further reduced, and occurrence of pelvic abscess can be prevented. The European Society of Human Reproduction and Embryology (ESHRE) recommends routine prophylactic administration of antibiotics post-ovum pick-up in cases on endometrioma.[25]
- *Diagnosing occult or early-stage malignancy:* Risk of malignancy in endometrioma as documented in two largest series is reported as to be 0.8 and 0.9%.[26,27] Thus, it concludes that even if the risk is very less but it is possible to progress to malignancy. There an association of endometrioma and ovarian cancer of clear cell is documented in many prospective and retrospective studies.[28] Surgery helps to avail the histological diagnosis. With good annual ultrasound along with help of Doppler studies a stringent follow-up can be kept but still that cannot replace histological diagnosis available in surgery.
- Preventing risk of rupture or torsion of OMA in later future
- *Prevention of pregnancy related complications associated with endometrioma/endometriosis:* It is postulated that patients with existing endometrioma are prone to preterm labor and placenta previa in pregnancy. In patient with endometrioma/endometriosis, the delayed implantation can lead to spontaneous pregnancy loss, intrauterine growth restriction (IUGR), placenta previa, and placental insufficiency. Also due to premature decidual senescence, there is increased risk of preterm delivery and small for gestational age babies.[29] Even though the association has been seen between endometriosis and pregnancy complication, there is no clear evidence that prophylactic surgery will prevent these complications.

RISKS ASSOCIATED WITH SURGERY FOR ENDOMETRIOMA BEFORE IN VITRO FERTILIZATION

- *Increase cost and complications associated with surgery:* Laparoscopy is the preferred method for surgical intervention for endometrioma due to vast expertise available, short hospital stay, and early recovery. Despite its advantages, it is still associated with complications.
- *Loss of normal ovarian tissue during surgery:* The preferred method for addressing endometrioma is excision[30] and it is associated with risk of removal of normal ovarian tissue. Studies concluded due to thick ovarian capsule and associated difficulty in surgery, primordial follicles are seen in >50% of endometriotic tissue removed.[25] Inadvertent removal of normal ovarian tissue along with primordial follicles is probably attributed to the pathogenic theory of endometrioma cyst being pseudocyst with wall being the inverted ovarian cortex. Study concluded cystectomy done for endometrioma even if done with accurate precautions and precision still can lead to significant removal of normal ovarian tissue. The thickness of normal ovarian tissue correlated the size on endometrioma and cyst wall diameter.[31] Laparoscopic stripping technique is found to be associated with loss of ovarian tissue seen in specimens, which is 10 times higher in endometrioma when compared to benign ovarian masses.[32]

  Factors associated with higher loss of normal ovarian tissue postsurgery are:
  - Young patients associated with small size of cyst[33]
  - Associated difficulty in finding cleavage between endometriotic tissue and normal ovary, and fibro-elastic ovaries with the OMA[33]
  - Surgical tissue if it is taken near the ovarian hilum
- *Reduced ovarian responsiveness post-endometrioma surgery:* IVF success depends on ovarian responsiveness, number of mature eggs obtained, and number of embryos formed. Ovarian response can be reduced after excision of endometrioma due to removal of normal ovarian tissue. In a meta-analysis, it was found that post surgery the dose of gonadotropins required for ovarian stimulation was found to be high in patients with previous surgery for endometrioma. Peak estradiol and metaphases II eggs were found to be lower in the operated ovary. Study by Gupta et al. found that relatively fewer follicles 0.9 [95% confidence interval (CI): 21.4 and 20.3] and fewer oocytes 1.69 [95% CI: (–3.16 and –0.23)] were retrieved from the affected ovary when compared to unaffected ovary.[34] Post-endometrioma surgery retrieval of fewer oocytes was seen than the unaffected contralateral ovary.[35]
- *Ovarian damage mediated by surgery:* Surgery by stripping technique causes damage to the ovary by removal of normal ovarian tissue[36] and also combine damage due to electrocoagulation leading to vascular compromise and local inflammation. All factors together leads to reduced ovarian function, stroma, and its vascularity. There is approximately 2.4% risk of ovarian failure in patients operated of bilateral endometrioma.[37]
- *Reduction in serum anti-Müllerian hormone (AMH):* Serum AMH was found to be lower in patients with stage IV endometriosis associated with bilateral endometrioma in comparison to unilateral endometrioma.[38] AMH was not found to be affected by laterality or size of endometrioma in one study.[39] Literature thus suggests to measure serum AMH before going for surgery and documenting it, and using it for decision-making and counseling. Studies have shown fall of ovarian reserve by documenting serum AMH post-endometrioma surgery more in bilateral endometrioma.[40] More decline in serum AMH was found when endometrioma was beyond 5 cm in size.[41] AMH value can be influenced by function of the other normal gonad and it represents both the ovaries. Some studies suggested fall in AMH is seen to be sustained up to 6–9 months postsurgery[41] with maximum recovery seen 3 months postsurgery.[42]
- *Reduction in antral follicle count (AFC):* AFC may not be a reliable marker as it is difficult to assess and count them preoperatively due to presence of the cyst. Some studies suggest that AFC can be more reliable than AMH as it is not affected by laterality, and they found rise in AFC despite fall in AMH 6 months postsurgery.[41]
- *Effect of ovarian surgery on ovarian reserve:* Postsurgery reduction in ovarian reserve (AMH and AFC) can be attributed to surgical technique per se where normal ovarian tissue is destroyed or it can be attributed to postsurgical edema, ischemia, inflammation, and vascular injury.[43,44] Long-term postsurgical vascular

injury is responsible for further reduction in the ovarian reserve.[42,45]

ENDOMETRIOMA AND IN VITRO FERTILIZATION

There are different school of thoughts and evidence available. Extensive evidence suggested that the presence of OMA affected ovarian responsiveness to superovulation at the time of ART.[46,47] Study done by Somigliana et al. concluded that patients with unilateral endometrioma had reduced AFC, reduced number of follicles, and less mature oocytes available. Thus, they concluded that endometrioma is associated with reduced ovarian responsiveness.[48] While other retrospective study found no effect of presence of unilateral endometrioma in terms of number of follicles formed or oocytes retrieved when compared to patients without endometrioma. Further, they found no relation of number or size of endometrioma in terms of ovarian response.[49] A meta-analysis by Hamdan et al. concluded that even though number of oocytes retrieved were less and the cycle cancellation rates were higher in patients with endometrioma undergoing IVF without any surgical intervention, but there was no difference in clinical pregnancy rate and live birth rates when compared to those who did not underwent endometrioma surgery before the IVF cycle.[46]

Various studies have varied conclusion on effect of surgery on ovarian response for patients going for IVF postsurgery. On one hand a study by Benaglia et al. reported 12 out of 93 patients did not show any difference in ovarian response in patients with unilateral endometrioma who underwent surgical correction while on other hand Hong et al. demonstrated no difference in IVF outcome in patients with reduced ovarian reserve postsurgery to patients with reduced ovarian reserve without surgery.[50,51]

The systematic review that compared IVF outcome in patients with endometrioma with prior surgery and without any prior IVF surgical correction, concluded both groups had similar clinical pregnancy rates, live birth rate, and number of oocytes retrieved.[46]

The European Society of Human Reproduction and Embryology guidelines recommend to avoid surgical correction of endometrioma before IVF as it does not improve the outcome and suggested that any surgical correction decision should be based on ovarian reserve. Further, they concluded that specific value of ovarian reserve test for decision-making needs proper research.[25]

In vitro fertilization treatment related to temporary exposure to estrogen in patients with endometrioma/endometriosis did not show to increase in disease progression or recurrence. IVF treatment does not affect the course of endometrioma disease.[52]

SURGERY FOR ENDOMETRIOMA

Endometrioma surgery can be more harmful in terms of reduction in ovarian reserve in certain group of patients, cases with history of previous surgery, and bilateral endometrioma. Postsurgery presence of primordial follicle seen in histology tissue suggests possible risk of future reduction in ovarian reserve. Studies suggest various ovarian tissue parts [hilum, intermediate part of cyst wall, and cyst adhesion site) seen on histology will predict loss of ovarian reserve. Tissue at ovarian hilum mainly was found to contain primary and secondary follicles, while tissue at cyst adhesion site and intermediate ovarian cyst tissue comprised of primordial follicles or tissue with no follicles.[53]

It is very important to go through literature to study if surgery offered benefits as compared to harm offered. Various techniques available for addressing endometriotic cysts are excision/stripping, drainage of the cyst, vaporization, and coagulation. Higher risk of reduction of ovarian reserve is seen in cases where surgery is done with stripping technique and in patients with bilateral endometrioma. Study randomized patients with bilateral endometrioma to surgical options of stripping and coagulation. They found postintervention ovarian response, AFC, and ovarian volume significantly reduced in the stripping group when compared to coagulation groups.[54]

Similarly, study demonstrated that AMH did not decrease in patients who underwent ablation procedure done in three-step approach [laparoscopic drainage followed by 3 months course of gonadotropin-releasing hormone (GnRH) analog that reduced cyst to 50% of its size followed by second-look laparoscopic CO_2 laser vaporization] when compared to stripping technique. AFC was found to be significantly higher in post three-step procedure as compared to no significant change seen postcystectomy.[55]

Considering effect on ovarian reserve of the stripping technique, Donnez et al. proposed more conservative

Flowchart 1: Individualized decision in current era whether to plan surgery or direct IVF.[17,61]

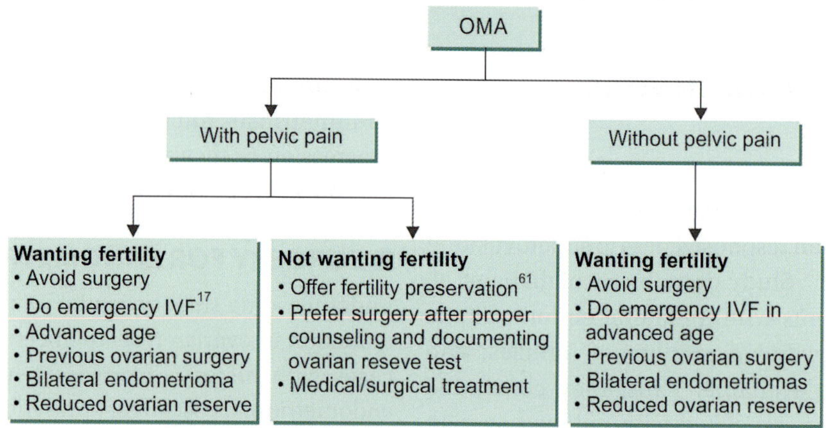

(IVF: in vitro fertilization; OMA: ovarian endometrioma)

surgical approach that combines benefits of both stripping and ablation technique. Surgery opts to excise large part of endometrioma by stripping technique and using conservative ablation technique when approaching to the hilum of the ovary. This thus preserves most of the ovarian pool of primordial follicles. After 6 months of follow-up, the authors did not find any statistical difference between AFC and ovarian volume between operated and contralateral normal ovary. The authors found this combined surgical approach reported 41% spontaneous pregnancy rate with 2% recurrence of the cyst, after mean follow-up of 8.3 months. However, the authors did not report conception rate after IVF treatment, thus more studies are needed before applying this technique before IVF treatment.[56]

Conservative surgical techniques should be opted to restrict postsurgical reduction on ovarian reserve. Following measures can be used:

- Avoiding stripping technique near hilum where maximum blood vessels are present.
- Tissue sparing conservative approach where traditional cystectomy is done for tissue which is away from the ovary and CO_2 laser is used for 10–20% of the tissue near to ovarian hilum.
- When using bipolar cautery, caution should be used applied by limiting coagulation time, applying only when concave area is under vision, and avoiding blind cauterization.

Garcia-Velasco conducted case-control study comparing patients with endometrioma who directly went for IVF and those who underwent laparoscopic cystectomy. They found no difference in mature oocytes retrieved, fertilization, implantation rate, and pregnancy rate, and thus the authors concluded surgical excision does not offer any improvement and nor does it compromise fertility.[57]

Prospective randomized study compared patients with endometrioma who went for direct intracytoplasmic sperm injection (ICSI) and those who underwent ovarian surgery and did ICSI treatment 3 months postsurgery. The postovarian surgery group when compared to direct IVF group had longer IVF cycle stimulation (14 days vs. 10.8 days), needed high follicle-stimulating hormone (FSH) requirements (4,575 IU vs. 3,675 IU) and had lower number of oocytes retrieved (7.8 vs. 8.6). There was no difference in the fertilization and implantation rates in both groups.[58]

Study concluded that surgery if done for bilateral endometrioma significantly impaired IVF outcome as had high rate of poor response, cycle cancelation, lower mature oocytes, and less embryos formed.[59]

In vitro fertilization treatment is now widely accepted approach for infertile women and surgical pretreatment does not seem to be necessary for managing OMA pre-IVF.[60]

In the era of individualized treatment, decision of surgery to do or not to do should be combined with symptoms, desire for fertility, previous surgery, unilateral or bilateral endometrioma, and existing ovarian reserve test value **(Flowchart 1)**.

Direct IVF treatment can be considered in patients who desire fertility, are not having painful symptoms, who are not willing for surgical option and who have coexistent adenomyosis.[62]

Objectives to decide the plan of management should be based on “do no harm by avoiding unnecessary ovarian surgeries to avoid further reduction in the ovarian reserve". Secondly, target is to perform surgery once in lifetime and do at appropriate time. Assisted reproductive technique (ART) can be considered as first line in specific group of patients and surgery can be reserved to later date when fertility is planned, patient is having painful symptoms and there is no or less fear of falling ovarian reserve. Going directly for IVF treatment helps to avoid surgical complications, reduces cost, and reduced time to pregnancy, especially in women in small endometrioma. Endometrioma <3 cm does not reduce the IVF treatment success and in these patients proceeding directly to IVF is more beneficial. It is very vital to offer fertility preservation for patients with OMA not wanting for immediate fertility.

CONCLUSION

Ovarian endometriomas are the most common presentation in endometriosis and affect fertility by mechanical stretching of ovarian cortex, oxidative stress, and inflammation and fibrosis of the tissue. The surgical approach is most common way to deal with them prior to IVF and of the surgical approach stripping of ovarian wall is the most preferred technique. But, both endometrioma and its surgical correction are associated with loss of ovarian volume and ovarian tissue. Studies have concluded neither surgical correction improves IVF outcome and nor the endometrioma adversely affects IVF outcome. It is practical to consider direct IVF treatment is patients with advanced age, low ovarian reserve, bilateral endometrioma, or previous endometrioma surgery. Surgical approach can be considered in patients after proper counseling of fall in ovarian reserve postsurgery. Surgery can also be considered prior to IVF to improve access to the follicles, prevent risk of ovarian abscess, rupture, and torsion and also to avail histological diagnosis to rule out malignancy. Endometrioma excision prior to IVF treatment is not mandatory as its removal does not improve the IVF outcome. Risk versus benefits evaluation and individualized treatment is needed. Fertility preservation should be offered to all patients with OMA not planning immediate fertility and counseling should be done with help of ovarian reserve tests.

Further studies and meta-analysis are needed to compare expectant management versus surgical approach in patients going for IVF treatment. Further research is needed to compare outcome of various surgical options in terms of ovarian reserve postsurgery.

REFERENCES

1. Giudice LC. Clinical practice. Endometriosis. N Engl J Med. 2010;362:2389-98.
2. Redwine DB. Ovarian endometriosis: a marker for more extensive pelvic and intestinal disease. Fertil Steril. 1999;72:310-5.
3. Jenkins S, Olive DL, Haney AF. Endometriosis: pathogenetic implications of the anatomic distribution. Obstet Gynecol. 1986;67:335-8.
4. Collins JA, Burrows EA, Wilan AR. The prognosis for live birth among untreated infertile couples. Fertil Steril. 1995;64:22-8.
5. Olive DL, Stohs GF, Metzger DA, Franklin RR. Expectant management and hydrotubations in the treatment of endometriosis-associated infertility. Fertil Steril. 1985; 44:35-41.
6. Miller JE, Ahn SH, Monsanto SP, Khalaj K, Koti M, Tayade C. Implications of immune dysfunction on endometriosis associated infertility. Oncotarget. 2017;8:7138-47.
7. Ahn SH, Monsanto SP, Miller C, Singh SS, Thomas R, Tayade C. Pathophysiology and immune dysfunction in endometriosis. Biomed Res Int. 2015;2015:795976.
8. Pellicer A, Oliveira N, Ruiz A, Remohi J, Simon C. Exploring the mechanism(s) of endometriosis-related infertility: an analysis of embryo development and implantation in assisted reproduction. Hum Reprod. 1995;10 Suppl 2:91-7.
9. Missmer SA, Hankinson SE, Spiegelman D, Barbieri RL, Marshall LM, Hunter DJ. Incidence of laparoscopically confirmed endometriosis by demographic, anthropometric, and lifestyle factors. Am J Epidemiol. 2004;160:784-96.
10. Practice Committee of the American Society for Reproductive Medicine. Endometriosis and infertility: a committee opinion. Fertil Steril. 2012;98:591-8.
11. Vercellini P. Endometriosis: What pain it is? Semin Reprod Endocrinol. 1997;15:251-6.
12. Ahmad G, O'Flynn H, Duffy JM, Phillips K, Watson A. Laparoscopic entry techniques. Cochrane Database Syst Rev. 2012;(2):CD006583.
13. Kitajima M, Defrere S, Dolmans MM, Colette S, Squifflet J, Van Langendonckt A, et al. Endometriomas as a possible cause of reduced ovarian reserve in women with endometriosis. Fertil Steril. 2011;96:685-91.
14. Ryan IP, Tseng JF, Schriock ED, Khorram O, Landers DV, Taylor RN. Interleukin-8 concentrations are elevated in peritoneal fluid of women with endometriosis. Fertil Steril. 1995;63:929-32.
15. Taketani Y, Kuo TM, Mizuno M. Comparison of cytokine levels and embryo toxicity in peritoneal fluid in infertile women with untreated or treated endometriosis. Am J Obstet Gynecol. 1992;167:265-70.

16. Halme J, Becker S, Hammond MG, Raj MH, Raj S. Increased activation of pelvic macrophages in infertile women with mild endometriosis. Am J Obstet Gynecol. 1983;145:333-7.
17. de Ziegler D, Borghese B, Chapron C. Endometriosis and infertility: pathophysiology and management. Lancet. 2010;376:730-8.
18. Garrido N, Navarro J, Remohı J, Simon C, Pellicer A. Follicular hormonal environment and embryo quality in women with endometriosis. Hum Reprod Update. 2000;6:67-74.
19. Garrido N, Navarro J, Garcıa-Velasco J, Remohı J, Pellicer A, Simon C. The endometrium versus embryonic quality in endometriosis related infertility. Hum Reprod Update. 2002;8:95-103.
20. Sanchez AM, Vigano P, Somigliana E, Panina-Bordignon P, Vercellini P, Candiani M. The distinguishing cellular and molecular features of the endometriotic ovarian cyst: from pathophysiology to the potential endometrioma-mediated damage to the ovary. Hum Reprod Update. 2014;20:217-30.
21. Kitajima M, Khan KN, Hiraki K, Inoue T, Fujishita A, Masuzaki H. Changes in serum anti-Mullerian hormone levels may predict damage to residual normal ovarian tissue after laparoscopic surgery for women with ovarian endometrioma. Fertil Steril. 2011;95:2589-91.e1.
22. Somigliana E, Vigano P, Filippi F, Papaleo E, Benaglia L, Candiani M, et al. Fertility preservation in women with endometriosis: for all, for some, for none? Hum Reprod. 2015;30:1280-6.
23. Giudice LC, Evers JL, Healy DL. Endometriosis: science and practice. London: Blackwell; 2012.
24. Benaglia L, Somigliana E, Iemmello R, Colpi E, Nicolosi AE, Ragni G. Endometrioma and oocyte retrieval-induced pelvic abscess: a clinical concern or an exceptional complication? Fertil Steril. 2008a;89:1263-6.
25. Dunselman GA, Vermeulen N, Becker C, Calhaz-Jorge C, D'Hooghe T, De Bie B, et al. ESHRE guideline: management of women with endometriosis. Hum Reprod. 2014;29(3):400-12.
26. Mostoufizadeh M, Scully R. Malignant tumors arising in endometriosis. Clin Obstet Gynecol. 1980;23:951-63.
27. Stern RC, Dash R, Bentley RC, Snyder MJ, Haney AF, Robboy SJ. Malignancy in endometriosis: frequency and comparison of ovarian and extraovarian types. Int J Gynecol Pathol. 2001;20:133-9.
28. Kobayashi H, Sumimoto K, Moniwa N, Imai M, Takakura K, Kuromaki T, et al. Risk of developing ovarian cancer among women with ovarian endometrioma: a cohort study in Shizuoka, Japan. Int J Gynecol Cancer. 2007;17:37-43.
29. Leone Roberti Maggiore U, Ferrero S, Mangili G, Bergamini A, Inversetti A, Giorgione V, et al. A systematic review on endometriosis during pregnancy: diagnosis, misdiagnosis, complications and outcomes. Hum Reprod Update. 2016;22:70-103.
30. Brosens IA, Van Baller P, Puttermens PJ, Deprest J. Reconstruction of the ovary containing large endometriomas by an extraovarian endosurgical technique. Fertil Steril. 1996;66:517-21.
31. Roman H, Tarta O, Pura I, Opris I, Bourdel N, Marpeau L, Sabourin JC. Direct proportional relationship between endometrioma size and ovarian parenchyma inadvertently removed during cystectomy, and its implication on the management of enlarged endometriomas. Hum Reprod. 2010;25(6):1428-32.
32. Matsuzaki S, Houlle C, Darcha C, Pouly JL, Mage G, Canis M. Analysis of risk factors for the removal of normal ovarian tissue during laparoscopic cystectomy for ovarian endometriosis. Hum Reprod. 2009;24(6):1402-6.
33. Romualdi D, Franco Zannoni G, Lanzone A, Selvaggi L, Tagliaferri V, Gaetano Vellone V, et al. Follicular loss in endoscopic surgery for ovarian endometriosis: quantitative and qualitative observations. Fertil Steril. 2011;96(2):374-8.
34. Gupta S, Agarwal A, Agarwal R, Loret de Mola JR. Impact of ovarian endometrioma on assisted reproduction outcomes. Reprod Biomed Online. 2006;13(3):349-60.
35. Ferrero S, Scala C, Tafi E, Racca A, Venturini PL, Leone Roberti Maggiore U. Impact of large ovarian endometriomas on the response to superovulation for in vitro fertilization: A retrospective study. Eur J Obstet Gynecol Reprod Biol. 2017;213:17-21.
36. Biacchiardi CP, Piane LD, Camanni M, Deltetto F, Delpiano EM, Marchino GL, et al. Laparoscopic stripping of endometriomas negatively affects ovarian follicular reserve even if performed by experienced surgeons. Reprod Biomed Online. 2011;23(6):740-6.
37. Busacca M, Riparini J, Somigliana E, Oggioni G, Izzo S, Vignali M, et al. Postsurgical ovarian failure after laparoscopic excision of bilateral endometriomas. Am J Obstet Gynecol. 2006;195:421-5.
38. Hwu YM, Wu FS, Li SH, Sun FJ, Lin MH, Lee RK. The impact of endometrioma and laparoscopic cystectomy on serum anti-Müllerian hormone levels. Reprod Biol Endocrinol. 2011;9:80.
39. Kim JY, Jee BC, Suh CS, Kim SH. Preoperative serum anti-mullerian hormone level in women with ovarian endometrioma and mature cystic teratoma. Yonsei Med J. 2013;54(4):921-6.
40. Kwon SK, Kim SH, Yun SC, Kim DY, Chae HD, Kim CH, et al. Decline of serum antimüllerian hormone levels after laparoscopic ovarian cystectomy in endometrioma and other benign cysts: a prospective cohort study. Fertil Steril. 2014;101(2):435-41.
41. Celik HG, Dogan E, Okyay E, Ulukus C, Saatli B, Uysal S, et al. Effect of laparoscopic excision of endometriomas on ovarian reserve: serial changes in the serum antimüllerian hormone levels. Fertil Steril. 2012;97(6):1472-8.
42. Alborzi S, Keramati P, Younesi M, Samsami A, Dadras N. The impact of laparoscopic cystectomy on ovarian reserve

in patients with unilateral and bilateral endometriomas. Fertil Steril. 2014;101(2):427-34.
43. Li CZ, Liu B, Wen ZQ, Sun Q. The impact of electrocoagulation on ovarian reserve after laparoscopic excision of ovarian cysts: a prospective clinical study of 191 patients. Fertil Steril. 2009;92:1428-35.
44. Hachisuga T, Kawarabayashi T. Histopathological analysis of laparoscopically treated ovarian endometriotic cysts with special reference to loss of follicles. Hum Reprod. 2002;17:432-5.
45. Goodman LR, Goldberg JM, Flyckt RL, Gupta M, Harwalker J, Falcone T. Effect of surgery on ovarian reserve in women with endometriomas, endometriosis and controls. Am J Obstet Gynecol. 2016;215:589.e1-589.e6.
46. Hamdan M, Dunselman G, Li TC, Cheong Y. The impact of endometrioma on IVF/ICSI outcomes: a systematic review and meta-analysis. Hum Reprod Update. 2015;21(6):809-25.
47. Bourdon M, Raad J, Dahan Y, Marcellin L, Maignien C, Even M, et al. Endometriosis and ART: a prior history of surgery for OMA is associated with a poor ovarian response to hyperstimulation. PLoS One. 2018;13(8):e0202399.
48. Somigliana E, Infantino M, Benedetti F, Arnoldi M, Calanna G, Ragni G. The presence of ovarian endometriomas is associated with a reduced responsiveness to gonadotropins. Fertil Steril. 2006;86:192-6.
49. Esinler I, Bozdag G, Arikan I, Demir B, Yarali H. Endometrioma ≤3 cm in diameter per se does not affect ovarian reserve in intracytoplasmic sperm injection cycles. Gynecol Obstet Invest. 2012;74:261-4.
50. Benaglia L, Somigliana E, Santi G, Scarduelli C, Ragni G, Fedele L. IVF and endometriosis-related symptom progression: insights from a prospective study. Hum Reprod. 2011;26:2368-72.
51. Hong SB, Lee NR, Kim SK, Kim H, Jee BC, Suh CS, et al. In vitro fertilization outcomes in women with surgery induced diminished ovarian reserve after endometrioma operation: Comparison with diminished ovarian reserve without ovarian surgery. Obstet Gynecol Sci. 2017;60(1):63-8.
52. Coccia ME, Rizzello F, Gianfranco S. Does controlled ovarian hyperstimulation in women with a history of endometriosis influence recurrence rate? J Womens Health (Larchmt). 2010;19:2063-9.
53. Esinler I, Bozdag G, Aybar F, Bayar U, Yarali H. Outcome of in vitro fertilization/intracytoplasmic sperm injection after laparoscopic cystectomy for endometriomas. Fertil Steril. 2006;85(6):1730-5.
54. Var T, Batioglu S, Tonguc E, Kahyaoglu I. The effect of laparoscopic ovarian cystectomy versus coagulation in bilateral endometriomas on ovarian reserve as determined by antral follicle count and ovarian volume: a prospective randomized study. Fertil Steril. 2011;95(7):2247-50.
55. Tsolakidis D, Pados G, Vavilis D, Athanatos D, Tsalikis T, Giannakou A, et al. The impact on ovarian reserve after laparoscopic ovarian cystectomy versus three-stage management in patients with endometriomas: a prospective randomized study. Fertil Steril. 2010;94(1):71-7.
56. Donnez J, Lousse JC, Jadoul P, Donnez O, Squifflet J. Laparoscopic management of endometriomas using a combined technique of excisional (cystectomy) and ablative surgery. Fertil Steril. 2010;94(1):28-32.
57. Garcia-Velasco JA, Mahutte NG, Corona J, Zúñiga V, Gilés J, Arici A, et al. Removal of endometriomas before in vitro fertilization does not improve fertility outcomes: a matched, case-control study. Fertil Steril. 2004;81(5):1194-7.
58. Demirol A, Guven S, Baykal C, Gurgan T. Effect of endometrioma cystectomy on IVF outcome: a prospective randomized study. Reprod Biomed Online. 2006;12(5): 639-43.
59. Somigliana E, Arnoldi M, Benaglia L, Iemmello R, Nicolosi AE, Ragni G. IVF-ICSI outcome in women operated on for bilateral endometriomas. Hum Reprod. 2008;23(7): 1526-30.
60. Suganuma N, Wakahara Y, Ishida D, Asano M, Kitagawa T, Katsumata Y, et al. Pretreatment for ovarian endometrial cyst before in vitro fertilization. Gynecol Obstet Invest. 2002;54 (Suppl 1):36-40; 41-42.
61. Somigliana E, Benaglia L, Paffoni A, Busnelli A, Vigano P, Vercellini P. Risks of conservative management in women with ovarian endometriomas undergoing IVF. Hum Reprod Update. 2015;21:486-99.
62. Ballester M, d'Argent EM, Morcel K, Belaisch-Allart J, Nisolle M, Daraï E. Cumulative pregnancy rate after ICSI-IVF in patients with colorectal endometriosis: results of a multicentre study. Hum Reprod. 2012;27(4):1043-9.

36

Chapter

When to Transfer? Day 3 Versus Day 5 Embryo Transfer

Runa Acharya

INTRODUCTION

The field of assisted reproduction has grown by leaps and bounds since its inception and since the birth of first in vitro fertilization (IVF) baby in 1978. Multiple new technologies have emerged to enhance the success rates. Pregnancy rate following assisted reproductive technology (ART) is approximately 40–60%, with live birth rates (LBRs) per embryo transfer cycle of approximately 30–40%.[1] The success rates have improved over the last decade due to better media, consistent advanced laboratory technology, and improvements in cryopreservation techniques. Various options have been proposed to increase the success rates further and one such strategy has been prolonged embryo culture.

DAY 3 VERSUS DAY 5

Human embryos are usually transferred either on day 3 (cleavage stage) **(Fig. 1)** or day 5 (blastocyst stage) **(Fig. 2)**. Initial attempts at blastocyst transfer failed to demonstrate an increase in either implantation or pregnancy rate because of poor embryo survival due to inadequate extended culture conditions.[2] However, the improvement in culture conditions have allowed for successful extended culture and acceptable rates of blastocyst formation.[3] In the present era, extending the embryo culture to day 5 or 6 may increase the success rate of ART. The reasons behind improved success rates after blastocyst transfer are:

- Embryos implant in the uterus at blastocyst stage
- Extended embryo culture until day 5 could lead to better embryo selection that has demonstrated better outcomes.[4]
- Embryos at blastocyst stage have their own genomic control and have already passed the maternal to zygotic transition.[5]

However, despite the considerable progress in culture conditions, advances in technology and, keeping all the benefits of blastocyst transfer in mind, questions do arise

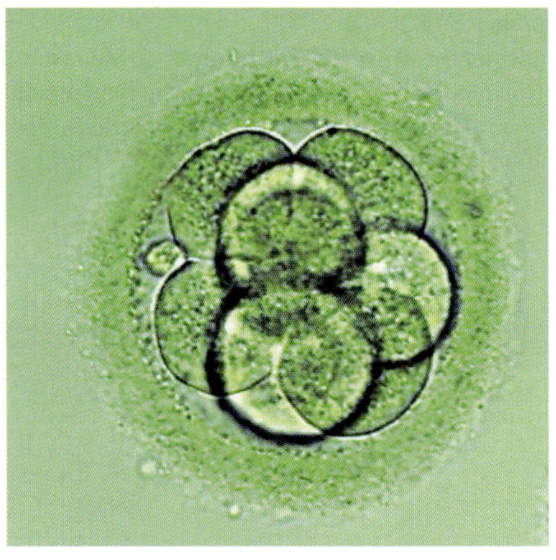

Fig. 1: Cleavage stage embryo.

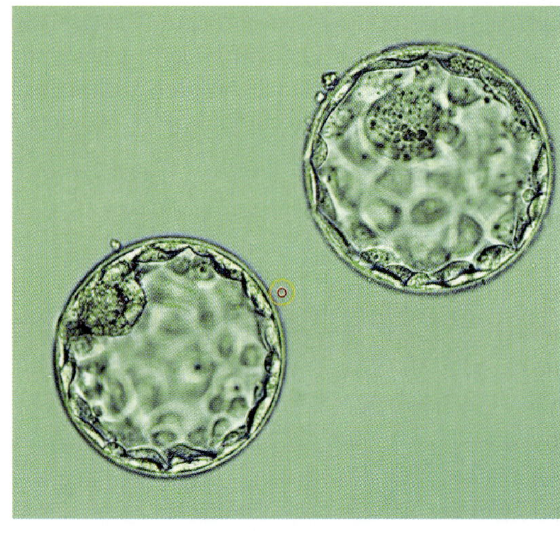

Fig. 2: Blastocyst.

as to whether day 5 transfer is appropriate for all patients and whether extending the duration of culture of some embryos for an additional 48 hours might compromise their implantation potential in a given subset of population.

In other words, are there some patients for whom the uterus is a better embryo incubator than that provided by our current technologies of extended culture in vitro?

In the gist of improving the pregnancy rate and LBR, the transfer of multiple embryos also results in the multiple births, which is the most common complication associated with ART. Multiple births are significantly related to increased adverse health outcomes for both mothers and neonates. The various complications associated with multiple births include preeclampsia, pregnancy-induced hypertension, diabetes, preterm delivery, low birth weight, intrauterine growth restriction, and prematurity, thus increasing maternal and neonatal morbidity and mortality.[6] The goal of ART is to achieve a successful pregnancy and healthy take-home baby. Another advantage with single-blastocyst transfer is the reduction the incidence of multiple pregnancies.

Single-embryo transfer (SET) has been instituted as a governmental policy in many countries. The reason for adopting such a policy is to avoid multiple pregnancies. Thus, the IVF centers dealing with SET have focused on identifying top-quality embryos and designating the optimal time for its transfer. In other words, an embryo with the highest chance of implantation should be selected to achieve satisfactory pregnancy rates. Hence, the prolongation of embryo culture to day 5 requires a relatively high number of top-quality embryos on day 3. Good-quality cleavage-stage embryos increase the likelihood of good-quality blastocyst embryos, provided the culture conditions are excellent.

Cleavage embryos are classified as top-quality embryos if they have six to eight cells on day 3, with <20% anucleate fragments according to the Cummin's criteria.[7] **(Fig. 1)**. Embryos graded III or IV include those that have less than six cells on day 3 and no <20% fragmentation are called poor quality **(Fig. 3)**. Blastocyst quality is graded on day 5 or 6 according to the degree of blastocoel expansion, inner cell mass (ICM), and trophectoderm (TE) cells.[8] Blastocysts of grade ≥3BB on day 5 or 6 are defined as good-quality embryos **(Fig. 2)**. In case of very few embryos of average to good quality, advancement to blastocyst would be a tricky decision, keeping the possibility of developmental arrest with no embryo left for transfer versus the chance that the same embryo may develop better in natural uterine environment. Another concern which influences the success rates is embryo selection, which is far from dependent on the skill set of the embryologist and is known to have observer bias. With newer technologies involving artificial intelligence this bias may be overcome. However, selection of the best embryo is a crucial step in embryo transfer cycles.

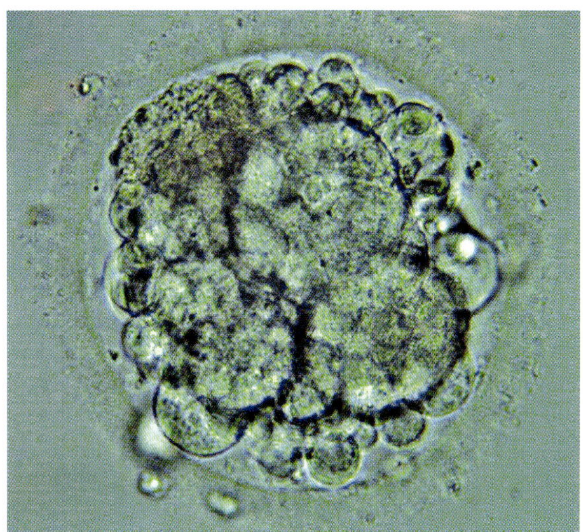

Fig. 3: Day 3 embryo with fragmentation.

DAY 3 VERSUS DAY 5: LITERATURE REVIEW

The chances of blastocyst transfer again is dependent on few clinical factors apart from the laboratory factors. Age has not been shown to have any effect on blastocyst formation; however, advanced age is reportedly independent factor associated with decline in implantation and pregnancy rates, keeping the aneuploidy rates in mind. Rather, the chances of blastocyst transfer have been reported to depend on the number of oocytes.[9]

Over the last two decades, improvements in laboratory equipment, culture media, and other techniques, there has been a consistent and reliable laboratory results in terms of blastocyst formations. The evolution from Hams F10, G1, G2 sequential media to the newer ones, which are one-step culture media (e.g., Origio, Irvine scientific, Quinn's Vitrolife) have improved blastocyst formation rates. Even with fewer embryos, blastocyst advancements are attempted in many well-equipped laboratories across the globe.

The transfer of two blastocysts at day 5 was more favorable than two embryos at day 3 in a cohort of 164 infertile women in a randomized controlled trial (RCT).

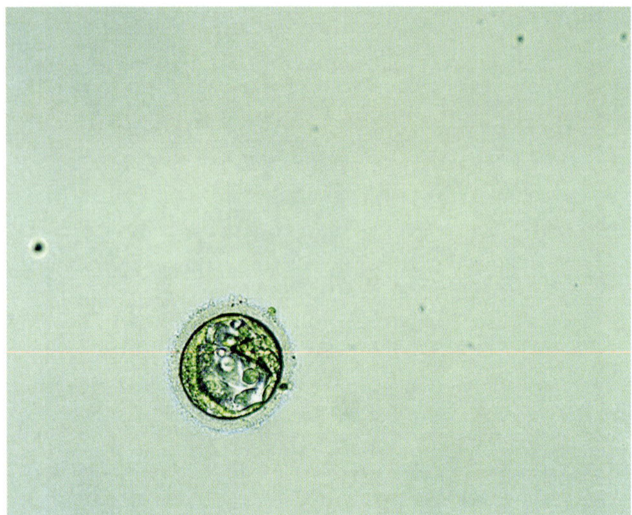

Fig. 4: Poor quality blastocyst.

It was observed that transfer at blastocyst stage resulted in significantly higher pregnancy (51.3% vs. 27.4%) and live birth (47.5% vs. 27.4%) rates than the transfers at the cleavage stage. Yet, the twinning rate was statistically similar for the day 3 and day 5 transfers (36.8% vs. 30.4%).[10] In accordance with this result, a prospective randomized study indicated that single-blastocyst transfers had significantly higher pregnancy rate (35.6% vs. 23.7%) than the single cleavage-stage embryo in a cohort of 227 infertile women aged <36 years, and who were on their first or second IVF trials.[11]

A retrospective cohort study including 6,077 single vitrified-thawed embryo transfers found significant increase in LBR and birth weight after transfer of single good-quality embryo on day 5 and day 6 compared with transfer of single good-quality embryo on day 3 in the vitrified embryo transfer cycles. However, no significant differences were seen in birth weight between transfer of single poor-quality embryo on day 5 and 6, **(Fig. 4)** and transfer single good-quality embryo on day 3.[6]

Contrary to the study above, another prospective randomized study reported that day 3 and day 5 transfers yielded statistically similar overall implantation (21% vs. 23%), pregnancy (39% vs. 39%), and twinning (11.9% vs. 15%) rates in a cohort of 201 infertile women.[12] Likewise, a prospective randomized study conducted on a total 190 Turkish women by Hatırnaz et al. in 2017 demonstrated that the in spite of the fact that the number of grade I embryos were significantly higher in day 5 transfers than in day 3 transfers (p = 0.001), day 3 and day 5 embryo transfers had statistically similar implantation (47.4% vs. 45.3%), clinical pregnancy (46.3% vs. 44.2%), twinning (4.2% vs. 8.4%), and LBRs (36.8% vs. 34.7%) (p = 0.779, p = 0.771, p = 0.183, and p = 0.649, respectively). The LBRs in singleton pregnancies conceived after day 3 and day 5 embryo transfers were statistically similar (p = 0.594).[13]

In fact, a prospective observational study showed that about 50% of embryos conceived in 224 IVF/ICSI (intracytoplasmic sperm injection) cycles were exposed to developmental arrest at the blastocyst stage.[14] Advocates of blastocyst culture maintain that the increased implantation rate, in conjunction with a policy to replace fewer embryos, may allow maintenance of the overall chance of pregnancy but reduce the costly multiple birth rate. Critics of the approach express concern at the increased incidence of women failing to have embryos for transfer. The cost of the treatment mode must be weighed against the odds of a healthy take-home baby. Also, extended embryo culture has reported an increase in embryo transfer cancellations due to a failure in embryos developing into blastocysts on the day of transfer, a failure to have extra embryos for freezing, the requirement of an excellent culture system, an increase in monozygotic twinning, and altered sex ratio.[5,15]

According to Cochrane Database Systematic Review, which included 27 RCTs comprising 4,031 women, the inference was that in fresh embryo transfers the clinical pregnancy rate (CPR) and LBR were higher in the blastocyst transfer compared to that of cleavage-stage transfer (39–46% vs. 36% and 32–42% vs. 29% respectively). However, when cumulative pregnancy rates per couple after one oocyte retrieval was compared between two groups there was no difference noted. Multiple pregnancy rates remained the same in both the groups. They also noted that in blastocyst group there was 1% chance of women who would have no embryos to transfer. The comparisons between fresh and frozen were not clear from these studies. So, the conclusion was though there could be a benefit favoring blastocyst transfer in fresh cycles, it is not clear whether the day of transfer has any impact on cumulative live birth and pregnancy rates.[16]

Recently a retrospective analysis showed transferring embryos at day 3 may provide the same benefits as day 5 blastocyst transfers to patients. However, more embryos (day 3) were required to be transferred to achieve these comparable results with no significant differences in clinical pregnancy, implantation, multiple pregnancy rates or LBRs.[17]

Most reports of day 5 transfers relate to selected populations of patients, who are good prognosis and also at a greatest risk of high-order multiple gestations; but would day 5 pregnancy rates be similar in poor prognosis patients.[18] A retrospective analysis of ART cycles was performed by Racowsky et al. comparing outcomes of day 3 and day 5 transfers in patients with no 8-cell embryos on day 3, 1–3 8-cell embryos on day 3, and 3 or more 8-cell embryos on day 3.[18] Interestingly, they found 0% and 33% pregnancies resulted from day 5 versus day 3 transfers in patients with no 8-cell embryos on day 3. With 1 or 2 8-cell embryos on day 3, ongoing and high-order multiple rates were not different between day 3 and day 5 transfers. With 3 or more 8-cell embryos, day 5 transfer resulted in a decrease in multiple gestations but no difference in ongoing pregnancy rates compared with day 3 transfer. This study concluded that with no 8-cell embryos on day 3, a day 3 transfer is warranted. However, with 1 or 2 8-cell embryos, any benefit of day 5 transfer appears to be equivocal. With 3 or more 8-cell embryos, day 5 transfer is recommended. Observations point out to the fact that extended culture conditions may be inadequate to support normal development of embryos in suboptimal slow-cleaving cohort and uterus may apparently be able to "rescue" some of the embryos in this cohort. So, it is very important to understand that subset of population who would benefit from day 3 embryo transfer over an enthusiastic advancement of culture that may lead to no blastocyst to transfer leaving a 0% chance of pregnancy.

CONCLUSION

Blastocyst transfer may have its own benefits of being associated with satisfactory pregnancy rates given the theory that morphological assessment on day 3 has limited predictive value for subsequent developmental process. Hence advancing the culture until day 5 appears to be a more sensible approach to select the best-quality embryo with the highest probability of successful implantation along with the added benefit of genetic testing. At the same time, keeping consideration of the fact that around 50% of embryos may undergo developmental arrest in this process and would have had a better chance of survival in in utero compared to in vivo environment, a diligent decision with individualized approach is needed. In cycles where several good-quality embryos are obtained on day 3, elective blastocyst transfer can be offered to maximize the probability of pregnancy. However, patients should be informed that there is a substantial risk of cycle cancellation as the embryo culture is extended and there is a possibility of no blastocyst formed. Individualized approach is necessary in decision-making, keeping all the clinical and embryological parameters in mind.

REFERENCES

1. Newman JE, Paul RC, Chambers GM. (2020). Assisted reproductive technology in Australia and New Zealand 2018.
2. Bolton VN, Wren ME, Parsons JH. Pregnancies after in vitro fertilization and transfer of human blastocysts. Fertil Steril. 1991;55:830-2.
3. Gardner DK, Vella P, Lane M, Wagley L, Schlenker T, Schoolcraft WB. Culture and transfer of human blastocysts increases implantation rates and reduces the need for multiple embryo transfers. Fertil Steril. 1998;69:84-8.
4. Gardner DK, Lane M. Blastocyst transfer. Clin Obstet Gynecol. 2003;46:231-8.
5. Johnson N, Blake D, Farquhar C. Blastocyst or cleavage-stage embryo transfer? Best Pract Res Clin Obstet Gynaecol. 2007;21:21-40.
6. Wang N, Zhao X, Ma M, Zhu Q, Wang Y. Effect of Day 3 and Day 5/6 Embryo Quality on the Reproductive Outcomes in the Single Vitrified Embryo Transfer Cycles. Front Endocrinol (Lausanne). 2021;12:641623.
7. Cummins JM, Breen TM, Harrison KL, Shaw JM, Wilson LM, Hennessey JF. A formula for scoring human embryo growth rates in in vitro fertilization: its value in predicting pregnancy and in comparison with visual estimates of embryo quality. J Vitro Fert Embryo Transf. 1986;5:284-95.
8. Gardner DK, Surrey E, Minjarez D, Leitz A, Stevens J, Schoolcraft WB. Single Blastocyst Transfer: A Prospective Randomized Trial. Fertil Steril. 2004;81:551-5.
9. Scolates MW, Zeilmaker GH. A prospective, randomized study of embryo transfer results after 3 or 5 days of embryo culture in in vitro fertilization. Fertil Steril. 1996;65:1245-8.
10. Papanikolaou EG, Camus M, Kolibianakis EM, Van Landuyt L, Van Steirteghem A, Devroey P. In vitro fertilization with single blastocyst-stage versus single cleavage-stage embryos. N Engl J Med. 2006;354:1139-46.
11. Zech NH, Lejeune B, Puissant F, Vanderzwalmen S, Zech H, Vanderzwalmen P. Prospective evaluation of the optimal time for selecting a single embryo for transfer: day 3 versus day 5. Fertil Steril. 2007;88:244-6.
12. Coskun S, Hollanders J, Al-Hassan S, Al-Sufyan H, Al-Mayman H, Jaroudi K. Day 5 versus day 3 embryo transfer: A controlled randomized trial. Hum Reprod. 2000;15:1947-52.
13. Hatırnaz Ş, Kanat Pektaş M. Day 3 embryo transfer versus day 5 blastocyst transfers: A prospective randomized controlled trial. Turk J Obstet Gynecol. 2017;14:82-8.

14. Zech NH, Lejeune B, Puissant F, Zech H, Vanderzwalmen S, Vanderzwalmen P. Single embryo transfer: selection on day 3 or day 5? A prospective observational study. Fertil Steril. 2005;84(Suppl 1):S266.
15. Ménézo YJ, Chouteau J, Torelló J, Girard A, Veiga A. Birth weight and sex ratio after transfer at the blastocyst stage in humans. Fertil Steril. 1999;72:221-4.
16. Glujovsky D, Farquhar C, Quinteiro Retamar AM, Alvarez Sedo CR, Blake D. Cleavage stage versus blastocyst stage embryo transfer in assisted reproductive technology. Cochrane Database Syst Rev. 2016;(6):CD002118.
17. Garbhini PG, Suardika A, Anantasika A, Adnyana IBP, Darmayasa IM, Tondohusodo N, et al. Day-3 vs. Day-5 fresh embryo transfer. JBRA Assist Reprod. 2023;27:163-8.
18. Racowsky C, Jackson KV, Cekleniak NA, Fox JH, Hornstein MD, Ginsburg ES. The number of eight-cell embryos is a key determinant for selecting day 3 or day 5 transfer. Fertil Steril. 2000;73:558-64.

Preimplantation Genetic Testing: Should it be done for all?

Garima Sharma

INTRODUCTION

In recent decades, the integration of molecular genetics into assisted reproductive technology (ART) has revolutionized the field, offering new possibilities for couples facing genetic risks. Traditional prenatal diagnostic techniques such as amniocentesis and chorionic villi sampling (CVS) have provided valuable information but also raised ethical concerns. Preimplantation genetic testing (PGT) emerges as a promising alternative, aiming to identify genetically normal embryos before implantation, thereby mitigating the need for difficult decisions postconception.

TERMINOLOGY

The history of PGT is intertwined with the rapid advancements in genetic technologies. Initially termed preimplantation genetic diagnosis (PGD), the field has evolved to encompass broader categories. With the advent of advanced genetic techniques, the terminology has transitioned to PGT, with subdivisions including preimplantation genetic testing-aneuploidy (PGT-A) for aneuploidies (formerly known as PGS), PGT-M for monogenic/single gene disorders (formerly PGD), and PGT-SR for chromosomal structural rearrangements (formerly PGS translocation).[1]

The transition from PGD to PGT reflects not only technological advancements but also a broader understanding of genetic testing's potential applications in ART. This evolution highlights the field's dynamic nature and its commitment to staying abreast of scientific progress while addressing clinical needs and ethical considerations. **Table 1** enlists the major historical events in the evolution of PGT.

HISTORY OF PREIMPLANTATION GENETIC TESTING

TABLE 1: Major historical events in the evolution of preimplantation genetic testing (PGT).

Name	*Year*	*Contribution*
Dr Robert Edwards and Dr Richard Gardner	1967	First described use of preimplantation genetic diagnosis (PGD) for sexing of rabbit blastocysts in Nature journal
Leeanda Wilton	1986	Initiated cleavage stage biopsy
Yuri Verlinsky	1988	Polar body biopsy
Audrey Muggleton-Harris	1988	Trophoectoderm biopsy
Elena Kontogianni	1989	PGD was first used for testing monogenic disorders and sex-linked disorders which showed polymerase chain reaction (PCR) for the Y chromosome from a blastomere

INDICATIONS OF PREIMPLANTATION GENETIC TESTING

The various indications for PGT are enumerated here:

- Higher age of female patient
- History of recurrent pregnancy loss
- Repeated in vitro fertilization (IVF) failure
- Severe male factor infertility
- Couples with family history of X-linked disorders carries 25% risk of having an affected embryo
- Carriers of autosomal recessive diseases, carries 25% risk of having an affected embryo
- Carriers of autosomal dominant diseases, carries 50% risk of having an affected embryo
- Human leukocyte antigen (HLA) matching[2]

SOURCES OF GENETIC MATERIAL FOR PREIMPLANTATION GENETIC TESTING

The choice of genetic material depends on factors, such as the stage of embryo development, the need for comprehensive testing, and ethical considerations regarding embryo manipulation. The genetic material can be obtained from:

- Polar bodies (PBs) from the oocyte/zygote stage
- Blastomeres from cleavage stage embryo
- Trophectoderm cells from blastocysts
- Blastocele fluid and culture medium as noninvasive method of PGT

Techniques: Polar Body, Blastomere, and Trophectoderm Biopsies

Preimplantation genetic testing encompasses a range of biopsy techniques, each tailored to specific clinical scenarios and genetic testing objectives. PB biopsy offers a noninvasive approach to preconception diagnosis, allowing for the identification of inherited diseases in oocytes before fertilization. This technique is particularly valuable in jurisdictions with restrictive embryo research laws or for couples with ethical considerations regarding embryo manipulation.

Blastomere biopsy, performed at the 6–8 cell stage, capitalizes on embryo totipotency, ensuring minimal impact on developmental potential. This technique allows for the comprehensive assessment of genetic abnormalities while preserving the embryo's viability for subsequent transfer. Trophectoderm biopsy at the blastocyst stage offers a more advanced approach to genetic testing, allowing for comprehensive assessment while minimizing the risk of harm to the inner cell mass, which forms the fetus.

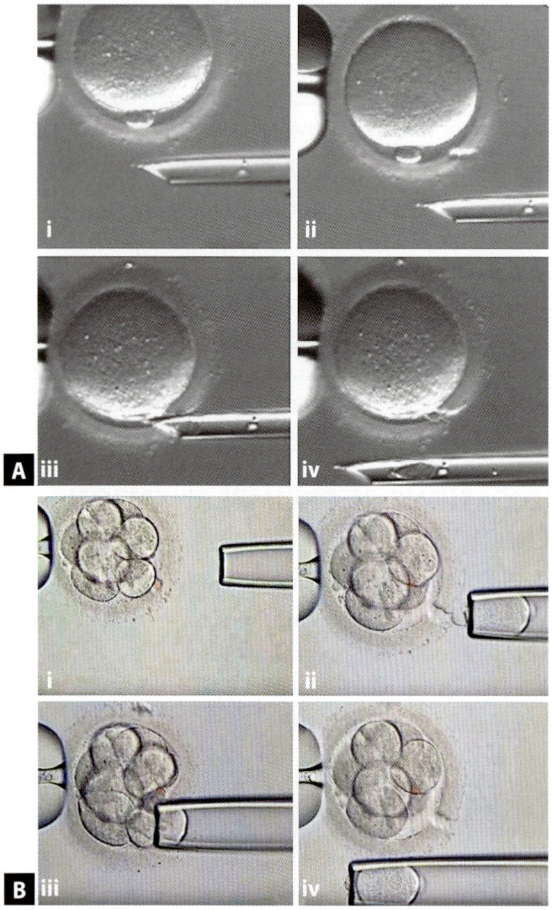

Figs. 1A and B: (A) Polar body (PB) biopsy. i: PB was kept at 6 o'clock; ii: Zona pellucida dissection with three laser impacts; iii: PB extrusion; iv: PB in micropipette. (B) Blastomere biopsy.

PREIMPLANTATION GENETIC TESTING-ANEUPLOIDY

Preimplantation genetic testing-aneuploidy represents a significant advancement in the field of reproductive medicine, offering hope to couples grappling with recurrent pregnancy loss and implantation failure. This technique aims to identify embryos with chromosomal abnormalities, known as aneuploidies, thereby enabling the selection of genetically normal embryos for transfer. Despite its potential benefits, PGT-A is not without challenges including the detection of mosaic embryos and the interpretation of results.

The identification of mosaic embryos, which contain both euploid and aneuploid cells, poses a significant challenge in PGT-A. The proportion of euploid and aneuploid cells within mosaic embryos can impact the likelihood of successful implantation and live birth, making accurate diagnosis and counseling essential. Additionally, the risk of misdiagnosis due to technical limitations underscores the importance of careful patient selection and counseling in PGT-A. Mosaic embryos may have a lower chance of pregnancy but there are also reports of healthy live births after a transfer of a mosaic embryo.

RECOMMENDATIONS AND FOLLOW-UP

Clinicians play a crucial role in guiding patients through the PGT process, from initial consultation to follow-up care. Proper counseling is essential to ensure that patients understand the limitations of PGT including the possibility of mosaic results and the potential risks associated with embryo biopsy. Priority should be given to transferring euploid embryos with careful consideration of the potential risks and benefits of transferring mosaic embryos.

Long-term follow-up is essential to assess the impact of PGT on neonatal outcomes and child development. Prenatal diagnosis should be offered to all patients who become pregnant following PGT, with options including invasive diagnostic tests such as CVS and amniocentesis, as well as noninvasive screening tests such as ultrasound scanning and cell-free fetal DNA testing. Postnatal confirmation may also be obtained through cord blood sampling, offering additional reassurance to patients and clinicians.

PREIMPLANTATION GENETIC TESTING-ANEUPLOIDY FOR ALL

The widespread adoption of PGT-A has sparked debate within the reproductive medicine community with proponents touting its potential benefits and skeptics raising concerns about its efficacy and safety.[3]

Supportive Arguments

Preimplantation genetic testing-aneuploidy is:

- Cost-effective, as it reduces costs related to multiple pregnancies, failed implantation, and miscarriage
- Accurate and does not harm embryo viability
- It is the future.
- It is more logical and appealing as patients want to check everything about the embryo health and make safety before transfer.
- Ideally, it forms an integrated part of fertility care

Arguments Against PGT-A for All

- Scientific papers and research shows that even after three decades, there are still doubts about PGT-A efficacy.
- Minimal or no improvement in pregnancy and live birth rate (LBR) reported in some patient categories
- There are reports of potential damage to the embryo and mosaicism
- Around 20–30% of samples analyzed with PGT-A might have a misdiagnosis (because of mosaicism and other technical problems), and unfortunately in such cases implantation is lost.
- There are specific indications for performing PGT. PGT-A is not for everybody.

Human Fertilization and Embryology Authority Ratings for PGT-A

Rated red for increasing chances of having a baby for *most fertility patients* as PGT-A is a selection tool which often reduces the number of embryos available for transfer and increases the time to conception

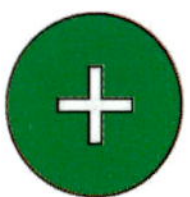

Green for *reducing the chances of miscarriage for most fertility patients*

- Gray for *reducing the chances of miscarriage for older women*
- There is insufficient high quality evidence to see effectiveness of using PGT-A in older women

- Gray for *improving chances of having a baby for older women*
- Again, due to lack of high quality evidence

Preimplantation genetic testing-aneuploidy is now mostly carried out at the blastocyst stage on day 5 or 6. But, there is no evidence to suggest from randomized controlled trials (RCTs) that PGT-A carried out at this stage is effective at improving chances of having a baby for most patients undergoing IVF.

IS THIS TREATMENT ADD-ON SAFE?

Preimplantation genetic testing-aneuploidy does not carry any additional known risks for the person who is undergoing fertility treatment. However, PGT-A is known to carry some risks for the embryo:

- The test may give the wrong result as false-positives or false-negatives (the incidence although is low).
- Healthy embryos may be discarded if the test result is not appropriate, meaning the couple may have fewer embryos for transfer.
- Viable embryos could be discarded in some cases due to reporting of mosaic embryos or because of the fact that not all embryos may be suitable for biopsy. There are reports of healthy live births after a transfer of a mosaic embryo.

- It is also possible that no embryos may be suitable if chromosomal abnormalities are detected in all the embryos tested.

A systematic review and meta-analysis by Simopoulou et al. on PGT-A including four RCTs concluded that PGT-A did not improve LBRs per patient in the general population.[4] However, PGT-A lowered miscarriage rate in the general population (RR: 0.45). The cumulative LBR per patient was improved by PGT-A. On performing an age-subgroup analysis, PGT-A improved LBR in women over the age of 35 years, whereas it appeared to be noneffective in younger women. Regarding optimal timing, only day-5 biopsy practice presented with improved LBR per embryo transfer (ET).

The American College of Obstetricians and Gynecologists (ACOG) committee opinion on PGT[5] states that the main purpose of preimplantation genetic testing-aneuploidy (known as PGT-A) is screening of the embryos for whole chromosome abnormalities. There is insufficient evidence to recommend the routine use of PGT-A in all infertile women. The ideal genetic testing platform to analyze all chromosomes has not yet been established. There are many challenges with PGT especially in detecting microdeletions and microduplications, de novo variants, and imprinting disorders. Another problem has been detection of mosaicism during PGT-A. Application of advanced genetic technologies, such as next-generation sequencing (NGS), has allowed mosaicism to be detected with greater sensitivity with an incidence as high as 20% of tested embryos. However, referral to a specialist with genetic training and expertise should be considered, and prenatal diagnosis with CVS or amniocentesis should be strongly encouraged and offered to couples with ongoing live pregnancy resulting from mosaic embryos. Traditional diagnostic testing or screening for aneuploidy should be offered to all patients who have had PGT-A, in accordance with recommendations. Large RCTs are needed to determine which patient cohorts, if any, may benefit from PGT-A.

The Preimplantation Genetic Diagnosis International Society (PGDIS) issued a position statement in 2016 on chromosome mosaicism. They suggested the range for defining an embryo as having chromosome mosaicism is if the amount of aneuploid DNA is between 20–80%. An embryo with <20% aneuploid deoxyribonucleic acid (DNA) is considered to be a euploid (normal) and ready for transfer. However, if it has >80% aneuploid DNA, it is considered to be an aneuploid (abnormal) and should not be transferred. If an embryo falls within the 20–80% range of aneuploidy, the transfer should only be considered after obtaining expert advice and genetic counseling. This standard has been followed by fertility clinics conducting PGT-A tests since 2016 without confirming the hypothesis that an embryo with 20–80% aneuploidy will be more likely to lead to chromosomal abnormalities and a lower possibility of a viable pregnancy.[6]

In 2019, the STAR study[7] was published which compared the LBR of patients who underwent PGT-A tests on their embryos before transfer for implantation, and patients whose embryos only underwent morphological assessment before transfer for implantation. The data revealed that there was no significant increase in LBRs or decrease in miscarriage rates among patients who performed PGT-A tests, compared to those who only performed morphological assessments.

CONCLUSION

Preimplantation genetic testing represents a significant advancement in reproductive medicine, offering hope to couples grappling with infertility and genetic risks. While its applications continue to expand, critical evaluation and ongoing research are imperative to optimize outcomes and ensure ethical practice in ART. By embracing evidence-based practice and prioritizing patient-centered care, clinicians can help patients navigate the complex landscape of genetic testing and make informed decisions about their reproductive options.

REFERENCES

1. Zegers-Hochschild F, Adamson GD, Dyer S, Racowsky C, de Mouzon J, Sokol R, et al. The International Glossary on Infertility and Fertility Care. Hum Reprod. 2017;32:1786-801.
2. Huang CC, Chang LJ, Tsai YY, Hung CC, Fang MY, Su YN, et al. A feasible strategy of preimplantation genetic diagnosis for carriers with chromosomal translocation: Using blastocyst biopsy and array comparative genomic hybridization. J Formos Med Assoc. 2013;112:537-44.
3. ESHRE PGT Consortium Steering Committee; Carvalho F, Coonen E, Goossens V, Kokkali G, Rubio C, et al. ESHRE PGT Consortium good practice recommendations for the organisation of PGT. Hum Reprod Open. 2020;2020(3):hoaa021.
4. Simopoulou M, Sfakianoudis K, Maziotis E, Tsioulou P, Grigoriadis S, Rapani A, et al. PGT-A: who and when? A systematic review and network meta-analysis of RCTs. J Assist Reprod Genet. 2021;38(8):1939-57.

5. Preimplantation Genetic Testing: ACOG Committee Opinion Summary, Number 799. Obstet Gynecol. 2020; 135(3):752-3.
6. PGDIS Newsletter. (2016). PGDIS position statement on chromosome mosaicism and preimplantation aneuploidy testing at the blastocyst stage.
7. Munné S, Kaplan B, Frattarelli JL, Child T, Nakhuda G, Shamma FN, et al. Preimplantation genetic testing for aneuploidy versus morphology as selection criteria for single frozen-thawed embryo transfer in good-prognosis patients: a multicenter randomized clinical trial. Fertil Steril. 2019;112(6):1071-79.e7.

Unexplained Infertility: Should In Vitro Fertilization be the First Line of Treatment?

Rohit Gutgutia

INTRODUCTION

Optimal treatment approach in couples with unexplained infertility (UI) remains one of the most enduring debates in reproductive medicine. Opinions have oscillated between the less expensive and less invasive intrauterine insemination (IUI) versus the more expensive but more sure option of in vitro fertilization (IVF) throughout the last two decades ever since IVF results have become more reliable and reproducible. As the European Society of Human Reproduction and Embryology (ESHRE) has released an update on unexplained infertility recently,[1] we thought it prudent to revisit the debate in light of the new document.

CONCEPT OF UNEXPLAINED INFERTILITY

Approximately 30% of infertile couple are considered to experienced "unexplained infertility" (2019 and 2020).[2,3] This controversial diagnosis is made when no abnormalities of the female and male reproductive systems are identified. Unexplained infertility is inevitably a diagnosis of exclusion, following otherwise "standard" investigations. The International Committee for Monitoring Assisted Reproductive Technologies (ICMART) defines unexplained infertility as "infertility in couple with apparently normal ovarian function, fallopian tubes, uterus, cervix, and pelvis, age ≤40 years and with adequate coital frequency; and apparently normal testicular, genitourinary anatomy, and a normal ejaculation."[4]

Before understanding the unexplained infertility, let us see the definition of infertility, which defines as a couple who is having regular, unprotected intercourse for at least 12 months and not having pregnancy (WHO, ICMART).[4]

In their seminal study, Wilcox et al. assessed prospectively in 221 women whether sexual frequency within the 6 days preceding ovulation could affect the probability of conception. The authors found that predicted conception rates did not alter significantly when comparing women who perform sexual intercourse daily, every other day, or twice during fertility window. Hence, in a couple seeking to conceive advice to having sexual intercourse at least every 2–3 days during fertility window to increase chances of conception.[5]

The guideline development group (GDG) of ESHRE for unexplained infertility 2023 recommends routinely taking a medical, reproductive, and sexual history from both the female and male partner.[6] Also, GDG recommends at least one basic semen analysis according to World Health Organization (WHO) criteria, performed by a laboratory which subscribes to an external quality protocol program. If the result from first basic is below the lower 5th percentile reference limit as per WHO criteria, a second analysis should be performed after 3 months interval.[7]

ASSESSMENT OF CAUSE OF INFERTILITY

Once the well-known and obvious causes of infertility have been excluded, the management of couples with unexplained infertility should follow clear protocols.[8] Studies of population of patients with infertility indicate that approximately 10–25% have unexplained infertility, 20–30% ovulatory dysfunction, 20–35% tubal damage, 10–50% sperm dysfunction, 5–10% endometriosis, 5% cervical mucus problems, and up to 5% coital dysfunction.[9]

DIAGNOSIS OF UNEXPLAINED INFERTILITY

According to ESHRE guidelines for unexplained infertility, following factors should be investigated.

Confirmation of Ovulation

There are various methods to detect ovulation like on the basis of menstrual history, menstrual history with single progesterone test, ultrasound, luteinizing urinary measurement, serial basal body temperature, changes in the characteristics of cervical mucus, etc.

In these all methods, ultrasound for follicular growth followed by rupture monitoring is the gold standard method. In the studies evaluation of urinary luteinizing hormone (LH) measurements, both the agreement (98–100%) and accuracy (97%) with ultrasound monitoring were very high.[10-13]

Recommendation of ESHRE guidelines: In the women with regular menstrual cycles, test for confirmation of ovulation is not routinely recommended. But, if confirmation is warranted, test such as urinary LH measurements, ultrasound monitoring, or midluteal progesterone measurement can be used.[1]

Oocyte/Corpus Luteal Quality

Few studies done to get correlation of midluteal phase progesterone level and endometrial biopsy with quality of oocytes/corpus luteal quality, but no difference was shown between fertile and nonfertile women in these parameters.[14,15]

Also, fertilization failure and euploid embryo with preimplantation genetic testing-aneuploidy (PGT-A) also cannot suggest about quality of oocyte.

Recommendation of ESHRE guidelines: In women investigated for fertility, midluteal phase serum progesterone level or endometrial biopsy is not recommended in the absence of other indication.[1]

Ovarian Reserve

To know ovarian reserve various tests are available like anti-Müllerian hormone (AMH), antral follicle count by ultrasound, day 3 follicle-stimulating hormone (FSH) and estradiol level, clomiphene citrate (CC) challenge test, ovarian volume, ovarian blood flow and inhibin B level, etc.

The term "ovarian reserve" refers to quantity of primordial follicles in a women's ovaries at a given time. Although the term has also been used in a broader sense to include quality of oocytes, it is difficult to assess the quality of oocytes during the diagnostic workup. The purpose of diagnostic workup is to identify any factor preventing pregnancy or decreasing spontaneous fecundity and to inform management strategy.

As long as the women maintain regular menstrual cycles, women with decreased ovarian reserve seem to have similar spontaneous pregnancy rate with women of similar age group with normal ovarian reserve.[16]

Recommendation of ESHRE guidelines: In women with regular menstrual cycle, ovarian reserve testing is not required to identify the etiology of infertility or to predict the probability of spontaneous conception over 6–12 months.[1]

Tubal Factor

In today's advance science, there are methods to check tubal patency like hysterosalpingo-contrast sonography [HyCoSy/HyFoSy (hysterosalpingo-foam sonography)], laparoscopy, chromopertubation, saline infusion sonography, hysterosalpingography (HSG), etc. From all these methods, laparoscopy is the gold standard test but also it is an invasive test so not used as a routine method.

High risk for tubal occlusion includes past *Chlamydia* infection, pelvic inflammatory disease (PID), peritonitis, known endometriosis, and/or pelvis surgery including salpingectomy for ectopic pregnancy.[17]

Recommendation of ESHRE guidelines: Hysterosalpingo-contrast sonography and hysterosalpingography are valid tests for tubal patency compared to laparoscopy and chromopertubation. HSG and HyCoSy are comparable in diagnostic capacity, thus selection of the technique depends on the preference of the clinician and patient.[1]

Uterine Factors

To detect most common congenital uterine anomalies and Müllerian anomalies 3D and 2D scans, magnetic resonance imaging (MRI) pelvis can be done. In a prospective cohort study, compared to 2D-US, the sensitivity and specificity of real-time 3D-US were significantly higher in both follicular and luteal phases.[18] There is no evidence in usefulness of MRI as a first-line test in confirming a normal uterine structure. Furthermore, MRI is expensive and time-consuming and should therefore be considered as a second-line diagnostic tool for the diagnosis of specific conditions.

Recommendation of ESHRE guidelines: Ultrasound, preferably 3D, is recommended to exclude uterine anomalies in women with unexplained infertility. MRI is not recommended as a first-line test to confirm a normal uterine structure and anatomy in women with unexplained infertility.[1]

Laparoscopy

Routine laparoscopy is not recommended in infertile women at low risk for tubal pathology but should be reserve for women with an abnormal HSG or those at risk for tuboperitoneal disease due to a history of PID, previous ectopic pregnancy, or clinically suspected or known endometriosis.[19]

Recommendation of ESHRE guidelines: Routine diagnostic laparoscopy is not recommended for the diagnosis of unexplained infertility. However, if mild or moderate endometriosis is diagnosed during laparoscopy incidentally, then it is not considered unexplained infertility any more.[1]

Cervical/Vaginal Factors

Few tests can be performed for cervical and vaginal factors such as postcoital test and vaginal microbiota testing but are not recommended for a routine under ESHRE guideline.[1] Vaginal microbiota testing could be considered in couples with unexplained infertility only in a research setting.[20]

Male Genitourinary Anatomy

Mean testicular volume is positively associated with sperm concentration and total sperm count. Epididymal mean head size is positively associated with normal sperm morphology and vas deferens mean size is positively associated with progressive motility.[21] Also, there is no additional benefit on performing scrotal color Doppler ultrasound on male partner with normal semen parameters and having undergone physical examination. It can be helpful to identify scrotal abnormalities and to assist in better understanding the pathophysiology of sperm abnormalities and male infertility.[21]

Recommendation of ESHRE guidelines: Testicular imaging is not recommended when semen analysis according to WHO criteria is normal.[1]

Male Additional Tests

Under GDG of ESHRE guidelines of unexplained infertility, it is a diagnosis of exclusion. In some patients, underlying sperm dysfunction may not be detected during a routine semen assessment of the ejaculate, which may appear to be normal regarding basic semen parameters. There are some adverse reproductive outcomes that have been identified during medical and reproductive history examination and may indicates use of further tests procedures specified in the WHO 6th edition Chapter 3 and 4 to assess sperm functions. Those are antisperm antibodies, deoxyribonucleic acid (DNA) fragmentation index, sperm chromatin condensation test, sperm aneuploidy screening, hormonal testing, human papillomavirus infection, and microbiology tests.

Recommendation of ESHRE guidelines: All these tests are not recommended when semen analysis is normal according to WHO criteria.[1]

Additional Tests for Systemic Conditions

Tests for autoimmunity like antisperm antibodies in serum, female celiac disease, thyroid antibodies, thrombophilia, oxidative stress test, genetic tests, vitamin D deficiency, prolactin levels, etc.

Recommendation of ESHRE guidelines: Testing for celiac disease in female with unexplained infertility can be considered. TSH measurement is considered good practice in preconception care. No additional thyroid evaluation in women is recommended if TSH is within the normal range. Body mass index (BMI) evaluation in women is considered good practice in preconception care. Rest all tests mentioned above are not recommended without an indication in couple of unexplained infertility.[1]

TREATMENT OPTIONS RECOMMENDATIONS AS PROPOSED BY THE ESHRE GUIDELINES

- *Expectant treatment:* The GDG advises to base the decision to start active treatment on prognosis in couples with unexplained infertility.
- *Active treatment:*
    - IUI with ovarian stimulation is recommended as a first-line treatment for couples with unexplained infertility.[22-26]
    - IVF is probably not recommended over IUI with conditional ovarian stimulation in couples with unexplained infertility.[27,28] It is expected that the decision to use IVF is individualized by patient

characteristics, such as age, duration of infertility, previous treatment, and previous pregnancy.
- Intracytoplasmic sperm injection (ICSI) is not recommended over conventional IVF in couples with unexplained infertility.[29-31]

- *Mechanical-surgical procedures:*
  - Hysteroscopy for the detection and possible correction of intrauterine abnormalities not seen at routine imaging is not recommended.[32,33]
  - HSG (i.e., tubal flushing) with an oil-soluble contrast medium is preferable over a water-soluble contrast medium. Risks and benefits of tubal flushing with oil-soluble contrast medium should be discussed with all couples with unexplained infertility.[34]
  - Endometrial scratching should not be offered for unexplained infertility.[35-40]
- *Alternative therapeutic approaches:*
  - Adjunct oral antioxidant therapy to women undergoing fertility treatment is probably not recommended.[41]
  - Adjunct oral antioxidant therapy to males undergoing fertility treatment is probably not recommended.
  - Acupuncture in women is probably not recommended.[42]
  - Inositol supplementation in women is probably not recommended.[43]
  - Psychological support, including psychotherapy, is recommended for patients when needed.
  - A healthy diet and regular exercise, supported by behavioral therapy when necessary, are recommended.

DISCUSSION

The summary of recommendations as per ESHRE brings out very pointedly that structural assessment is prioritized over functional assessment as because functional assessment tools have not been developed or tested adequately enough. If we look at putative causes of unexplained infertility beyond the obvious structural factors, we realize that we have not been able to factor in functional factors even in the most recent attempt at trying to understand unexplained infertility. Below is the list of probable factors of unexplained infertility:

- *Ovarian and endocrine factors:*
  - Abnormal or dysfunctional follicular growth
  - Luteinized unruptured follicles and functional ovarian cysts
  - Hypersecretion of LH
  - Hypersecretion of prolactin in the presence of ovulation
  - Growth hormone deficiency or insensitivity
  - Cytological abnormality in oocytes
  - Genetic abnormality in oocytes
  - Antibodies to the zona pellucida
- *Peritoneal factors:*
  - Altered macrophage and immune activity
  - Mild endometriosis
  - Microbiome
- *Tubal factors:*
  - Abnormal peristaltic or cilial activity
  - Altered macrophage and immune activity
- *Endometrial factors:*
  - Abnormal secretion of endometrial proteins
  - Abnormal integrin/adhesion molecules
  - Abnormal T-cell and natural killer cell activity
  - Secretion of embryo toxic factors
  - Abnormality in uterine perfusion and contractility
  - Uterine microbiome
- *Cervical factors:*
  - Altered cervical mucus
  - Increased immunogenicity
  - Vaginal microbiome
- *General immune factors:* Altered cell-mediated immunity
- *Male factors:*
  - Reduction in motility, acrosome reaction, oocyte binding, and zona pellucida penetration
  - Ultra structural abnormality of head morphology
  - DNA fragmentation and genetic abnormality
  - Microbiome
- *Embryological factors:*
  - Poor quality embryo
  - Reduced progression of blastocyst in vitro
  - Abnormal or altered chromosomal complement.

As it is clear from the above list, we are as yet not competent to diagnose and therefore treat unexplained infertility by conventional means as the cause is not known or identifiable. To quote from the ESHRE guidelines, notwithstanding the importance and relevance of the topic, research data on many key aspects are scarce. As a basis for the current guideline, a formal literature review was conducted. Most studies on diagnosis were old with often incomplete reporting of methodology. Review of additional tests for establishing the diagnosis of unexplained infertility was plagued by heterogeneity of the study population and lack of standardization of assays. The literature on the diagnosis of a putative male cause for unexplained infertility was complicated by the interchangeable use of the terms unexplained and idiopathic male infertility.

So, to compensate for absence of treatment algorithms based on robust diagnostic and assessment tools, we have devised a simple IUI versus IVF approach to help couples with unexplained infertility conceive. The moot question is whether in today's scenario should IVF be considered as the first option?

Should In Vitro Fertilization be Considered as the First Option?

If we look at the ICMART definition of unexplained infertility, affected couples have 'apparently normal ovarian function, normal fallopian tubes, uterus, cervix and pelvis, adequate coital frequency, apparently normal testicular function, genitourinary anatomy, and a normal ejaculate" so obviously there seems to be no structural reason for infertility in these couples. It is one of the putative factors as detailed above or a situation where we have not been able to diagnose a structural factor correctly. Till we have more accurate methods to assess structural factors we need to base our decisions on what we have on table.

It is a fair argument to place that IVF has a role to play in treating or managing unexplained infertility. As a routine practice in IVF, we use gonadotropins to stimulate the ovaries to grow multiple follicles yielding multiple eggs at the time of follicle aspiration. While not really corrective, this method of multiplying available eggs we do overcome egg-related factors with quantity making up for quality. When we fertilize the eggs in the laboratory, we overcome subtle tubal factors too. There is a case that even undetectable sperm factors such as ability to bind and penetrate egg can be overcome with the act of forced fertilization with sperms with help of ICSI. As the resulting embryo development is monitored, we are able to select embryo/s which seem to do better in terms of rate of growth and other parameters and as these embryos are then replaced in the uterine cavity, usually under strict controlled environment, we may be taking care of endometrial receptivity issues too. So, with multiple such interventions, IVF does seem to be able to provide answers to the conundrum of unexplained infertility.

On the other hand, we have no idea how, if at all, IUI works in couples with unexplained infertility. IUI involves ovarian stimulation to ensure at least one mature follicle which is present at the time of placing processed sperms in the uterine cavity, most often supracervically at the expected time of ovulation.

So, the points at which the process of IUI may help are as follows:

- Correcting hormonal milieu by superovulation with ovulogens like CC but CC has not been shown to be superior to unstimulated IUI or expectant management in ovulatory women.
- Processing of sperms and optimizing their performance by laboratory methods of washing and removing foreign materials, which may impair their fertilizing ability.
- By placing sperms in the uterine cavity as IUI has shown better outcomes than intracervical placement of sperms in women undergoing insemination with donor sperms.
- Timing of insemination has also shown to be related to better outcomes.

A recent Cochrane review on IUI for unexplained subfertility looked at 15 trials with 2,068 women and concluded that "it is uncertain whether treatment with IUI with or without ovarian hyperstimulation (OH) compared to timed intercourse or expectant management with or without OH improves cumulative live birth rates with acceptable multiple pregnancy rates in couples with unexplained subfertility. However, treatment with IUI with OH probably results in a higher cumulative live birth rate compared to expectant management without OH in couples with a low prediction score of natural conception.

In spite of IVF scoring over IUI in terms of efficacy, most practices across the world keep performing IUI as the first step in treating couples with unexplained infertility. The probable reason is the perceived low cost and lower burden of treatment in IUI. On the other hand, most fertility physicians and embryologists and even some couples would prefer the tangible approach of IVF and screening of embryos before transfer as the logical approach in cases of unexplained infertility, especially where time to birth is a concern.

We can refer to FASTT trial where they effectively proved that both the time and costs per pregnancy were lower in women who were randomized into the fast-track route to IVF versus the conventional route where they were offered OH and IUI first.

CONCLUSION

There is no single answer to this debate. It is up to the couple who is the most important stakeholder and who needs to be decide on the route they need to take based on the available information.

The points they may want to consider are:

- If there is any reason where they cannot be advised IUI or IVF.
- Whether they want a trial of 2–3 IUIs before they choose IVF or they would want to proceed with IVF as the first step?
- They need to look at the costs and number of interventions needed even with IVF for a pregnancy to occur in similar circumstances.

REFERENCES

1. Guideline Group on Unexplained Infertility; Romualdi D, Ata B, Bhattacharya S, Bosch E, Costello M, et al. Evidence-based guideline: unexplained infertility. Hum Reprod. 2023;38(10):1881-90.
2. Infertility Workup for the Women's Health Specialist: ACOG Committee Opinion, Number 781. Obstet Gynecol. 2019;133(6):e377-e384.
3. Practice Committee of the American Society for Reproductive Medicine. Evidence-based treatments for couples with unexplained infertility: a guideline. Fertil Steril. 2020;113(2):305-22.
4. Zegers-Hochschild F, Adamson GD, Dyer S, Racowsky C, de Mouzon J, Sokol R, et al. The International Glossary on Infertility and Fertility Care, 2017. Hum Reprod. 2017; 32(9):1786-801.
5. Wilcox AJ, Weinberg CR, Baird DD. Timing of sexual intercourse in relation to ovulation. Effects on the probability of conception, survival of the pregnancy, and sex of the baby. N Engl J Med. 1995;333(23):1517-21.
6. Munro MG, Critchley HOD, Fraser IS; FIGO Menstrual Disorders Committee. The two FIGO systems for normal and abnormal uterine bleeding symptoms and classification of causes of abnormal uterine bleeding in the reproductive years: 2018 revisions. Int J Gynaecol Obstet. 2018;143(3):393-408. Erratum in: Int J Gynaecol Obstet. 2019;144(2):237.
7. World Health Organization. WHO laboratory Manual for the Examination and Processing of Human Semen, 6th edition. Geneva, Switzerland: WHO Press; 2021.
8. Siristatidis C, Bhattacharya S. Unexplained infertility: Does it really exist? Does it matter? Hum Repord. 2007;22:2084-7.
9. Hull MG, Glazener CM, Kelly NJ, Conway DI, Foster PA, Hinton RA, et al. Population study of causes, treatment, and outcome of infertility. Br Med J (Clin Res Ed). 1985;291(6510):1693-7.
10. Bischof P, Bianchi PG, Campana A. Comparison of a rapid, quantitative and automated assay for urinary luteinizing hormone (LH), with an LH detection test, for the prediction of ovulation. Hum Reprod. 1991;6(4):515-8.
11. Gregoriou O, Kassanos D, Vitoratos N, Papadias C, Zourlas PA. Clinical efficacy of LH-color: a new home ovulation test. Int J Gynaecol Obstet. 1990;32(2):141-3.
12. Guermandi E, Vegetti W, Bianchi MM, Uglietti A, Ragni G, Crosignani P. Reliability of ovulation tests in infertile women. Obstet Gynecol. 2001;97(1):92-6.
13. Martinez AR, Bernardus RE, Kucharska D, Schoemaker J. Urinary luteinizing hormone testing and prediction of ovulation in spontaneous, clomiphene citrate and human menopausal gonadotropin-stimulated cycles. A clinical evaluation. Acta Endocrinol (Copenh). 1991;124(4):357-63.
14. Hull MG, Savage PE, Bromham DR, Ismail AA, Morris AF. The value of a single serum progesterone measurement in the midluteal phase as a criterion of a potentially fertile cycle ("ovulation") derived from treated and untreated conception cycles. Fertil Steril. 1982;37:355-60.
15. Coutifaris C, Myers ER, Guzick DS, Diamond MP, Carson SA, Legro RS, et al. Reprint of: histological dating of timed endometrial biopsy tissue is not related to fertility status. Fertil Steril. 2019;112:e116-e124.
16. Hagen CP, Vestergaard S, Juul A, Skakkebæk NE, Andersson AM, Main KM, et al. Low concentration of circulating anti-Müllerian hormone is not predictive of reduced fecundability in young healthy women: a prospective cohort study. Fertil Steril. 2012;98:1602-1608.e1602.
17. Babay ZA, Al-Meshari A. The role of *Chlamydia trachomatis* infection in female infertility. Ann Saudi Med. 1993;13(5): 423-8.
18. Caliskan E, Ozkan S, Cakiroglu Y, Sarisoy HT, Corakci A, Ozeren S. Diagnostic accuracy of real-time 3D sonography in the diagnosis of congenital Mullerian anomalies in high-risk patients with respect to the phase of the menstrual cycle. J Clin Ultrasound. 2010;38(3):123-7.
19. Lavy Y, Lev-Sagie A, Holtzer H, Revel A, Hurwitz A. Should laparoscopy be a mandatory component of the infertility evaluation in infertile women with normal hysterosalpingogram or suspected unilateral distal tubal pathology? Eur J Obstet Gynecol Reprod Biol. 2004;114(1): 64-8.
20. Patel N, Patel N, Pal S, Nathani N, Pandit R, Patel M, et al. Distinct gut and vaginal microbiota profile in women with recurrent implantation failure and unexplained infertility. BMC Womens Health. 2022;22:113.
21. Lotti F, Frizza F, Balercia G, Barbonetti A, Behre HM, Calogero AE, et al. The European Academy of Andrology (EAA) ultrasound study on healthy, fertile men: Scrotal

ultrasound reference ranges and associations with clinical, seminal, and biochemical characteristics. Andrology. 2021;9:559-76.

22. Agarwal S, Mittal S. A randomised prospective trial of intrauterine insemination versus timed intercourse in superovulated cycles with clomiphene. Indian J Med Res. 2004;120(6):519-22.
23. Bhattacharya S, Harrild K, Mollison J, Wordsworth S, Tay C, Harrold A, et al. Clomifene citrate or unstimulated intrauterine insemination compared with expectant management for unexplained infertility: pragmatic randomised controlled trial. BMJ. 2008;337:a716.
24. Ayeleke RO, Asseler JD, Cohlen BJ, Veltman-Verhulst SM. Intra-uterine insemination for unexplained subfertility. Cochrane Database Syst Rev. 2020;3(3):CD001838.
25. Harira M. Use of Letrozole versus clomiphene-estradiol for treating infertile women with unexplained infertility not responding well to clomiphene alone, comparative study. Middle East Fertil Soc J. 2018;23:384-7.
26. Ibrahim MI, Moustafa RA, Abdel-Azeem AA. Letrozole versus clomiphene citrate for superovulation in Egyptian women with unexplained infertility: a randomized controlled trial. Arch Gynecol Obstet. 2012;286(6):1581-7.
27. Pandian Z, Gibreel A, Bhattacharya S. In vitro fertilisation for unexplained subfertility. Cochrane Database Syst Rev. 2015;2015:CD003357.
28. Nandi A, Raja G, White D, Tarek ET. Intrauterine insemination + controlled ovarian hyperstimulation versus in vitro fertilisation in unexplained infertility: a systematic review and meta-analysis. Arch Gynecol Obstet. 2022;305: 805-24.
29. Bhattacharya S, Hamilton MP, Shaaban M, Khalaf Y, Seddler M, Ghobara T, et al. Conventional in-vitro fertilisation versus intracytoplasmic sperm injection for the treatment of non-male-factor infertility: a randomised controlled trial. Lancet. 2001;357:2075-9.
30. Foong SC, Fleetham JA, O'Keane JA, Scott SG, Tough SC, Greene CA. A prospective randomized trial of conventional in vitro fertilization versus intracytoplasmic sperm injection in unexplained infertility. J Assist Reprod Genet. 2006;23(3):137-40.
31. Dang VQ, Vuong LN, Luu TM, Pham TD, Ho TM, Ha AN, et al. Intracytoplasmic sperm injection versus conventional in-vitro fertilisation in couples with infertility in whom the male partner has normal total sperm count and motility: an open-label, randomised controlled trial. Lancet. 2021;397:1554-63.
32. Casini ML, Rossi F, Agostini R, Unfer V. Effects of the position of fibroids on fertility. Gynecological endocrinology. Gynecol Endocrinol. 2006;22(2):106-9.
33. Seyam EM, Hassan MM, Mohamed Sayed Gad MT, Mahmoud HS, Ibrahim MG. Pregnancy Outcome after Office Microhysteroscopy in Women with Unexplained Infertility. Int J Fertil Steril. 2015;9(2):168-75.
34. Wang R, Watson A, Johnson N, Cheung K, Fitzgerald C, Mol BWJ, et al. Tubal flushing for subfertility. Cochrane Database Syst Rev. 2020;10:CD003718.
35. Parsanezhad ME, Dadras N, Maharlouei N, Neghahban L, Keramati P, Amini M. Pregnancy rate after endometrial injury in couples with unexplained infertility: A randomized clinical trial. Iran J Reprod Med. 2013;11(11): 869-74.
36. Senocak GC, Yapca OE, Borekci B. Comparison of pregnancy rates between patients with and without local endometrial scratching before intrauterine insemination. J Gynecol Obstet Hum Reprod. 2017;46(9):687-90.
37. Ghuman NK, Raikar S, Singh P, Gothwal M, Yadav G. Improving reproductive outcomes of intrauterine insemination: Does endometrial scratch injury help? A randomised controlled trial. Eur J Obstet Gynecol Reprod Biol. 2020;253:225-31.
38. Jafarabadi MN, Bagheri M, Ebrahimi Z, Shariat M, Haghollahi F. Endometrial scratching effect on pregnancy rate in intrauterine insemination cycles: a randomized controlled trial. Int J Women's Health Reprod Sci. 2020; 8:85-9.
39. Yildiz G, Kurt D, Mat E, Yildiz P. The effect of local endometrial injury on the success of intrauterine insemination. J Exp Clin Med (Turkey). 2021;38:521-4.
40. Wong TY, Lensen S, Wilkinson J, Glanville EJ, Acharya S, Clarke F, et al. Effect of endometrial scratching on unassisted conception for unexplained infertility: a randomized controlled trial. Fertil Steril. 2022;117:612-9.
41. Showell MG, Mackenzie-Proctor R, Jordan V, Hart RJ. Antioxidants for female subfertility. Cochrane Database Syst Rev. 2020;8:CD007807.
42. Guven PG, Cayir Y, Borekci B. Effectiveness of acupuncture on pregnancy success rates for women undergoing in vitro fertilization: A randomized controlled trial. Taiwan J Obstet Gynecol. 2020;59:282-6.
43. Montanino Oliva M, Buonomo G, Carra MC, Lippa A, Lisi F. Myo-inositol impact on sperm motility in vagina and evaluation of its effects on foetal development. Eur Rev Med Pharmacol Sci. 2020;24:2704-9.

Chapter

Endometrial Scratching: To Do or Not to Do?

Shrutika Thakkar, Sheetal Sawankar

INTRODUCTION

With the rise in infertility in society, more and more assisted reproductive techniques and procedures have been developed in the past decade or so. Despite accelerated research in the direction of increasing treatment success, implantation rates of assisted reproductive technology (ART) protocols have more or less staggered around the same figures. Many approaches have been suggested as means of enhancing the likelihood of implantation including the technique of "scratching the endometrium" prior to embryo transfer (ET). It was in 2003 that Barash et al. suggested that any kind of local injury to the endometrium, increased the uterine receptivity through a probable decidualization kind of response.[1] An exhaustive research and analysis of current literature is needed to investigate if there is any possible benefit from endometrial scratching.

ENDOMETRIAL "SCRATCHING": THE TECHNIQUE

Scratching of the endometrium prior to ET is usually done in the luteal phase of the cycle preceding in vitro fertilization (IVF) although many researchers have also studied doing the same procedure during the first few days of the menses. The procedure involves using a small catheter, 3 mm in width, known as the Pipelle® or an endometrial biopsy metal curette to make a scratch on the endometrium.[2] Usually the catheter/curette is inserted through the cervix up till the fundus, and then retracted in up-down or circular movements in order to stimulate the endometrium. When needed and as required, diagnostic means such as histopathology, immunological tests, and infection screens can also be carried out during the same procedure. This procedure usually does not require any pain relief/anesthesia or patient preparatory techniques and can be performed very easily as an outpatient-basis procedure. When an hysteroscopy operation is also being performed as part of the treatment protocol, the same procedure of scratching can be performed using hysteroscopic scissors.

SCIENTIFIC LOGIC BEHIND THE PROCEDURE

Intentional endometrial injury has been mooted to initiate the following responses at the cellular, immunological, and hormonal levels.

- The local injury induced by the procedure induces a decidualization response, which in turn increases the likelihood of implantation of the transferred embryo.[3]
- During the healing and repair process, it has been noted that there is a local increase in scavenger cells such as macrophages and dendritic cells. This results in a proinflammatory response with increase in cytokines such as tumor necrosis factor-alpha (TNF-α), growth-regulated oncogene-alpha, and macrophage-inflammatory protein-1 beta (MIP-1β), which are known to exert a positive effect on implantation.[3,4]
- The hyperestrogenic influence of ovarian stimulation during the IVF treatment on the endometrium may make it nonreceptive to the developing embryo.[5] The scratching, previously done, may suppress this disorganized and uninhibited proliferative response to high estrogen levels, positively impacting the embryo-endometrial synchrony.[5,6]

REVIEW OF LITERATURE

Due to the simplicity of the procedure to be performed and the apparent logical sense in performing endometrial scratching, there have been multiple research papers and study protocols that have been evaluated in an attempt to conclusively find out if this simple procedure can positively impact the IVF/IUI (intrauterine insemination) outcomes.

Dr Sarah Lensen from New Zealand in 2018 at the European Society of Human Reproduction and Embryology meeting, Barcelona, received the Clinical Science Award for oral presentation for her work on this very subject.[7] She also subsequently published her work in the New England Journal of Medicine.[8] As per the study, data was collected from 1,364 women (690 in the scratching arm vs. 674 in the control group), who had undergone ET after IVF during the fresh embryo or cryo-thawed cycle. All those who had any recent exposure to disruptive intrauterine instrumentation (e.g., hysteroscopy) were excluded from the study. Study subjects were randomly assigned in a 1:1 ratio to either Pipelle biopsy between day 3 of the cycle preceding the ET cycle and day 3 of the ET cycle or no intervention. It was reported that there was no increase in live birth rates after endometrial scratching.

This publication led to multiple meta-analyses on the same subject, critically evaluating the possibility of any benefit from performing endometrial scratching in IVF patients. A systematic review and meta-analysis was published in 2022 by Metwally et al.[9] that evaluated the benefit of performing endometrial scratching in women undergoing first-time IVF treatment. A total of 12 studies were made part of this study and evidence was gathered to find out whether endometrial scratching improves pregnancy outcomes, including live birth rates, for women in their first IVF cycles. The evidence gathered led to a recommendation that clinicians will not yield any positive outcome on live birth rates, miscarriage rates from performing this procedure in women undergoing their first IVF cycle.[9]

The timing of endometrial scratching vis-à-vis improvement in implantation rates was reported as crucial in a meta-analysis research study conducted by Maged et al.[10] An increase in multiple pregnancy rate as well as implantation rate was reported when the procedure was performed in the follicular phase of the cycle preceding the stimulation cycle. This same observation was not reported when the scratch was performed during the follicular phase of the same cycle of stimulation, the luteal phase, or both follicular and luteal phases. It is speculated that the endometrial scratch made in the preceding cycle resulted in an improvement in implantation rates, because it resulted in a longer healing time and therefore yielded more beneficial effects.[10] When the scratching was performed during the follicular phase in the same cycle of stimulation, probably sufficient time was not available to achieve healing of the endometrium, thereby not yielding positive outcomes.

As endometrial scratching is considered to enhance chances of embryo implantation, the benefit of this procedure in women with one or more previous ART failure has been a matter of controversy and has also been studied extensively. A meta-analysis conducted by Kang et al.[11] reviewed 16 articles on the subject and concluded that improvement in pregnancy rates and live birth rates without increasing miscarriage or multiple pregnancy rates, was evidently seen in the scratching group. According to this study, an intentional injury to the endometrium performed during the endometrial scratching procedure causes better synchronization of the embryo and the endometrium and even overcomes the disorder caused by controlled ovarian hyperstimulation done in IVF.

Not only has endometrial scratching been studied in IVF but also in IUI cycles. However, there is conflicting evidence with regard to the effect of endometrial scratching in improving pregnancy outcomes among women with previous IUI failure. It was reported in a systematic review and meta-analysis by Baradwan et al.[12] that there was a significant improvement in the biochemical and clinical pregnancy rates among women with previous IUI failure after performing the endometrial scratch. This finding very clearly points to the fact that more research is definitely needed on this subject.

CONCLUSION

These conflicting results of most of the research studies point out that the main limitation in the existing research is the substantial methodological heterogeneity in the various studies conducted especially with regard to the timing, number, and intensity of endometrial scratch.

The ease and simplicity of the endometrial scratch procedure has perhaps been the main reason for its rapid adoption into routine clinical practice, initially without the support of good-quality research. To be able to conclusively opine on the effect of scratching in regard to implantation, pregnancy, and live birth rates, it is prudent to accurately ascertain the precise patient profile that would benefit from this intervention. It seems logical to believe that scratching may be able to enhance the receptivity of the endometrium, but studies are limited by the fact that a number of other pathologies may be responsible for implantation failure. Present research shows that unselected, infertile women may benefit less from endometrial scratching; however, scratching may be a successful measure for enhancing the chances of implantation in women with recurrent implantation failure.

As this procedure is associated with significant pain to the patient, and as most guidelines do not point to a clear benefit arising out of endometrial scratching, patients should definitely be informed that the evidence pointing toward any benefit is inconclusive at the moment.

REFERENCES

1. Barash A, Dekel N, Fieldust S, Segal I, Schechtman E, Granot I. Local injury to the endometrium doubles the incidence of successful pregnancies in patients undergoing in vitro fertilization. Fertil Steril. 2003;79(6):1317-22.
2. Günther V, von Otte S, Maass N, Alkatout I. Endometrial “Scratching” An update and overview of current research. J Turk Ger Gynecol Assoc. 2020;21(2):124-9.
3. Li R, Hao G. Local injury to the endometrium: its effect on implantation. Curr Opin Obstet Gynecol. 2009;21(3): 236-9.
4. Gnainsky Y, Granot I, Aldo PB, Barash A, Or Y, Schechtman E, et al. Local injury of the endometrium induces an inflammatory response that promotes successful implantation. Fertil Steril. 2010;94(6):2030-6.
5. Ubaldi F, Bourgain C, Tournaye H, Smitz J, Van Steirteghem A, Devroey P. Endometrial evaluation by aspiration biopsy on the day of oocyte retrieval in the embryo transfer cycles in patients with serum progesterone rise during the follicular phase. Fertil Steril. 1997;67:521-6.
6. Fatemi HM, Popovic-Todorovic B. Implantation in assisted reproduction: a look at endometrial receptivity. Reprod Biomed Online. 2013;27:530-8.
7. Lensen SO, Armstrong D, Napier S, Sadler E, Hennes L, Stadelmann A, et al. (2018). Endometrial scratching by pipelle biopsy in IVF (the PIP study): a pragmatic randomised controlled trial. ESHRE, Barcelona 2018, 34. Annual conference, 2018. Abstract O-139.
8. Lensen S, Osavlyuk D, Armstrong S, Stadelmann C, Hennes A, Napier E, et al. A Randomized Trial of Endometrial Scratching before In Vitro Fertilization. N Engl J Med. 2019; 380:325-34.
9. Metwally M, Chatters R, White D, Hall J, Walters S. Endometrial scratch in women undergoing first-time IVF treatment: a systematic review and meta-analysis of randomized controlled trials. Reprod Biomed Online. 2022; 44(4):617-29.
10. Maged AM, El-Mazny A, Lasheen Y, El-Nassery N. Endometrial scratch injury in infertile women undergoing in vitro fertilization cycles: a systematic review and meta-analysis. J Int Med Res. 2023;51(7):3000605231175365.
11. Kang Y, Wang Z, Yang Y, Liang H, Duan X, Gao Q, et al. Impact of endometrial scratching on reproductive outcome in patients: a systematic review and meta-analysis. Medicine (Baltimore). 2022;101(33):e30150.
12. Baradwan S, Alshahrani MS, AlSghan R, Alkhamis WH, Alsharif SA, Alanazi GA, et al. The Effect of Endometrial Scratch on Pregnancy Rate in Women with Previous Intrauterine Insemination Failure: A Systematic Review and Meta-analysis of Randomized Controlled Trials. Reprod Sci. 2023;30(5):1399-407.

Addendum

Assisted Reproductive Technology Act
Rahul Wani

Assisted Reproductive Technology Act

Rahul Wani

INTRODUCTION

The Assisted Reproductive Technology (ART) Act, 2021 provides for the regulation and supervision of the ATR clinics and the ART banks, prevention of misuse, and safe and ethical practice of ART services.

The Act intends to protect the affected women and children from exploitation, support the oocyte donor with an insurance cover, regulate multiple embryo implantations, and protect the children born through ART.

The Act, further, aims to regulate cryopreservation of sperm, oocytes, and embryo and intends to provide for preimplantation genetic testing (PGT) for preexisting, heritable, or genetic diseases.

ORIGIN OF THE ACT

The world's first test tube baby, Louise Brown, was born on 25th July 1978. About 2 months later, the world's second and India's first IVF baby, Kanupriya alias Durga, was born in Kolkata. Since then, the field of ART has grown exponentially. India has become one of the major centers of ART resulting in multitude of legal, ethical, and social issues and there were no standardizing protocols available.

The Law Commission presented its 228th Report in 2009 which stated that an active legislative intervention is required to facilitate correct uses of the new technology, i.e., ART and legalization of surrogacy.

NECESSITY OF THE ACT

According to the Statement of Objects and Reasons (SOR) of the Act, the ART has grown rapidly in the last few years and India has registered the highest growth in the ART centers and the number of ART cycles performed every year.

Assisted reproductive technology, including in vitro fertilization (IVF), has given hope to many persons suffering from infertility but introduced a plethora of legal, ethical, and social issues.

As per the background note on the Act furnished by the Ministry, India has become one of the major centers of this global fertility industry over the years, with reproductive medical tourism becoming a significant activity. Clinics in India offer nearly all the ART services—gamete donation, intrauterine insemination (IUI), IVF, intracytoplasmic sperm injection (ICSI), PGT, and gestational surrogacy.

The reproductive segment of the Indian medical tourism market is valued at >$450 million a year and was forecast by the Indian Council of Medical Research (ICMR) to be a 6 billion dollar a year market value in 2008. India's fertility industry is an integral part of the country's growing medical tourism industry, which experienced 30% growth in 2000 and 15% growth between 2005 and 2010. Despite so much activity in India, there is no standardization of protocols yet and reporting is still very inadequate. Furthermore, there were only guidelines of ART, and no law existed. This presented with host of legal and ethical issues.

Legal and Ethical Issues of Assisted Reproductive Technology

- Noncoital reproduction
- *Treatment for infertile couple:* Mixing of gametes
- Single?
- Same sex couples?
- Legal rights of the child
- Abandonment of child
- Exploitation of donors
- Commercialization
- Exploitation of surrogates
- Sex selection

Considering all the above issues, legislation was required and came to being as per below mentioned sequence of events:

- ART gazetted on 20th December 2021
- Notified on 20th January applicable from 25th January 2022
- Surrogacy Act gazetted on 25th December 2021
- Notified on 20th January applicable from 25th January 2022
- ART rules notified on 7th June 2022
- Surrogacy rules notified on 21st June 2022
- Regulations yet to be framed by National Board.

IMPORTANT DEFINITIONS IN THE ACT

Assisted Reproductive Technology Procedures

It means "all techniques that attempt to obtain a pregnancy by handling the sperm or the oocyte outside the human body and transferring the gamete or the embryo into the reproductive system of a woman."

Assisted Reproductive Technology Bank

It means "an organization which shall be responsible for collection of gametes, storage of gametes, and embryos and supply of gametes to the ART clinics or their patients."

Assisted Reproductive Technology Clinic

It means "any premises equipped with requisite facilities and medical practitioners registered with the National Medical Commission for carrying out the procedures related to the ART."

Commissioning Couple

It means "an infertile married couple who approach an ART clinic or ART bank for obtaining the services authorized of the said clinic or bank."

Infertility

It means "the inability to conceive after 1 year of unprotected coitus or other proven medical condition preventing a couple from conception."

Woman

It means "any woman above the age of 21 years who approaches an ART clinic or ART bank for obtaining the authorized services of the clinic or bank."

PROCEDURES FOR REGISTRATION

- Every clinic or bank which is conducting ART, partly or exclusively shall, within a period of 60 days from the date of establishment of the National Registry, apply for registration.
- Provided that such clinics and banks shall cease to conduct any such counseling or procedures on the expiry of 6 months from the date of commencement of this Act, unless such clinics and banks have applied for registration and is so registered separately or till such application is disposed of, whichever is earlier.

Grant of Registration

- Within a period of 30 days the appropriate authority:
  - Must grant registration subject to the provisions of this Act and the rules and regulations made thereunder, and provide a registration number to the applicant.
  - Reject the application for reasons to be recorded in writing, if such application does not conform to the provisions of this Act or the rules or regulations. Applicant should be given an opportunity of being heard in the matter.
- If the appropriate authority fails to grant the registration or reject the application, the appropriate authority shall, within a period of 7 days from the expiry of the said period of 30 days, provide a reason for the failure to process the application.
- The registration granted under this section shall be valid for a period of 5 years from the date of registration granted by the appropriate authority.
- The certificate of registration shall be displayed by the clinic or bank at a conspicuous place and such certificate shall contain the duration of validity of such registration.

Suspension or Cancellation of Registration

- The appropriate authority on receipt of a complaint, or suo moto issue a notice to the clinic or bank to show cause, why its registration should not be suspended or canceled?
- After giving a reasonable opportunity of being heard to the clinic or bank, the appropriate authority is satisfied that there has been a breach of the provision of this Act or the rules or regulations or if the data obtained from them periodically do not satisfy the provisions of this

Act, the rules and regulations, it may, without prejudice to any criminal action, suspend its registration for such period as it may deem fit or cancel its registration.

Appeal Against Rejection, Suspension, or Cancellation of Registration

- Within a period of 30 days from the date of receipt of the communication relating to order of rejection of application, suspension or cancellation of registration passed by the appropriate authority an appeal against such order can be made to:
  - The state government, where the appeal is against the order of the appropriate authority of a state.
  - The central government, where the appeal is against the order of the appropriated authority of a union territory.

DUTIES OF CLINIC AND BANKS

- Eligibility of couple to avail the ART procedures should be confirmed.
- The clinics shall obtain donor gametes from the banks and such banks shall ensure that the donor has been medically tested for such diseases.
- Professional counseling to commissioning couple and woman about all the implications and chances of success of ART procedures in the clinic.

Success Rates of Procedures

Disclose specifically to the patient in writing if the success rate of a treatment/procedure/surgery is low.

Mrs Balwinder Kaur vs. Sidharth Charitable Hospital and Others:

- The hospital stated in defense that the success rate of IVF is only 40%. The court rejected this defense as the hospital did not place on record any document to show that the patient was made aware about the percentage of success rates.
- Inform the commissioning couple and woman of the advantages, disadvantages, and cost of the procedures, their medical side effects, and risks including the risk of multiple pregnancy.
- Arrive at an informed decision on such matters that would most likely be the best for the commissioning couple.
- Shall make commissioning couple or woman, aware of the rights of a child born through the use of ART.
- Information about the commissioning couple, woman, and donor shall be kept confidential except in a medical emergency at the request of the commissioning couple to whom the information relates, or by an order of a court of competent jurisdiction.
- Grievance cell should be formed to deal with grievances of the clients.

WHO CAN AVAIL ASSISTED REPRODUCTIVE TECHNOLOGY SERVICES?

- Woman above the age of 21 years and below the age of 50 years
- Man above the age of 21 years and below the age of 55 years

Duties when Performing Procedures

- Clinics shall issue to the commissioning couple or woman a discharge certificate stating details of the ART procedure performed on the commissioning couple or woman shall not perform any treatment or procedure without:
  - Written informed consent of all the parties seeking ART
  - Insurance coverage of such amount as may be prescribed for a period of 12 months in favor of the oocyte donor
  - Insurance should be in place before stimulation.
- The clinics and banks shall not cryopreserve any human embryos or gamete without specific instructions and consent in writing from all the parties seeking ART, as to what should be done with the gametes or embryo's in case of death or incapacity of any of the parties.
- The clinic shall not use any human reproductive material to create a human embryo or use an in vitro human embryo for any purpose without the specific consent in writing of all the concerned persons to whom the ART relate.
- Commissioning couple may withdraw his or her consent before the procedure is carried out.
- Parties include the commissioning couple or woman and the donor.

Records

- Clinics and banks shall maintain detailed records of all donor's oocytes, sperm, or embryos used or unused, the manner and technique of their use in such manner as may be prescribed.

- Clinics and banks shall, as and when the National Registry is established, submit by online:
  - Information available with them in regard to progress of the commissioning couple or woman
  - Information about number of donors (sperm and oocyte), screened, maintained, and supplied within a period of 1 month from the date of receipt of such information
  - Shall be maintained for at least a period of 10 years, upon the expiry of which the clinic and bank shall transfer the records to a central database of the National Registry.

Duties when using Gametes and Embryos

- The clinics shall retrieve oocytes in such manner as may be specified by regulations.
- Not >3 oocytes or embryos may be placed in the uterus of a woman during the treatment cycle in such manner as may be specified by regulations.
- A woman shall not be treated with gametes or embryos derived from >1 man or woman during any one treatment cycle.
- A clinic shall never mix semen from two individuals for the procedures specified under this Act.
- The embryos shall not be split and used for twinning to increase the number of available embryos.
- The collection of gametes posthumously shall be done only if prior consent of the commissioning couple is available in such manner as may be prescribed.
- The clinic shall not use ovum that is derived from a fetus, in any process of IVF.

PREIMPLANTATION GENETIC TESTING

- The PGT shall be used to screen the human embryo for known, preexisting, heritable, or genetic diseases only.
- "Preimplantation genetic diagnosis," means the genetic diagnosis when one or both genetic parents, has a known genetic abnormality and testing is performed on an embryo to determine if it also carries a genetic abnormality.
- "Preimplantation genetic testing" means a technique used to identify genetic defects in embryos created through IVF before pregnancy.

PRECONCEPTION AND PRENATAL DIAGNOSTIC TECHNIQUE PROHIBITION

- Shall not offer to provide a couple or woman with a child of a predetermined sex.
- It is prohibited for anyone to do any act, at any stage, to determine the sex of the child to be born through the process of ART to separate, or yield fractions enriched in sperm of X or Y variations.
- A person shall not knowingly provide, prescribe, or administer anything that shall ensure or increase the probability that an embryo shall be of a particular sex, or that shall identify the sex of an in vitro embryo, except to diagnose, prevent or treat a sex-linked disorder or disease.

ASSISTED REPRODUCTIVE TECHNOLOGY BANK AND DONOR GAMETES

The screening of gamete donors, the collection, screening, and storage of semen; and provision of oocyte donor, shall be done only by a bank registered as an independent entity under the provisions of this Act.

Donors

- Obtain semen from males between 21 years of age and 55 years of age, both inclusive.
- Obtain oocytes from females between 23 years of age and 35 years of age.
- Examine the donors for such diseases, as may be prescribed.
- A bank shall not supply the sperm or oocyte of a single donor to >1 commissioning couple.
- An oocyte donor shall donate oocytes only once in her life and not >7 oocyte shall be retrieved from the oocyte donor.
- All unused oocytes shall be preserved by the banks for use on the same recipient, or given for research to an organization registered under this Act after seeking written consent from the commissioning couple.
- The gamete of a donor or embryo shall be stored for a period of not >10 years and at the end of such period such gamete or embryo shall be allowed to perish or be donated to a research organizations registered under this Act.
- A bank shall obtain all necessary information in respect of a sperm or oocyte donor including the name, Aadhaar number, address, and any other details of such donor.
- Shall undertake in writing from such donor about the confidentiality of such information.

Transfer of Gametes

The sale, transfer or use of gametes, zygotes and embryos, or any part thereof or information related thereto, directly or indirectly to any party within or outside India shall be prohibited except in the case of transfer of own gametes and embryos for personal use with the permission of the National Board.

Offences and Penalties

- Shall not issue, publish, distribute, communicate or cause to be issued, published, distributed or communicated any advertisement in any manner including internet, regarding facilities of sex-selective ART.
    - Contravention leads to 5 years imprisonment but may extend to 10 years or with fine which shall not be <1,000,000 rupees but may extend to 25,000,000 rupees or with both.
- Abandon, disown or exploit or cause to be abandoned, disowned or exploited in any form the child or children born through ART
- Sell human embryos or gametes, run an agency, a racket or an organization for selling, purchasing or trading in human embryos or gametes
- Import or help in getting imported in whatsoever manner, the human embryos or human gametes
- Exploit the commissioning couple, woman, or the gamete donor in any form
- Transfer human embryo into a male person or an animal
- Sell any human embryo or gamete for the purpose of research
- Use any intermediates to obtain gamete donors or purchase gamete donors
    - Shall be punishable with a fine which shall not be <500,000 rupees but may extend to <1,000,000 rupees for the first contravention and for subsequent contravention, shall be punishable with imprisonment for a term which shall not be <3 years but may extend to 8 years and with fine which shall not be <1,000,000 rupees but may extend to <2,000,000 rupee
- Whoever contravenes any of the provisions of this Act or any rules will be punished as per above-mentioned punishment.
- National Board, State Board, or Any officer authorized can lodge a complaint
- Offences are Cognizable and bailable.

LEVELS OF ASSISTED REPRODUCTIVE TECHNOLOGY CLINICS, STAFF, EQUIPMENT, AND FEES

Assisted Reproductive Technology Level 1

Assisted reproductive technology clinics, where only IUI procedure is carried out as part of treatment:

- *Staff:* Gynecologist
- *Equipment:*
    - Centrifuge
    - Microscope
    - Refrigerator
- *Fees:* Rupees 50,000

Assisted Reproductive Technology Level 2

- ART clinics, where the procedures, that attempt to obtain a pregnancy shall be carried out by any or all of the following, namely:
    - Surgical retrieval of gametes
    - Handling the oocyte outside the human body
    - Use sperms for fertilization of oocytes
    - Transfer of the embryo into the reproductive system of a woman
    - Carryout storage of gametes or embryos or perform any kind of procedure or technique involving gametes or embryos. Provided that such clinics may also undertake research.
- *Staff:*
    - Gynecologist
    - Anesthetist
    - Embryologist
    - Counselor
- *Equipment:*
    - Microscope
    - Incubator (minimum 02 in number)
    - Laminar airflow
    - Sperm counting chambers
    - Centrifuge
    - Refrigerator
    - Equipment for cryopreservation
    - Ovum aspiration pump
    - USG machine with transvaginal probe and needle guard
    - Test tube warmer
    - Anesthesia resuscitation trolley
- *Fees:* Rupees 200,000

Assisted Reproductive Technology Bank

- *Staff:* Registered medical practitioner
- *Equipment:*
    - Centrifuge
    - Microscope
    - Laminar flow
    - Incubator
- *Fees:* Rupees 50,000

CONCLUSION

- The Act provides for steep penalties for not following any of the provisions of the act, rules, or regulations
- Wide powers in the hands of appropriate authority
- Breach of any of the provisions can lead to suspension, cancellation, and/or criminal action
- Fortunately, there is no presumption in case of deficiency of record keeping.

Index

Page numbers followed by *b* refer to box, *f* refer to figure, *fc* refer to flowchart, and *t* refer to table.

F

G